HEALTHIEST
Places to Live

Where You Live Makes a Difference

How High Natural Amenities and Altitude Help You Lose Weight

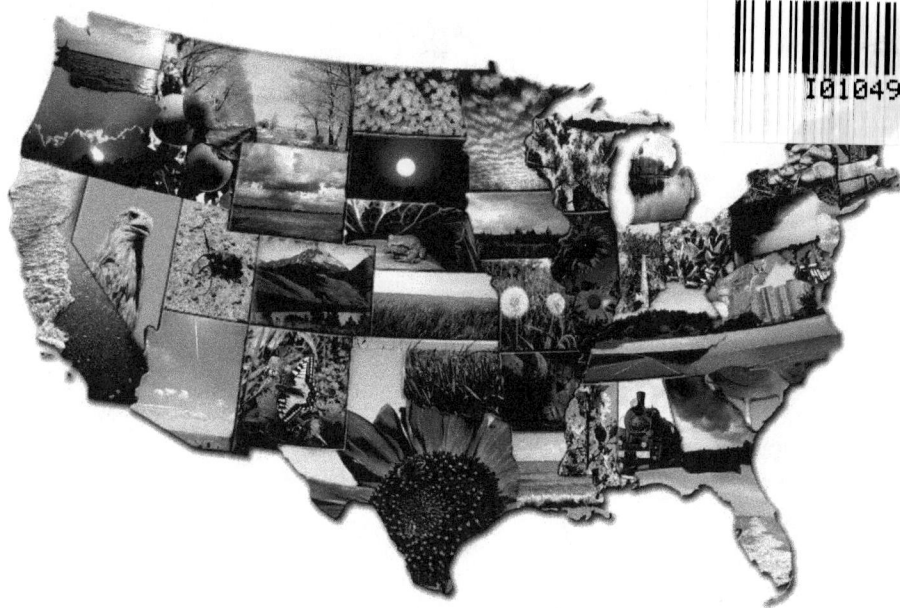

The Blue Book on the Correlation Between Natural Amenities, Altitude, Obesity, Diabetes, Inactivity and Longevity for 3,108 Counties

PEGGY FORNEY

The information in this book is provided to assist the reader in making informed life choices. This book is not intended as a substitute for medical advice. Before making any decisions based on information contained in this book, you should consult your personal physician. The author shall not be liable or responsible for any loss or damage allegedly arising from any information or suggestion in this book.

For Megan and Ashley

So that you and your families can have better lives

TABLE OF CONTENTS

ABOUT THE AUTHOR

You do not sell a fundamental change on the merits of the fundamental change.–Peggy June Forney

Peggy Forney spent twenty-three years working as marketing professional at Mountain Bell, AT&T, US WEST, and Qwest. She has a bachelor's degree in merchandising/marketing and a master's degree in technology management. US WEST was the first Regional Bell Operating Company to implement voice messaging. US WEST was also first to offer DSL (high-speed Internet). Peggy was there. Her passion is enabling fundamental change.

INTRODUCTION

The definition of insanity is doing the same thing over and over again and expecting different results. —Albert Einstein (1879–1955)

It's lean times for the diet industry.[1] A 2015 Marketdata report says the value of the US weight loss market actually declined in 2014 by 1.1 percent, to $59.8 billion.[2] Perhaps this is a good trend. Research studies reveal that many people who diet don't achieve significant long-term weight loss.

The graph on the following page is a five-year weight loss chart from a study conducted by the American Society for Clinical Nutrition titled "Long-term weight-loss maintenance: a meta-analysis of US studies" that analyzed results from twenty-nine weight loss studies. Even though the graph is a little hard to read, what's not hard to read is that most people who lose weight will regain a substantial amount. At year one, weight loss ranged from approximately 6 kilograms to 17 kilograms, or 13 to 37 pounds. At year five, the average (dotted triangle line in the middle) weight loss appears to be just over 2 kilograms, or approximately 5 to 6 pounds.

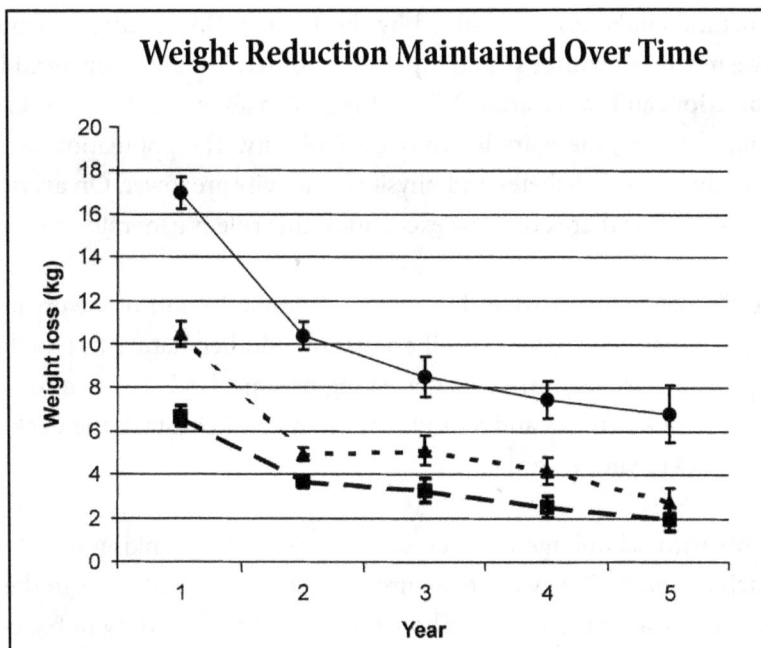

Weight Reduction Maintained Over Time

For the 78.6 million adult Americans who are obese,[4] 5 to 6 pounds of long-term weight loss is not a viable solution. So, until our weight loss industry invents a "magic obesity pill" or a "miracle altitude simulation device" or a Walt Disney-style "physical entertainment complex," another option is to leverage Mother Nature. Both natural amenities, as defined by the United States Department of Agriculture (USDA), and altitude can do what the weight loss industry has failed to do: enable the overweight or obese individual to lose a significant amount of weight without regaining most or all of it back over time.

What is significant long-term weight loss? It depends on the individual but, in my personal case, it was 90 pounds. In my case, it was also about halting the progression of diabetes and heart disease. By leveraging Mother Nature, I was able to achieve significant long-term weight loss and halt the progression of these diseases. In the process, I regained my health and freedom. Here is what my primary care physician of thirty years has to say:

> *Peggy's inspirational weight loss and success at halting the progression of diabetes and heart disease make me wish I had more patients like her.*
> —Eric H. Leder, MD

What are natural amenities? As defined by the 1999 USDA Natural Amenities Scale, they are: **warm winter, winter sun, temperate summer, low summer humidity, topographic variation,** and **water area.**[5] Where there is an abundance of natural amenities and/or a high altitude, there are lower rates of obesity. The population as a whole is slimmer and the rates of diabetes and physical inactivity are lower. On average, people also live longer. While there are a few exceptions, this rule is generally true.

Leveraging Mother Nature is what this book is all about. It's sort of the organic version of weight loss. Regardless of your specific situation, Mother Nature has a solution, and this book provides the road map. Just as eating organic foods is not a total solution, neither are natural amenities and altitude. But they can help stack the deck. They can help tip the scales in your favor.

Many parents with school-age children carefully scrutinize ranking data for schools' academic achievement. They want to assure their children have access to the very best education. Some will even purchase a home based on the proximity of high-achieving schools. By placing their child in a favorable educational environment, they can increase the chances for success.

The same is true for high natural amenities and high altitude. High scores in these areas generally mean lower obesity, lower diabetes, more physical activity, and a longer life span. Living where there are high natural amenities and high altitude is very similar to picking a good school. The student must still do the homework and take the tests, but the deck has been stacked in their favor. So why not live in a high achieving place to tip the scales in your favor?

This blue book provides the facts and data to help overweight and obese individuals make informed choices. It compiles research from multiple government sources and scientific publications and presents all the information in one location. The decision is yours, but now you can make your choices with facts and data in hand. Rather than depend upon glossy marketing brochures to help you decide where to live, you now can make your decisions based upon the numbers.

For retiring baby boomers, this resource guide delivers the skinny on where you might want to move for your golden years. Since your primary motivator is not "the job," you can pick and choose freely among the very best places to maximize your health and freedom. This blue book will examine Leadville, Colorado, as the benchmark case study, but there are literally hundreds of other high-altitude and/or high-natural-amenity counties and communities in the United States. Choose a high achieving county and you've improved your chances for success.

Like food, altitude is one of those things that are good for you…up to a point. However, once a certain threshold is crossed, it can become detrimental to your health. The altitude threshold varies greatly from individual to individual. While most healthy individuals can benefit from living at high altitude, there are some who will find that living at a lower altitude is a better choice. And if someone is already suffering from certain chronic health conditions (COPD, emphysema, cystic fibrosis, heart failure, arrhythmias, pulmonary hypertension, congenital heart problems, etc.), high altitude can make things worse. Even your genes may play a role in determining how you react to high altitude. Chapters 2 and 4 discuss altitude in more detail.

If you are sensitive to high altitude, there are a large number of low-altitude, high-amenity counties that have low obesity rates. For example, the coastline of California has relatively low obesity rates, as do both coastlines of Florida. So if access to golf and the ocean twelve months a year is your definition of paradise, many counties in these two states can make an excellent choice. If you want to live in the mountains but at lower altitudes, there are the Appalachian Mountains in the eastern United States. Since both high natural amenities and high altitude are correlated with lower obesity rates, the choice is yours.

CHAPTER 1

How High Natural Amenities and Altitude Help You Lose Weight

Every man is the creature of the age in which he lives; very few are able to raise themselves above the ideas of the time. —Voltaire (1694–1778)

In 2002 I moved to Leadville, Colorado. Being extremely obese at 10,152 feet was especially difficult. Climbing stairs would leave me completely breathless and drained. I was always hot, and I couldn't do any sort of physical activity without being in complete misery.

Because I was so heavy, I had lost my personal freedom and my health was beginning to suffer. By the time I turned fifty-two, I was diagnosed with insulin resistance (a physiological condition in which the natural hormone insulin becomes less effective at lowering blood sugars).[1] This meant I was well on my way to becoming a type 2 diabetic, and my high cholesterol levels required the prescription medication Lipitor.

But moving to Leadville had a completely unexpected side effect. I quit gaining weight! I didn't initially lose weight, but I stopped gaining without changing what I ate. Why? What was it about Leadville that caused me to turn it around? Why were there so many slim people living here?

Here's what I discovered: As a general rule, people who live where there are lots of natural amenities weigh less, have less diabetes, and are more physically active than people who live where there are few natural amenities. On average, they also live longer. How do I know this? Because I matched up data from a number of US government sources

1

and scientific publications that clearly show this correlation. Let's start with these two government sources.

1. A 1999 United States Department of Agriculture (USDA) Natural Amenities Scale that rates all the counties in the lower forty-eight states for natural amenities. The scale is a measure of the physical characteristics of a county area that enhance the location as a place to live. (The USDA report does not include Alaska or Hawaii.) Each county in the lower forty-eight states is rated according to natural amenities such as climate, topography, and water area that reflect environmental qualities most people prefer. **The six measures are warm winter, winter sun, temperate summer, low summer humidity, topographic variation, and water area.**[2]

    The total number of USDA-rated counties in this book is 3,108. The USDA rates the counties numerically, from +11.17 for the county having the most natural amenities to −6.40 for the county having the fewest. Because the USDA numbers can be a little difficult to decipher, I ranked the counties from 1 to 3,108, with 1 rated highest for natural amenities by the USDA and 3,108 rated lowest.

2. The Centers for Disease Control and Prevention (CDC) data that tracks obesity, diabetes, and leisure-time physical inactivity rates at the county level. When I did my research in 2012, the most recent year for which data were posted was 2009. Here is what the CDC has to say.

    The prevalence of obesity, diabetes, and leisure-time physical inactivity by county was estimated using data from CDC's Behavioral Risk Factor Surveillance System (BRFSS) and data from the US Census Bureau's Population Estimates Program. The BRFSS is an ongoing, monthly, state-based telephone survey of the adult population. The survey provides state-specific information on behavioral risk factors and preventive health practices. Respondents were considered,

    -   to have diabetes if they responded "yes" to the question, "Has a doctor ever told you that you have diabetes?" Women who indicated that they only had diabetes during pregnancy were not considered to have diabetes.

    -   To be obese if their body mass index was 30 or greater. Body mass index (weight [kg]/height [m]2) was derived from self-report of height and weight.

- To be physically inactive if they answered "no" to the question, "During the past month, other than your regular job, did you participate in any physical activities or exercises such as running, calisthenics, golf, gardening, or walking for exercise?"[3]

Here's an average of the fifty lowest-obesity-rated counties compared to the fifty highest-obesity-rated counties. The average rates of obesity, diabetes, and leisure-time physical inactivity are more than 200 percent higher in counties that have fewer natural amenities compared to those counties with more natural amenities.

AVERAGE OBESITY	AVERAGE AMENITY RATING	AVERAGE % OBESITY	AVERAGE % DIABETES	AVERAGE % INACTIVE
50 LOWEST Obesity Rated Counties	282 (high) out of 3,108	17.3%	5.4%	15.8%
50 HIGHEST Obesity Rated Counties	1,840 (low) out of 3,108	41.2% (238% higher)	13.9% (257% higher)	34.3% (217% higher)

Colorado dominates the fifty lowest-obesity-rated counties with twenty-nine counties. Mississippi, with sixteen counties and Alabama, with eleven counties, dominate the fifty highest-obesity-rated counties. Below are the numbers for the two counties with the lowest and highest obesity rates in the country. The rates of obesity, diabetes, and leisure-time physical inactivity are 336 percent to 426 percent higher in the county that has fewer natural amenities.

COUNTY & STATE	AMENITY RATING	% OBESITY	% DIABETES	% INACTIVE
Routt County, Colorado	90 (high) out of 3,108	13.5%	3.8%	11.1%
Green County, Alabama	1,469 (low) out of 3,108	47.9% (355% higher)	16.2% (426% higher)	37.3% (336% higher)

There is also a big correlation between life expectancy and high natural amenities ranking, obesity rate, diabetes rate, and leisure-time physical inactivity. To determine this, I compiled data from a June 15, 2011 study done by the Institute of Health Metrics and Evaluation at the University of Washington in Seattle titled, "Falling behind:

life expectancy in US counties from 2000 to 2007 in an international context."[4] Then I added it to the USDA Natural Amenities Scale data.

I identified the top five and bottom five longevity counties for both men and women. When I averaged them, here is what I found. While there are a couple of anomalies regarding natural amenities rating, the correlation between the other variables is stunning. On average, men live 14.6 years longer and women live 10.9 years longer in counties with higher natural amenities. Their obesity, diabetes, and leisure-time physical inactivity rates help explain why.

Average of Five Highest Longevity and Five Lowest Longevity Counties

MEN	AVERAGE LONGEVITY (YEARS)	AVERAGE AMENITY RATING	AVERAGE OBESITY RATE	AVERAGE DIABETES RATE	AVERAGE INACTIVITY RATE
HIGHEST	80.7	866 (high)	18.6%	6.4%	15%
LOWEST	66.1	2235 (low)	39%	14.2%	36.9%

WOMEN	AVERAGE LONGEVITY (YEARS)	AVERAGE AMENITY RATING	AVERAGE OBESITY RATE	AVERAGE DIABETES RATE	AVERAGE INACTIVITY RATE
HIGHEST	84.8	420 (high)	17.8%	6%	14.3%
LOWEST	73.9	2200 (low)	40.8%	14.3%	35.4%

Now you may ask why obesity, diabetes, and leisure-time physical inactivity are emphasized by the CDC as health indicators. It's because these three factors are highly correlated with each other and so many serious health issues in the United States.

This correlation with health is especially true for diabetes. Diabetes can affect many parts of the body and is associated with serious complications, such as heart disease, stroke, blindness, kidney failure, and lower-limb amputation. People with diabetes may have or develop other complications or conditions, such as nerve disease, non-alcoholic fatty liver disease, periodontal (gum) disease, hearing loss, erectile dysfunction, depression, and complications of pregnancy, among others. In 2003-2006, after adjusting for population age differences, rates of death from all causes were about 1.5 times higher among adults aged 18 years or older with diagnosed diabetes than among adults without diagnosed diabetes.[5]

While I was conducting my obesity research utilizing the 1999 USDA Natural Amenities Scale data and the CDC 2009 obesity, diabetes, and leisure-time physical inactivity data, I noticed something odd. California has the top ten natural amenities rated counties in the United States, but it doesn't have the very lowest obesity rates. The obesity rates are low, but Colorado is the leanest state in the country, with twenty-nine of the fifty leanest counties. So 45 percent of Colorado's sixty-four counties are in the top fifty from a low-obesity standpoint. The average Natural Amenities Scale rating of these twenty-nine Colorado counties is 104 (high) out of 3,108 (low).

But if natural amenities were the whole story, California should win the low-obesity game. When you rate the lower forty-eight states by natural amenities, California has not only the top ten counties in the country, but thirty of the top fifty counties. In comparison, Colorado has only ten counties in the top fifty when rated by natural amenities. There must be another variable operating, and I predicted it was high altitude. But I could find no research to substantiate my high altitude hypothesis. It turns out the research was published the following year.

A doctor by the name of Jameson D. Voss, MD, was the lead researcher of a 2013 study titled "Association of elevation, urbanization and ambient temperature with obesity prevalence in the United States." This research combined several publicly available national datasets and used actual self-reported height and weight. Here are the research publication conclusions.

> Obesity prevalence in the United States is inversely associated with elevation and urbanization, after adjusting for temperature, diet, physical activity, smoking and demographic factors.[6]

Dr. Voss was even more specific in a blog he authored.

> **Recently, we've identified a strong association between obesity prevalence and altitude within the US.** Our findings were surprising because they indicated the magnitude of this association was large and the pattern of association exhibited a curvilinear dose response in 500 meter [1,640'] categories of altitude. **There was a 4–5 fold increase in obesity prevalence at low altitude as compared with the highest**

altitude [9,843'–11,450'] category after controlling for diet, activity level, smoking, demographics, temperature, and urbanization.[7]

Now take a look at the color maps on the back cover of this book. My research utilized the 1999 USDA Natural Amenities Scale map and the CDC 2009 County-Level Estimates of Obesity Among Adults ≥ 20 map. Dr. Voss's blog utilized the US Topographic map and the same CDC map.

The green colors on the USDA Natural Amenities Scale map indicate high natural amenities. The brown and white colors on the US Topographic map show higher altitude. The white indicates the highest altitude. Compare these two maps with the CDC 2009 County-Level Estimates of Obesity Among Adults ≥ 20 map.

Look at Florida. It has virtually no altitude, but it has lots of natural amenities and lower obesity rates. Look at the Appalachian Mountains. While there are relatively few natural amenities, there is moderate altitude and lower obesity rates. The California coastline has low elevation but high natural amenities and lower obesity rates. The maps clearly show that, separately, high natural amenities and high altitude are each correlated with lower obesity rates. Together, they explain why Colorado, with both high natural amenities and high altitude, is the leanest state in the United States.

Higher altitude linked with lower obesity rates may make some logical sense, especially in light of Dr. Voss's recent research. But why are higher natural amenities also correlated with lower obesity rates? **The six measures that make up the USDA Natural Amenities Scale are warm winter, winter sun, temperate summer, low summer humidity, topographic variation, and water area.** Each of the six USDA measures involves environmental conditions that are pleasant to our senses. It's easy to be physically active when you are surrounded by wonderful weather and beautiful scenery. Getting outside and being surrounded by Mother Nature becomes a whole lot more inviting. With high natural amenities and high altitude, Mother Nature delivers the very best natural weight loss program in the world. It's sort of the organic version of weight loss. Here's what the CDC has to say about being physically active.

> Physical activity can improve health. People who are physically active tend to live longer and have lower risk for heart disease, stroke, type 2 diabetes, depression, and some cancers. Physical activity can also help with weight control, and may improve academic achievement

in students. About 1 in 5 (21%) adults meet the 2008 [CDC] Physical Activity Guidelines.[8]

So here is a fundamental change concept to wrap your brain around. We're always told we need to get more physical exercise. Rather than engage in physical exercise, it's much easier and more fun to engage in *physical entertainment*. The biggest difference between physical exercise and *physical entertainment* is the goal. The primary goal of physical exercise is the exercise. The primary goal of *physical entertainment* is the entertainment. This may sound like a shallow play on words, but the difference between the two is huge. Most of us exercise because it is good for us, not because it is incredibly pleasurable. The result is that most of us aren't physically active on a regular basis, especially when it's hot and muggy or cold and damp. With high natural amenities, Mother Nature helps us want to engage in *physical entertainment*. Here is my personal story of how I discovered the concept of *physical entertainment*.

In 2002 I was extremely obese when I moved to Leadville, Colorado. I fell in love with the area because it is absolutely beautiful, and living here made me feel truly alive. One of the county's crown jewels is the paved twelve-mile Mineral Belt bike trail, which loops around the mining district. At the top, the elevation is 10,606 feet!

But I was too obese to ride my bike. I couldn't hike or snowshoe on the wonderful mountain trails that are everywhere. I couldn't ski at the eight world-class ski areas that are less than an hour's drive from Leadville. I was too fat to bend over and fasten ski boots even if I could have found ski clothes that were big enough.

In March, 2004 I changed what I was eating and began the long journey toward normal weight. Although there was a good indoor pool nearby, I wouldn't be seen dead in it because felt I was too fat to wear a swimsuit and was not thrilled at doing pool laps for exercise. So I didn't engage in any physical activity from March through May. But by June, I had lost about eighteen pounds, so I decided to try and get on my twenty-year-old bike. With many stops and shaky legs, I finally completed the twelve-mile loop around the Mineral Belt trail. I was completely exhausted but thrilled!

I got back on the bike again and again. It was during the long, six-mile uphill climbs on the Mineral Belt trail that I questioned why I continued to get on my bike. The rides were physically very difficult, but I began to look forward to them. Why? Because the environment and scenery are stunning. As you slowly grind up the first six miles, you are able to see the beautiful trees, flowers, and occasional wildlife. You can smell the high mountain forest in all its glory. And the sun at 10,000+ feet and the pure, dry air at 70 degrees create an exquisite experience that you cannot adequately describe.

Then, as you swoop down the final six miles, you feel the cool, fresh mountain air on your skin and in your lungs. It was wonderful, and I came to feel deprived if the weather occasionally didn't cooperate. And the rides got easier and easier. Pretty soon I was pedaling that bike all the way around the twelve-mile loop without stopping even once. In the process, I finally figured out that, for me, this was not physical exercise but *physical entertainment*.

By late fall, I had lost almost forty pounds. Since I live where there are so many world-class ski areas within minutes, I decided to investigate the possibility of learning how to ski. Imagine my amazement to discover that the season pass prices for many of these ski areas are complete bargains! If you ski fifty days a year, the daily cost can be less than $10!

So in the fall of 2004, I decided I was going to take a huge risk and try to become a skier. At age fifty-three, it took a lot of courage for me to actually take this step in my life, because I didn't know how to ski. I went out and bought extra-large ski clothing on sale and joined the nearby Copper Mountain Over the Hill Gang for fifty-plus-year-old skiers.[9] There was guided skiing, lessons, lots of emotional support, and many friendships to be found in Copper OHG.

Once I learned how to ski and was not so afraid, I was able to experience the *physical entertainment* of skiing. I have never tried heroin or cocaine, but I am now addicted to another white powder. It's called snow. Over time my skiing ability improved significantly, and in 2013 I became a Level 1 Certified PSIA (Professional Ski Instructors of America) ski instructor.

So I don't exercise. But, in my perfect world, there would be a hundred days of perfect biking weather and a hundred days of perfect snow conditions for skiing. That leaves 165 days to hike, snowshoe, cross-country ski, and kayak, or not engage in any *physical entertainment* at all.

Now just a bit of clarification is in order. I'm not a *physical entertainment* animal. I never have been much of an athlete and, compared to many, I'd say I'm a bit of a wimp. I bike short distances but on a very frequent basis. I do the same thing when I hike. And my ski day may be over by noon unless skiing conditions are great. This *physical entertainment* concept is about cherishing the journey, not arriving at the destination. You need to occasionally stop, smell the flowers, and embrace the scenery.

While my personal story involves a county ranked high in both natural amenities and altitude, a similar story can play out in all counties ranked high in natural amenities. It can also play out in all high-altitude counties. Both high natural amenities and high altitude can literally tip the scales.

But there are a few exceptions to the rule. For example, Montgomery County, Maryland, has a low obesity rate of 18.1 percent, a low natural amenities rating of 1,859, and a mean altitude of 404 feet. And Arlington County, Virginia, has a low obesity rate of 19.4 percent, a low amenity rating of 2,674, and a mean altitude of 207 feet.

The biggest exception is the Big Apple. New York County has a very low 15.2 percent obesity rate, a low natural amenities rating of 1,682, and a mean altitude of 48 feet. Based on natural amenities, altitude, and demographics, New Yorkers should have a much higher obesity rate.

Yes, New York, Montgomery, and Arlington Counties are very urban, very educated, and have extremely high median household incomes, but that doesn't totally account for the low obesity rates. So here's another possibility that may contribute to this anomaly: Most New Yorkers don't climb into their cars to go to work and go shopping because driving and parking a car in New York City is not for the timid or poor. New York's massive public transportation system requires most folks to walk a little *every day*, even if it's not always for pleasure. So perhaps even this low level of *daily* physical activity may result in lower obesity rates over the long haul. At this point we don't really know, and science doesn't yet have all the answers.

In addition to the obesity research that Dr. Voss has done, there is a 2011 *Journal of Epidemiology and Community Health* research publication titled "Altitude, life expectancy and mortality from ischaemic heart disease, stroke, COPD and cancers: national population-based analysis of US counties." Here is what the article says.

> After adjustment, altitude had a beneficial association with IHD mortality and a harmful association with COPD...Of the 20 counties with the highest life expectancy, 11 for men and five for women are in Colorado and Utah, all at mean elevations of 1,819 m [5,968'] or higher. Men and women who lived in counties at a higher altitude in the USA had a longer life expectancy.[10]

While those with chronic lung diseases such as COPD, emphysema, and cystic fibrosis generally do better at lower altitudes, there's a surprise: asthma. Here's what the Institute for Altitude Medicine in Telluride, Colorado, has to say.

> Persons with asthma do better at high altitude, contrary to some opinions. Pollution is less and dust mites, a very common allergen, don't live at high altitude. Overall there is evidence that those plagued with asthma, in particular allergic asthma, do better at altitude than at sea level.[11]

The Asthma Center, Allergic Disease Associates, in Philadelphia, offers additional information.

> Studies in the United States have shown that 30–40% of all asthmatics and the majority of patients with hayfever are allergic to dust mites. Atopic dermatitis is also commonly triggered by mite sensitivity... They thrive when the temperature is warm (70–90 degrees) and when the relative humidity is 75–80%. Dust mites cannot survive when the relative humidity falls below 40% or at very high altitudes (greater than 9,000 feet elevation) or when it is too cold.[12]

Now let's pause for a moment and put all this information together. Lake County, Colorado, is rated by the USDA as the #1 high-altitude county for natural amenities. At 10,152 feet, Leadville is the highest-altitude incorporated city in the United States. In addition, the county has unpolluted, dry air with high temperatures that generally don't exceed 70 degrees. So, based upon the latest scientific research, Lake County offers an environment that is associated with lower obesity, lower ischemic heart disease, higher longevity, and better breathing for those plagued with asthma and allergies. Leadville/Lake County may just be the healthiest place in America!

But there are those in the medical community who are not quite ready to say that high altitude is correlated with improved health. Perhaps the study results might be slanted because bad health could force some folks to move to a lower altitude. Perhaps the results are skewed because the unhealthy don't move to high altitudes in the first place. Unlike weight, which is more straightforward because it's quantitative, "health" is very complex and nebulous, so it's difficult to pinpoint direct quantitative correlation or causation.

It can take a while for the medical community to adopt a fundamental change in its thinking. For example, it took about twenty-five years for Barry Marshall and Robin Warren to be awarded the Nobel Prize for their discovery that peptic ulcer disease is caused by bacteria, not excess stomach acid.[13] And the high-altitude-equals-health debate could take just as long. The bottom line is our medical professionals and research scientists don't yet know everything they need to know. Here is what Dr. Voss has to say about his obesity-altitude research.

> While it is always important to remember correlation does not prove causation, in this case, we already know hypoxia causes anorexia and weight loss based on well controlled interventional data. This effect is biologically plausible based on the relationship between hypoxia and leptin signaling, norepinephrine and sympathetic tone, non-erythroid erythropoietin receptor signaling, and the metabolic demands at high altitude. We hope additional research will help clarify the mechanisms and long term health effects of either high altitude residence or normobaric hypoxia [simulated altitude].[14]

Until our scientific community conducts more research and develops additional empirical explanations, the best option we have is to leverage Mother Nature. One of these days we may be able to take a "magic obesity pill" or utilize a "miracle altitude simulation device" or even patronize a Walt Disney–style "physical entertainment complex" to minimize our weight and maximize our health, but today we don't have these things. However, we do have Mother Nature.

This is not the first time humans have leveraged Mother Nature. For example, history shows that, in the early 20th century, there were seventeen tuberculosis sanatoriums in the Pikes Peak region of the Rocky Mountains alone.

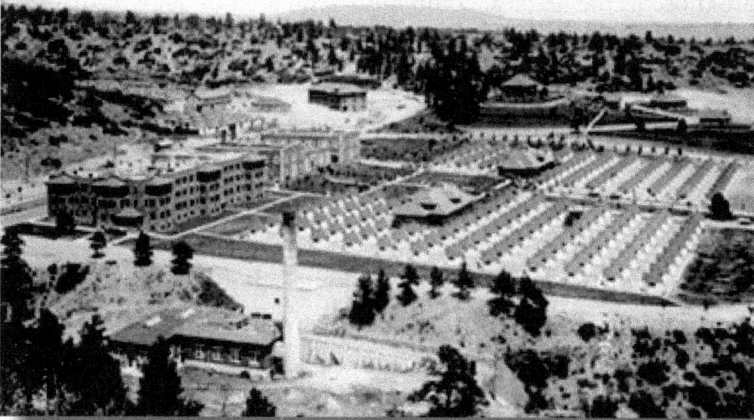

The Woodmen Sanatorium, complete with individual cabins shaped like tepees to maximize air circulation, Colorado Springs, Colorado. *Photograph courtesy the Colorado Springs Pioneers Museum.*[15]

According to the CDC, tuberculosis was once the leading cause of death in the United States.[16] Like obesity, tuberculosis used to be an intractable epidemic. Like obesity, there was no cure except Mother Nature's healing geography. Until our scientific community comes up with a better long-term solution for obesity, Mother Nature's natural amenities and altitude offer the best weight loss program in the world.

The maps on the back cover of this book and the 3,108 county listings by amenity and obesity provide the information that can help us come up with strategies to minimize our weight and maximize our health. There's no one right answer for everyone. But there is a right answer for each of us that can now be based on facts and data rather than on fancy marketing brochures.

Again, here's the graph that was featured in the Introduction to this book. It is a five-year weight loss chart from a research study conducted by the American Society for Clinical Nutrition titled "Long-term weight-loss maintenance: a meta-analysis of US Studies" that analyzed results from 29 weight loss studies. Even though the graph is a little hard to read, what's not hard to read is that most people who lose weight will regain a substantial amount. At year one, weight loss ranged from approximately 6 kilograms to 17 kilograms, or 13 to 37 pounds. At year five, the average (dotted triangle line in the middle) weight loss appears to be just over 2 kilograms, or approximately 5 to 6 pounds.

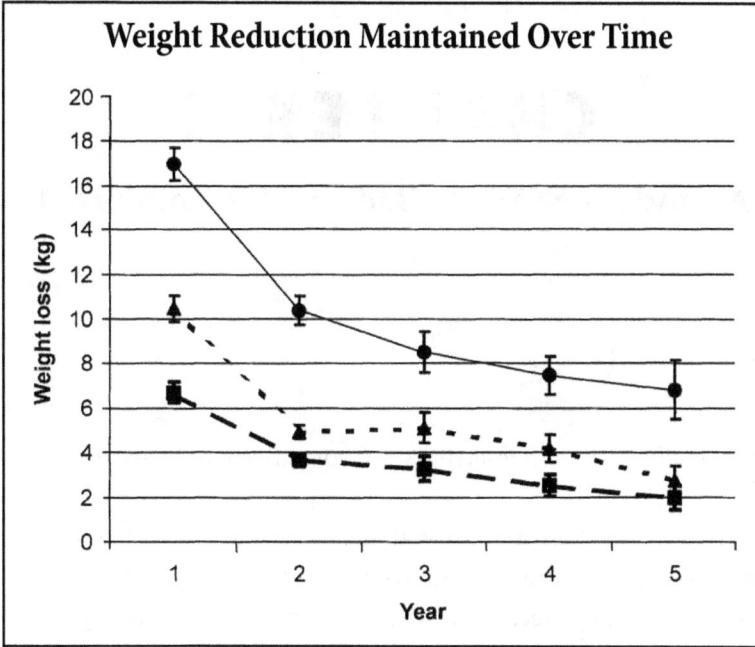

Weight Reduction Maintained Over Time

[chart: Weight loss (kg) vs. Year, showing three declining lines from year 1 to year 5] [17]

Like many overweight and obese people, I couldn't seem to lose weight and keep it off. Moving to Leadville helped tip the scales and, in 2010, my doctor quit prescribing Lipitor for high cholesterol. While my weight still fluctuates some on the low end, leveraging Mother Nature's high natural amenities and high altitude helped me be successful. Mother Nature helped me beat the odds, and I've regained my health and freedom.

> *Peggy's inspirational weight loss and success at halting the progression of diabetes and heart disease make me wish I had more patients like her.*
> —Eric H. Leder, MD

CHAPTER 2

Altitude Is NOT the Bad Guy We Think He Is

All great truths begin as blasphemies. —George Bernard Shaw (1856–1950)

Most folks don't associate high altitude with the word good. Realizing that high altitude can actually be good for many of us who struggle with our weight involves a fundamental change in our thinking. Decades will pass before some folks change their thinking on the subject.

But knowledge can help us begin the change. So here is what Wikipedia has to say on the subject of acclimatization to altitude.

> The human body can adapt to high altitude through both immediate and long-term acclimatization. At high altitude, in the short term, the lack of oxygen is sensed by the carotid bodies, which causes an increase in the breathing rate (hyperventilation). However, hyperventilation also causes the adverse effect of respiratory alkalosis, inhibiting the respiratory center from enhancing the respiratory rate as much as would be required. Inability to increase the breathing rate can be caused by inadequate carotid body response or pulmonary or renal disease.
>
> In addition, at high altitude, the heart beats faster; the stroke volume is slightly decreased; and non-essential bodily functions are suppressed, resulting in a decline in food digestion efficiency (as the

body suppresses the digestive system in favor of increasing its cardio-pulmonary reserves).

Full acclimatization, however, requires days or even weeks. Gradually, the body compensates for the respiratory alkalosis by renal excretion of bicarbonate, allowing adequate respiration to provide oxygen without risking alkalosis. It takes about four days at any given altitude and can be enhanced by drugs such as acetazolamide. Eventually, the body has lower lactate production (because reduced glucose breakdown decreases the amount of lactate formed), decreased plasma volume, increased hematocrit (polycythemia), increased RBC mass, a higher concentration of capillaries in skeletal muscle tissue, increased myoglobin, increased mitochondria, increased aerobic enzyme concentration, increase in 2,3-BPG, hypoxic pulmonary vasoconstriction, and right ventricular hypertrophy. Pulmonary artery pressure increases in an effort to oxygenate more blood.

Full hematological adaptation to high altitude is achieved when the increase of red blood cells reaches a plateau and stops. The length of full hematological adaptation can be approximated by multiplying the altitude in kilometers by 11.4 days. For example, to adapt to 4,000 meters (13,000 ft) of altitude would require 45.6 days. The upper altitude limit of this linear relationship has not been fully established.[1]

Leadville's altitude is 10,152 feet, or 3,094 meters. So if you've been living at sea level, full hematological adaptation to Leadville's altitude will require approximately 35 days. I always tell folks who inquire that it takes about a month to fully get your altitude legs. Since I moved to Leadville, my annual physicals always show my hematocrit (red blood cell) levels to be above normal because I live at high altitude.

Now let me provide you with my low-tech explanation of what might be going on at high altitude. I call it my "combustion engine theory." Each motor/engine/furnace will react differently, but a general rule of thumb is that, for every 1,000 feet of altitude increase, anything combustion loses approximately 3 percent of its power.[2] At 10,000 feet, that's 30 percent.

Lots of civilian and military aircraft fly in and out of the Lake County Airport. Sometimes there are strange-looking cars with their identities concealed on the road bearing

Michigan manufacturer license plates. They're conducting high-altitude performance testing because aircraft and cars that perform well at sea level can turn into gutless wonders at high altitude. And all the natural gas furnaces I put in the seven homes I built in Lake County were significantly derated for the altitude. That means a bigger furnace is required to adequately heat the square footage of a given-size house.

Although we humans aren't machines, we still metabolize food a little like machines. So maybe we humans have to physiologically work 30 percent harder at 10,000 feet than at sea level to just breathe and move. Perhaps altitude helps tip the scales. If so, it may partially explain why folks who live at high altitudes weigh less.

The bottom line is that the scientists and researchers don't yet know exactly why high altitude is correlated with low obesity. But the USDA Natural Amenities Scale map, the US Topographic map, and the CDC 2009 County-Level Estimates of Obesity among Adults ≥ 20 map on the back cover of this book clearly show that high natural amenities and/ or high altitude go hand-in-hand with lower obesity rates. Together, high altitude and high natural amenities are correlated with the lowest obesity rates in the United States.

Now let's discuss acute mountain sickness (AMS). As a ski instructor at Ski Cooper (elevation 10,500–11,700 feet), I frequently saw what I term "Houston green." Many wonderful ski tourists from Houston, who are accustomed to living at about 50 feet above sea level, fly via high-speed jet into Denver. They then rent a car and immediately drive to over 10,000 feet. All this happens in a few short hours, so a certain percentage will develop AMS and turn sort of green. AMS feels like a bad hangover.[3] Symptoms can include headache, queasiness, tiredness, and trouble sleeping.[4] And no, these symptoms are not limited to tourists from Houston. Anyone who comes from a very low altitude and goes immediately to a very high altitude is a candidate for AMS.

According to the National Institutes of Health (NIH), acute mountain sickness is caused by reduced air pressure and lower oxygen levels at high altitudes. Here is what the NIH has to say.

> The faster you climb to a high altitude, the more likely you will get acute mountain sickness. You are at higher risk for acute mountain sickness if:
>
> - You live at or near sea level and travel to a high altitude
> - You have had the illness before.[5]

AMS is not to be taken lightly. While it's just a temporary inconvenience for many folks, there are a few who will need medical attention. According to the NIH, severe cases may even result in death due to lung problems or brain swelling, called cerebral edema.[6] Additional terms you may see are HACE, for high-altitude cerebral edema, and HAPE, for high-altitude pulmonary edema.

To put things into perspective, altitude is sort of like peanut butter. The peanut butter and jelly sandwich is the epitome of an all-American food. But for the few who are allergic, peanut butter can sicken or even kill. The same is true for AMS.

The scientific community has been hard at work to tease out why certain people and even certain animals are more affected by altitude than others. Scientists have known for some time that certain people are inherently more susceptible to altitude sickness than others and that this susceptibility is heritable. Preliminary studies suggest that a group of six genes predicts who will get altitude sickness with greater than 90 percent accuracy, and research continues to fit more puzzle pieces together.[7]

Cows also get AMS. Scientists have been searching for the genes that determine which cows develop altitude sickness, also known as brisket disease, when they graze in the Rocky Mountains. Because tens of thousands of cows die in the western United States from brisket disease annually, ranchers would like nothing more than to strip the responsible genes from the breeding population.[8]

The bottom line is that AMS is not necessarily caused because you're in terrible shape or because you're old. In fact, healthy older folks are actually a little less susceptible to AMS than younger people are.[9] And, like eye and hair color, our genes may be partially responsible for the way we react to altitude.

However, if folks are already suffering from certain chronic conditions like COPD, heart failure, arrhythmias, congenital heart problems, emphysema, pulmonary hypertension, and cystic fibrosis, a lower altitude may be in order.[10] My nearest neighbor is a registered nurse who makes a living delivering oxygen, and he tells me that high altitude can make certain types of chronic conditions even worse. So if you've got existing health issues, just take his expert opinion into consideration. Maybe a low-altitude, high-natural-amenity county might be a better option, and there are lots of counties to choose from. Yes, swimming in the ocean and golfing twelve months a year is a tough life, but someone's got to do it.

Here is a vacation tip gleaned from in-the-know folks who live at high altitude. A retired physician friend of mine makes a point of staying a night or two in Denver when he flies back from his month-long bicycling vacations in France. And the Institute for Altitude Medicine in Telluride, Colorado, recommends "an overnight stay at an intermediate altitude such as Denver or preferably a bit higher prior to further ascent into the mountains."[11] So if you are coming to Colorado from very low altitude, an evening flight into Denver with an overnight stopover at a moderate altitude is a very good vacation strategy.

CHAPTER 3

A Case Study: Why Leadville, Colorado is #1 in the United States

I have always thought Leadville was missing the mark as the next obesity resort. —A medical doctor and altitude researcher

Historic Leadville, Colorado, with a population of 2,602,[1] is truly a diamond in the rough. It doesn't glitter and it's not flashy. Downtown currently has too many vacant storefronts, and the roads in and out of Leadville conceal the true wealth of what is here. Leadville's wealth of high natural amenities and high elevation is right under our feet, but many folks just can't see it.

The majority of Lake County's 7,290 residents live near the city of Leadville.[2] Fifteen miles south of Leadville is the rural enclave of Twin Lakes, with a population of 171.[3] As the name suggests, Twin Lakes overlooks two breathtaking alpine lakes.

Again, the 1999 USDA Natural Amenities Scale rates the lower forty-eight US counties on **warm winter, winter sun, temperate summer, low summer humidity, topographic variation,** and **water area.** Leadville/Lake County has everything except a Bermuda shorts winter.

While California has Colorado beat for high natural amenities, Colorado is the state with the highest altitude. In addition, many Colorado counties are also highly rated for natural amenities. As a result, Colorado is the leanest state in the United States. Here are the top twenty US counties as rated by the USDA Natural Amenities Scale.

Top 20 Counties Ranked by Natural Amenity

(High Amenity Ranking = Low Number)

STATE	COUNTY	AMENITY RANKING	USDA RATING	CDC % OBESITY	CDC % DIABETES	CDC % INACTIVE	MEAN ALTITUDE
CA	Ventura	1	11.17	22.9	6.8	16.8	2,690'
CA	Humboldt	2	11.15	25.9	8.1	18.9	1,754'
CA	Santa Barbara	3	10.97	19.9	6.6	15.8	1,823'
CA	Mendocino	4	10.93	22.6	6.3	17	1,827'
CA	Del Norte	5	10.75	27.2	7.6	18.1	2,189'
CA	San Francisco	6	10.52	17.2	7.3	17	236'
CA	Los Angeles	7	10.33	21.4	7.7	18.9	2,265'
CA	San Diego	8	9.78	22.8	7.3	17.4	1,975'
CA	Monterey	9	9.24	22.3	7.3	16	1,464'
CA	Orange	10	8.74	20.5	7.1	16.4	725'
CO	Lake	11	8.52	17.7	5.1	18.9	10,931'
CA	Santa Cruz	12	8.49	19.5	6.1	12.4	939'
CA	Contra Costa	13	8.36	24.2	6.9	17.3	486'
CA	Calaveras	14	8.27	25.6	6.7	19.3	2,430'
CA	Mariposa	15	8.25	24.1	7.2	19.4	3,637'
CA	Mono	16	8.21	20.3	6.5	13.6	7,760'
CA	San Mateo	17	8.19	19.8	6.5	16.1	669'
CA	Marin	18	8.14	15	5.4	12.1	426'
CO	Summit	19	8.08	15.1	4.7	12.3	10,481'
CA	Sonoma	20	7.93	22.7	6.1	14.2	729'

If high natural amenities and high altitude result in lower obesity, why don't the CDC percentages show Lake County as having the lowest obesity rate? Because the CDC numbers are raw percentages. This means that the numbers will be somewhat skewed because of differences in the demographic makeup (race, income, education level, etc.) of the population. Let's review Dr. Voss's altitude research study statement again.

> Obesity prevalence in the United States is inversely associated with elevation and urbanization, after adjusting for temperature, diet, physical activity, smoking and demographic factors.[4]

Lake County currently serves as a bedroom community for rich Summit and Eagle Counties to the north. These two counties have the huge, glitzy ski resorts of Vail, Beaver Creek, Copper Mountain, Keystone, and Breckenridge. In these two counties, wealthy second-home owners have driven the cost of housing up so high that the middle-income wage earner can't afford to live there. The cost of housing is much lower in Lake County, so many workers commute from Leadville.

Since Lake County and adjacent Summit County are similar in natural amenities and altitude, we'll compare their respective demographics. (Eagle County is lower in altitude and is rated lower for natural amenities, so we won't use it for comparison.)

According to 2013 US Census Bureau numbers, Lake County's population is 7,290, with 58.7 percent categorized as white and 38.4 percent categorized as Hispanic. Median household income, 2009–2013, is $44,610, and 28.1 percent of its inhabitants have a bachelor's degree or higher. In contrast, adjacent Summit County's population is 28,755, with 82.6 percent categorized as white and 14.4 percent categorized as Hispanic. Median household income, 2009–2013, is $63,697, and 47.7 percent of all residents have a bachelor's degree or higher.[5] As you can see, the demographics of Lake County and Summit County are considerably different. In addition, many Lake County residents live approximately 500 to 1,000 feet higher than many Summit County residents.

After adjusting for urbanization and demographic factors, Lake County's adjusted obesity rate is probably lower than adjacent Summit County's very low obesity rate of 15.1 percent. The bottom line is to take the CDC percentages with a grain of salt. You will need to do some homework to estimate the impact that demographics and urbanization may have on a particular county or community. The US Census Bureau website (www.quickfacts.census.gov) provides the details for all US counties.

Now let's take a peek at the future. Although the United States has historically been a youth-driven culture, the number one consumer age demographic is now baby boomers. But here's a stunning statistic. According to the AARP, only about 10 percent of advertising dollars are currently being directed at baby boomers because Madison Avenue remains youth obsessed.[6] This could be a very costly mistake for some unaware companies. Here are the AARP numbers.

The number one consumer age demographic is now baby boomers.

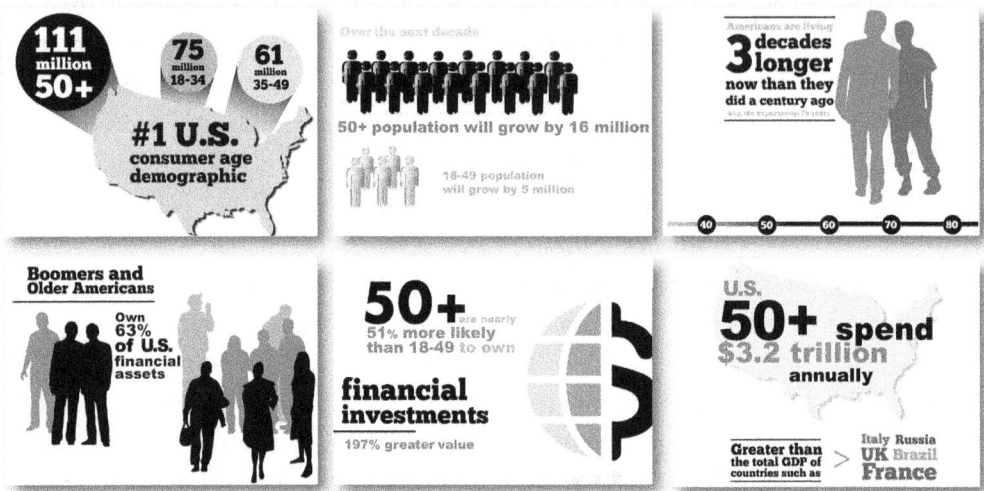

111 million 50+
75 million 18-34
61 million 35-49
#1 U.S. consumer age demographic

Over the next decade
50+ population will grow by 16 million
18-49 population will grow by 5 million

3 decades longer now than they did a century ago
Americans are living

40 50 60 70 80

Boomers and Older Americans Own 63% of U.S. financial assets

50+ are nearly 51% more likely than 18-49 to own **financial investments** 197% greater value

U.S. **50+ spend $3.2 trillion** annually
Greater than the total GDP of countries such as > Italy Russia UK Brazil France

7

According to a March 11, 2015, report published by the Center for Western Priorities (CWP),[8] there are 70,000 baby boomers reaching the age of retirement each week, and this will continue until 2030. The CWP says that between 2000 and 2010, more than 500,000 seniors migrated into western counties, both from outside of the western United States and from other western counties. What are these seniors seeking? High natural amenities! With them they are bringing accumulated wealth, investment income, and aging-related payments. This nonlabor income is one of the fastest-growing sources of income in the western United States.[9]

The influx of retirees is also an important job creator. According to an analysis by the University of Georgia, it takes only 1.8 in-migrating retirees to create one job; in other words, for every 100 retirees relocating to a new community, about 55 new jobs are generated.[10] Thus, seniors relocating to western states created nearly 300,000 jobs between 2000 and 2010.[11] In the sweepstakes to attract relocating retirees, America's spectacular public lands, with their high natural amenities, provide a unique and enduring competitive advantage to western towns and cities.[12] With bragging rights as the USDA #1 high-altitude county and also the highest-altitude incorporated city in the United States, Leadville/Lake County has an unbeatable, unique, and enduring competitive advantage. But, as with all fundamental change, it can take some time for folks to recognize what Leadville/Lake County has to offer.

Now, based upon the recent explosion of retirees in adjacent counties, Leadville/Lake County will probably soon experience a similar increase of baby boomers. Here's what has happened: In neighboring Summit (Frisco) and Eagle (Vail) Counties, the boomers have definitely been booming! According to the US Census Bureau, between 1990 and 2000, Summit County, with 180.3 percent growth, experienced the largest increase in residents age 65+ in the United States. Eagle County was number five in the nation, with 135.2 percent growth.[13] Here's what the retiree growth in Frisco and Vail looks like.

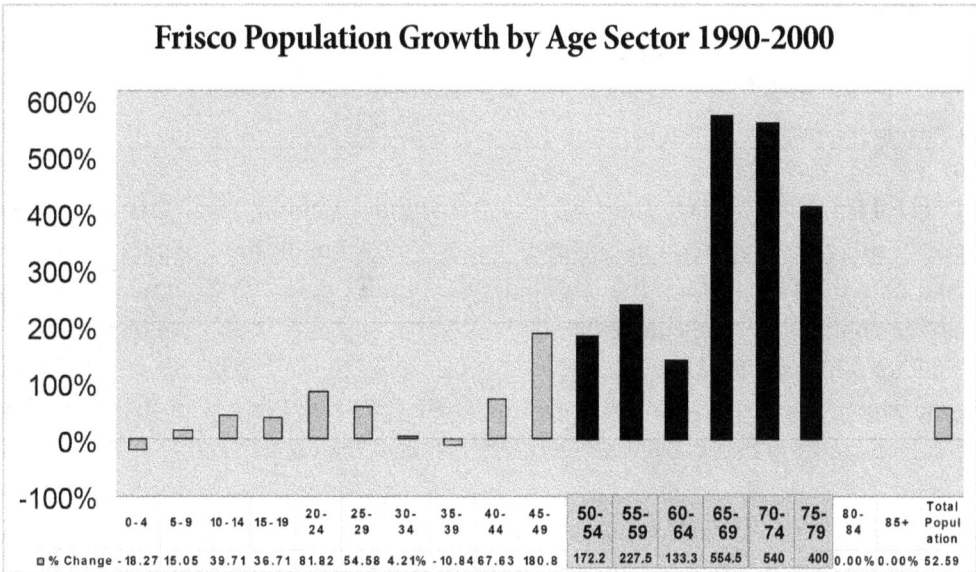

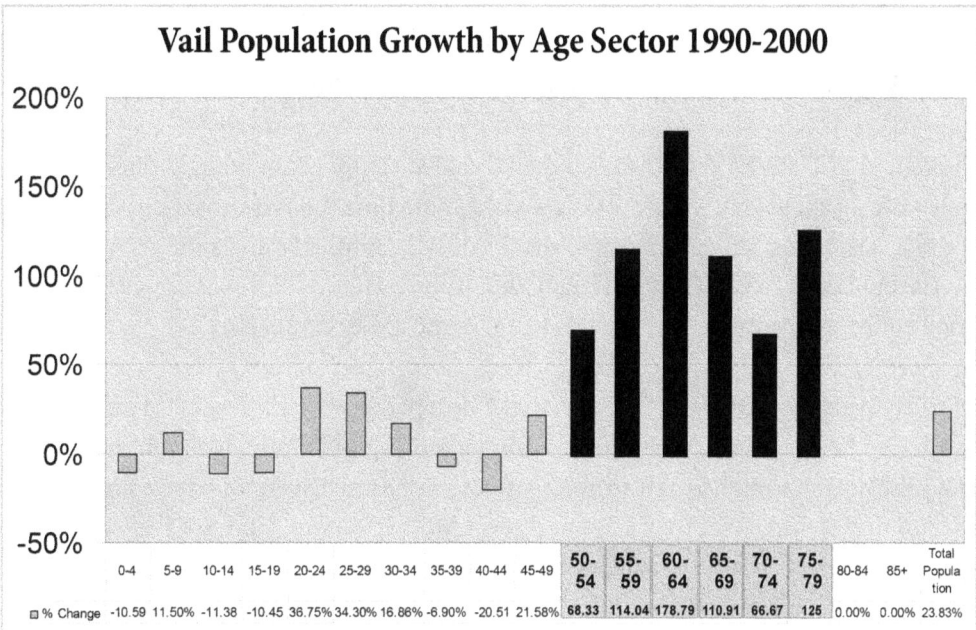

Frisco Population Growth by Age Sector 1990-2000

	0-4	5-9	10-14	15-19	20-24	25-29	30-34	35-39	40-44	45-49	50-54	55-59	60-64	65-69	70-74	75-79	80-84	85+	Total Population
% Change	-18.27	15.05	39.71	36.71	81.82	54.58	4.21%	-10.84	67.63	180.8	172.2	227.5	133.3	554.5	540	400	0.00%	0.00%	52.59

Vail Population Growth by Age Sector 1990-2000

	0-4	5-9	10-14	15-19	20-24	25-29	30-34	35-39	40-44	45-49	50-54	55-59	60-64	65-69	70-74	75-79	80-84	85+	Total Population
% Change	-10.59	11.50%	-11.38	-10.45	36.75%	34.30%	16.86%	-6.90%	-20.51	21.58%	68.33	114.04	178.79	110.91	66.67	125	0.00%	0.00%	23.83%

14

Leadville/Lake County hasn't yet seen the same large growth in the baby boomer population. Why? Partly it's because Vail and Frisco are adjacent to multiple huge, glitzy ski resorts that have multimillion-dollar advertising budgets. In contrast, Leadville/Lake County has small back-in-time Ski Cooper, another diamond in the rough. (Ski Cooper is owned as a nonprofit by Lake County so it hasn't gone the route of the large commercial ski resorts.) Compared with Summit County, Lake County's advertising is minimal. Another reason Leadville/Lake County has not yet seen the same type of growth is that there is an abundance of ridiculous myths. You often hear, "It's too cold!" "It's too high!" "It's too far away!" or "Winter driving is awful!" As with the rest of this book, here are the facts.

MYTH: IT'S TOO COLD! The 1999 USDA Natural Amenities Scale lists the thirty-year mean January temperature for each county. According to the scale, there are 370 counties in the United States that are colder than Lake County. In Colorado, there are thirteen counties that are colder than Lake County. So Lake County is comparatively balmy for a high-altitude mountain county. According to the USDA, it's even warmer in the winter than neighboring Summit and Eagle Counties. But if your idea of cold is 75 degrees and you hate snow, there are better choices than Lake County.

MYTH: IT'S TOO HIGH! Leadville's altitude is 10,152 feet. That's 1,077 feet higher than Summit County's Frisco at 9,075 feet and 552 feet higher than Breckenridge at 9,600 feet. It's sort of like $9.99 versus $10.00. That extra digit just looks big. But now scientists and medical doctors are saying that higher altitude is correlated with lower obesity, lower ischemic heart disease, higher longevity, and many other health benefits. So thinking that Leadville/Lake County is too high in altitude is just simply outdated.

MYTH: IT'S TOO FAR AWAY! I frequently ski at Copper Mountain. Although it's 23 miles away, I am able to leave my house at the same time the Frisco folks are getting on the bus. Yes, I must drive 30 miles to drink coffee at Starbucks and shop at Walmart in Frisco, but I don't mind. The local Leadville City on a Hill coffee house serves incredibly good coffee. And a little planning takes care of most everything else.

MYTH: WINTER DRIVING IS AWFUL! Compared with Highways 24 and 91 into Leadville, the Interstate 70 corridor in Summit and Eagle Counties is a nightmare, especially during the winter. This is primarily due to nonlocal drivers who have not learned, as local drivers have, that they need to respect Mother Nature. Here are the winter road closure numbers (due to accidents or bad weather) for 2014. On I-70, the Vail Pass area had fifty-eight closures and the Eisenhower Tunnel area had thirty-four closures.

Officer's Gulch (between Frisco and Copper Mountain) had twenty-five closures. In contrast, Highway 24 (between Leadville and Minturn) had six closures. Highway 91 (between Leadville and Copper Mountain) had two closures.[15] And here is something most nonlocals don't realize: traveling from Leadville, the closures on I-70 don't impact you if you want to ski at Copper Mountain, Vail, Beaver Creek, or Ski Cooper. While thousands of skiers are stranded along I-70, you're skiing in fresh powder!

Number of Road Closures Due to Accidents 2014

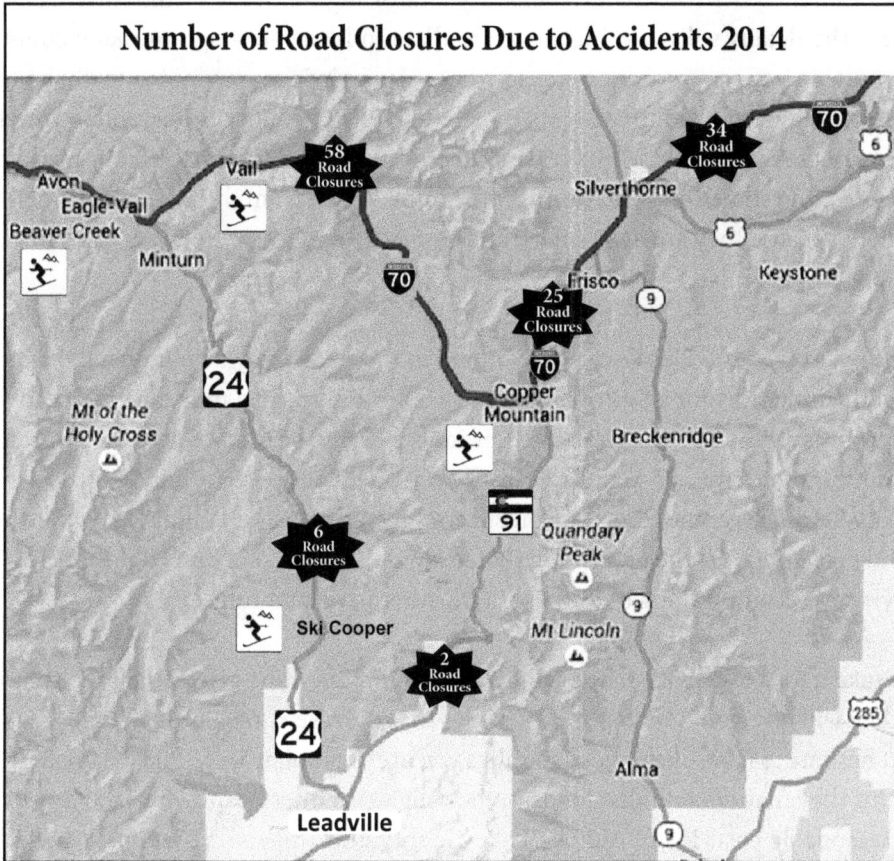

Now let's take a peek at what may happen down the road. Leadville/Lake County's future resides in its youth, the millennial and Gen X generations. Unlike the neighboring wealthy counties where there has been a mass exodus due to the high cost of housing, there is still a healthy population of these young folks in Leadville/Lake County. In Eagle, Summit, and Pitkin Counties, these younger populations are even referred to as "the lost generation."[16]

Hopefully these bright young adults will have the vision and energy to preserve what makes this little piece of paradise special. Maybe more baby boomers arriving with their pension funds and retirement checks in hand will encourage the revitalization of downtown Leadville. Perhaps there will soon be more places for retirees to spend their money. New seniors will need new homes that require all sorts of maintenance, they'll eat at restaurants, they'll get their hair cut, they'll need medical care, and more.

Although Leadville has served as the benchmark example for this case study, communities in many other high-natural-amenity and/or high-altitude counties have similar stories. The details will vary, but there are diamonds in the rough in many counties. You must do your homework because what seems obvious may not actually be true. Like Leadville/Lake County, you can't really tell what a county is like unless you drill down to get the facts. You definitely won't get the information from the fancy marketing brochures, and sometimes you won't get the information from the locals. Many of them are there because they are darn smart, and some of them might not want to share their little piece of paradise.

On a final note, Leadville's days as a diamond in the rough may be numbered. Plans are currently under way for a $94 million luxury hotel and resort a mile north of Leadville. With rooms in the $300/night range, an indoor water park, three restaurants, and a convention center for 250 people, Leadville can't help but become a little more gentrified.[17] A Starbucks at the resort is almost certainly a given, and Walmart might even sit up and take notice. So the perception that Leadville is Too Cold! Too High! and Too Far Away! may become a thing of the past in the not too distant future.

Now take a look at chapters 4 through 7. The numbers won't give you all the answers, but they will give you a short list of counties that deserve your thorough investigation. Don't hesitate to investigate those counties you aren't familiar with. Like Leadville/Lake County, they may contain diamonds in the rough that offer healthy high-quality living at a reasonable cost. Like Leadville/Lake County, they may not contain all the man-made amenities such as big shopping malls and a Starbucks on every corner, but they have an abundance of natural amenities and/or altitude that can help you lose weight and regain your health and freedom. And here's something else to consider: driving a modest distance to access all those man-made amenities will help keep Mother Nature's natural amenities intact right outside your front door.

CHAPTER 4
Altitude Facts and Figures

Human beings, who are almost unique in having the ability to learn from the experience of others, are also remarkable for their apparent disinclination to do so. —Douglas Adams (1952–2001)

The county altitudes listed in this book are mean elevation. A mean elevation is the average of all the elevations within the county.

At this time, the United States Geological Survey (USGS) website does not post mean elevation by county. However, the website does provide a procedure to extract an elevation for the centroid of each county polygon using Environmental Systems Research Institute (ESRI) ArcGIS software.[1] The result is county mean elevation. This calculation was done by a bright young man named Steven Jay. He has a master of science degree in Land resources and Environmental Science and he used USGS and ESRI data and software.[2] While elevation results may vary slightly depending on parameters used, small differences aren't going to have much impact on your weight.

The following county and state altitude data pages will provide you with a list of counties that have mean elevations of 5,000 feet or more and the altitude ranges for each state. Some counties have wide elevation spans, while others don't. The same is true for the states. California has the widest span, with altitudes ranging from −279 feet to 14,505 feet. That's an altitude span of 14,784 feet! With this information, you can begin to narrow down your list of potential options.

To determine the actual altitude of a particular community that may interest you, just check a source such as Wikipedia. Here's an example. The mean elevation for Lake County, Colorado, is 10,931 feet. According to Wikipedia, the altitude for the city of Leadville is 10,152 feet.

Low-elevation counties have obesity rates all over the map, so to speak. A big indicator for low obesity in a low-elevation county is close proximity to an ocean. Inland lower-altitude counties will often have higher obesity rates.

The highest-altitude eastern counties are located in the Appalachian Mountain range. All of the very high altitudes in the United States are located in the western part of the country. In the West, there are sixty-one counties with a mean elevation of at least 7,000 feet. Colorado dominates this list with thirty-six counties and is also home to the twenty-one highest-altitude counties.

As a general rule, high altitude is also an indicator for high natural amenities. Only two counties with an elevation of 7,000 feet or more are not in the top 10 percent (311 counties) for high natural amenities. Only four counties with an elevation of 5,000 feet or more are not in the top 30 percent (932 counties).

Here are the number of counties by mean altitude.

MEAN ALTITUDE	NUMBER OF COUNTIES
≥8,000'	29
7,000'-7,999'	32
6,000'-6,999'	47
5,000'-5,999'	70
4,000'–4,999'	87
3,000'–3,999'	120
2,000'–2,999'	230
1,000'–1,999'	752
<1,000'	1,741
TOTAL	3,108

High-altitude counties are sort of like diamonds: lots of little diamonds/altitude and very few big diamonds/altitude. Of the 3,108 counties, 2,493, or 80 percent, are at less than 2,000 feet elevation. Many of these lower-altitude counties are in the eastern part of the United States. The 178 counties with mean altitudes of 5,000 feet or more start in Montana, Wyoming, Colorado, and New Mexico and extend west. Of course, not everyone is able or willing to follow the 19th-century advice "Go West young man, go West and grow up in the country."[3]

But altitude is a valuable tool that can help us manage our weight and maintain our health. Again, here are Dr. Voss's research findings.

> **Recently, we've identified a strong association between obesity prevalence and altitude within the US.** Our findings were surprising because they indicated the magnitude of this association was large and the pattern of association exhibited a curvilinear dose response in 500 meter [1,640'] categories of altitude. **There was a 4–5 fold increase in obesity prevalence at low altitude as compared with the highest altitude [9,843'–11,450'] category after controlling for diet, activity level, smoking, demographics, temperature, and urbanization.**[4]

The bad news is that there are only a small number of counties that have high altitude, and none of them are in the eastern part of the United States. Is there any good news? Yes. There are 78.6 million adult Americans who are obese, so there is a lot of money to be made on normobaric hypoxia (simulated altitude) medicine and equipment. Like air-conditioning, we can simulate high altitude. This is not something out of a science fiction movie.

To put this into perspective, here is an example of another product that was invented not too long ago. It's called the finger-pulse oximeter. This little contraption measures your blood oxygen saturation level and pulse rate. Just clip it on your finger sort of like a clothespin.

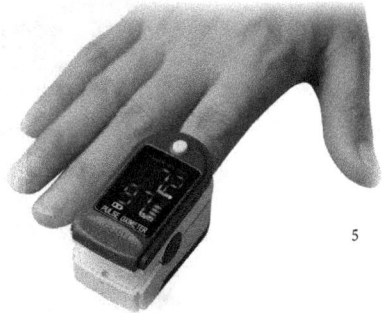

As with any new discovery in medicine or any fundamental change, it took a while for this new tool to catch on. Early on, few foresaw its value in anesthesiology, intensive care, and emergency situations. Currently, the portable pulse oximetry market is estimated at $200 million, with 9 to 11 percent compound annual growth.[6]

While the early versions of oximeters cost tens of thousands of dollars, the price recently dropped below $100. Today, you can buy a finger-pulse oximeter for less than

$20. There's even a new pulse oximeter being developed that can be wrapped around the wrist like a watch.[7]

The high-altitude simulation industry is no different, and there are already a few researchers and commercial companies tinkering in this field. The early use of altitude simulators has been primarily by athletes for training. The current school of thought is "live high, train low." The United States Olympic Committee has an Altitude Factsheet that discusses "sleep high, train low."[8] Olympic swimmer Michael Phelps prepared for the 2012 Summer Olympics by hitting the hay in a high-altitude sleeping chamber. The air Phelps slept in was the equivalent of the air at 8,500–9,000 feet.[9] Here's a picture.

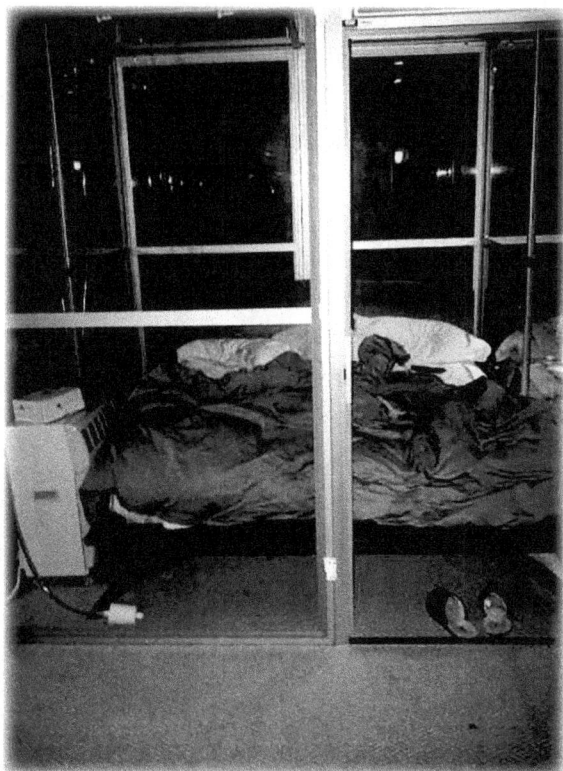

10

But today's high-altitude simulation equipment is very expensive. To achieve mass market status, the price point needs to drop and the availability and functionality need to rise. So, to borrow a phrase from NASCAR, "Ladies and gentlemen, start your engines."[11] It's invention time!

Altitude Statistics for Each State

ST*	State Information				County Information	
	Highest Elevation*	Lowest Elevation*	Mean Elevation*	Elevation Span*	Highest Elevation County in State**	Mean County Elevation**
AL	2,413 ft 736 m	sea level	500 ft 150 m	2,413 ft 736 m	DeKalb	1,216 ft 371 m
AR	2,753 ft 839 m	55 ft 17 m	650 ft 200 m	2,698 ft 822 m	Madison	1,651 ft 503 m
AZ	12,637 ft 3852 m	72 ft 22 m	4,100 ft 1250 m	12,565 ft 3830 m	Apache	6,554 ft 1998 m
CA	14,505 ft 4421 m	−279 ft −85 m	2,900 ft 880 m	14,784 ft 4506 m	Mono	7,760 ft 2365 m
CO	14,440 ft 4401 m	3,317 ft 1011 m	6,800 ft 2070 m	11,123 ft 3390 m	San Juan	11,344 ft 3458 m
CT	2,379 ft 725 m	sea level	500 ft 150 m	2,379 ft 725 m	Litchfield	914 ft 279 m
DC	409 ft 125 m	1.0 ft 0.3 m	150 ft 50 m	408 ft 124 m	Washington	139 ft 42 m
DE	447 ft 136 m	sea level	60 ft 20 m	447 ft 136 m	New Castle	90 ft 27 m
FL	345 ft 105 m	sea level	100 ft 30 m	345 ft 105 m	Gadsden	202 ft 62 m
GA	4,784 ft 1458 m	sea level	600 ft 180 m	4,784 ft 1458 m	Towns	2,551 ft 778 m
IA	1,671 ft 509 m	480 ft 146 m	1,100 ft 340 m	1,191 ft 363 m	Osceola	1,542 ft 470 m
ID	12,668 ft 3861 m	713 ft 217 m	5,000 ft 1520 m	11,955 ft 3644 m	Custer	7,615 ft 2321 m
IL	1,235 ft 376 m	280 ft 85 m	600 ft 180 m	955 ft 291 m	McHenry	873 ft 266 ft
IN	1,257 ft 383 m	320 ft 97 m	700 ft 210 m	937 ft 286 m	Randolph	1,083 ft 330 m
KS	4,041 ft 1232 m	679 ft 207 m	2,000 ft 610 m	3,362 ft 1025 m	Greeley	3,661 ft 1116 m
KY	4,145 ft 1263 m	257 ft 78 m	750 ft 230 m	3,888 ft 1185 m	Harlan	2,095 ft 638 m
LA	535 ft 163 m	−8.0 ft −2.4 m	100 ft 30 m	543 ft 166 m	Claiborne	202 ft 62 m
MA	3,489 ft 1063 m	sea level	500 ft 150 m	3,489 ft 1063 m	Berkshire	1,404 ft 428 m

ST*	State Information				County Information	
	Highest Elevation*	Lowest Elevation*	Mean Elevation*	Elevation Span*	Highest Elevation County in State**	Mean County Elevation**
MD	3,360 ft 1024 m	sea level	350 ft 110 m	3,360 ft 1024 m	Garrett	2,460 ft 750 m
ME	5,270 ft 1606 m	sea level	600 ft 180 m	5,270 ft 1606 m	Franklin	1,552 ft 473 m
MI	1,979 ft 603 m	571 ft 174 m	900 ft 270 m	1,408 ft 429 m	Iron	1,538 ft 469 m
MN	2,300 ft 701 m	600 ft 183 m	1,200 ft 370 m	1,700 ft 518 m	Pipestone	1,714 ft 522 ft
MO	1,772 ft 540 m	230 ft 70 m	800 ft 240 m	1,542 ft 470 m	Webster	1,411 ft 430 m
MS	807 ft 246 m	sea level	300 ft 90 m	807 ft 246 m	Tishomingo	527 ft 161 m
MT	12,807 ft 3904 m	1,804 ft 550 m	3,400 ft 1040 m	11,003 ft 3354 m	Beaverhead	7,078 ft 2157 m
NC	6,684 ft 2037 m	sea level	700 ft 210 m	6,684 ft 2037 m	Haywood	3,581 ft 1092 m
ND	3,508 ft 1069 m	751 ft 229 m	1,900 ft 580 m	2,757 ft 840 m	Bowman	2,974 ft 906 m
NE	5,427 ft 1654 m	840 ft 256 m	2,600 ft 790 m	4,587 ft 1398 m	Kimball	4,933 ft 1504 m
NH	6,288 ft 1917 m	sea level	1,000 ft 300 m	6,288 ft 1917 m	Coos	1,857 ft 566 m
NJ	1,803 ft 550 m	sea level	250 ft 80 m	1,803 ft 550 m	Sussex	806 ft 246 m
NM	13,167 ft 4013 m	2,844 ft 867 m	5,700 ft 1740 m	10,323 ft 3147 m	Taos	8,533 ft 2601 m
NV	13,147 ft 4007 m	482 ft 147 m	5,500 ft 1680 m	12,665 ft 3860 m	White Pine	6,825 ft 2080 m
NY	5,343 ft 1629 m	sea level	1,000 ft 300 m	5,343 ft 1629 m	Hamilton	1,985 ft 605 m
OH	1,549 ft 472 m	455 ft 139 m	850 ft 260 m	1,094 ft 333 m	Richland	1,195 ft 364 m
OK	4,975 ft 1516 m	289 ft 88 m	1,300 ft 400 m	4,686 ft 1428 m	Cimarron	4,139 ft 1262 m
OR	11,249 ft 3429 m	sea level	3,300 ft 1010 m	11,249 ft 3429 m	Lake	5,132 ft 1564 m
PA	3,213 ft 979 m	sea level	1,100 ft 340 m	3,213 ft 979 m	Somerset	2,193 ft 668 m

HEALTHIEST PLACES TO LIVE

| ST* | State Information | | | | County Information | |
---	Highest Elevation*	Lowest Elevation*	Mean Elevation*	Elevation Span*	Highest Elevation County in State**	Mean County Elevation**
RI	811 ft 247 m	sea level	200 ft 60 m	811 ft 247 m	Providence	362 ft 110 m
SC	3,560 ft 1085 m	sea level	350 ft 110 m	3,560 ft 1085 m	Pickens	1,122 ft 342 m
SD	7,244 ft 2208 m	968 ft 295 m	2,200 ft 670 m	6,276 ft 1913 m	Lawrence	4,968 ft 1514 m
TN	6,644 ft 2025 m	178 ft 54 m	900 ft 270 m	6,466 ft 1971 m	Johnson	2,915 ft 888 m
TX	8,751 ft 2667 m	sea level	1,700 ft 520 m	8,751 ft 2667 m	Jeff Davis	4,906 ft 1495 m
UT	13,534 ft 4125 m	2,180 ft 664 m	6,100 ft 1860 m	11,354 ft 3456 m	Summit	8,472 ft 2582 m
VA	5,729 ft 1746 m	sea level	950 ft 290 m	5,729 ft 1746 m	Grayson	3,015 ft 919 m
VT	4,395 ft 1340 m	95 ft 29 m	1,000 ft 300 m	4,300 ft 1311 m	Bennington	1,710 ft 521 m
WA	14,417 ft 4394 m	sea level	1,700 ft 520 m	14,417 ft 4394 m	Chelan	3,944 ft 1201 m
WI	1,951 ft 595 m	579 ft 176 m	1,050 ft 320 m	1,372 ft 418 m	Vilas	1,672 ft 510 m
WV	4,863 ft 1482 m	240 ft 73 m	1,500 ft 460 m	4,623 ft 1409 m	Pocahontas	3,215 ft 980 m
WY	13,809 ft 4209 m	3,100 ft 945 m	6,700 ft 2040 m	10,709 ft 3264 m	Sublette	8,045 ft 2452 m

*Wikipedia [12]
**USGS and ESRI [13]

178 Counties with a Mean Elevation of ≥5,000'

ST	County	Elevation in Feet	Amenity Ranking	ST	County	Elevation in Feet	Amenity Ranking
CO	San Juan	11344	31	CO	San Miguel	7943	108
CO	Hinsdale	10935	38	CO	Garfield	7893	214
CO	Lake	10931	11	UT	Duchesne	7792	220
CO	Mineral	10492	72	UT	Piute	7786	209
CO	Summit	10481	19	CA	Mono	7760	16
CO	Clear Creek	10296	37	CO	Alamosa	7744	573
CO	Pitkin	10010	54	CA	Alpine	7732	26
CO	Chaffee	9959	47	CO	Larimer	7725	77
CO	Park	9672	33	NM	Rio Arriba	7657	95
CO	Gunnison	9548	132	NM	Los Alamos	7655	305
CO	Gilpin	9303	36	ID	Custer	7615	881
CO	Grand	9259	25	UT	Sevier	7550	229
CO	Saguache	9206	137	UT	Daggett	7536	176
CO	Teller	9181	52	WY	Park	7529	202
CO	Eagle	9074	156	CO	Fremont	7525	143
CO	Custer	9062	78	CO	Huerfano	7507	100
CO	Rio Grande	9029	92	WY	Albany	7464	138
CO	Ouray	8980	57	CO	Boulder	7381	71
CO	Conejos	8951	123	WY	Lincoln	7381	111
CO	Jackson	8919	49	NM	Catron	7377	53
CO	Costilla	8861	130	UT	Sanpete	7311	166
NM	Taos	8533	189	WY	Carbon	7294	86
UT	Summit	8472	131	WY	Uinta	7249	272
CO	Dolores	8330	170	CO	Rio Blanco	7231	241
CO	Archuleta	8265	80	NM	Colfax	7214	226
CO	Routt	8197	90	NM	Mora	7166	96
WY	Sublette	8045	91	UT	Carbon	7129	294
WY	Teton	8044	87	NM	Cibola	7096	304
UT	Wasatch	8034	136	MT	Beaverhead	7078	247
CO	La Plata	7988	69	CO	Jefferson	7056	79

HEALTHIEST PLACES TO LIVE

ST	County	Elevation in Feet	Amenity Ranking	ST	County	Elevation in Feet	Amenity Ranking
WY	Fremont	7037	225	UT	Cache	6306	354
CO	Delta	6982	232	MT	Gallatin	6274	210
MT	Park	6960	237	UT	Utah	6264	135
CO	Montrose	6943	316	UT	Uintah	6258	244
NM	McKinley	6942	260	NV	Eureka	6211	491
ID	Lemhi	6928	1124	ID	Fremont	6163	315
NM	Santa Fe	6924	307	NV	Elko	6144	461
CO	Douglas	6876	104	WY	Hot Springs	6124	784
WY	Sweetwater	6869	355	MT	Granite	6118	419
CO	Mesa	6846	421	UT	Wayne	6110	855
NV	White Pine	6825	303	ID	Blaine	6103	318
UT	Rich	6822	119	ID	Bonneville	6090	472
CO	Montezuma	6813	167	WY	Natrona	6069	373
UT	Garfield	6778	200	NV	Douglas	6047	22
ID	Bear Lake	6769	235	NM	San Juan	6047	330
UT	Morgan	6736	221	AZ	Navajo	6016	495
CO	Moffat	6733	190	NV	Lander	6000	227
NM	Sandoval	6720	228	NM	Socorro	5989	293
MT	Deer Lodge	6664	598	WY	Laramie	5987	302
MT	Madison	6657	281	ID	Butte	5977	1389
AZ	Apache	6554	250	NM	Bernalillo	5967	216
ID	Teton	6512	498	CO	Elbert	5965	861
ID	Caribou	6494	298	CO	Las Animas	5947	239
ID	Valley	6466	154	NM	San Miguel	5930	218
MT	Silver Bow	6456	444	MT	Ravalli	5918	574
NM	Torrance	6455	197	AZ	Coconino	5914	134
CO	El Paso	6423	105	NV	Mineral	5872	73
ID	Clark	6414	1493	MT	Jefferson	5869	420
UT	Iron	6376	395	MT	Meagher	5861	329
UT	Beaver	6359	393	NM	Lincoln	5852	178
ID	Camas	6320	341	UT	Emery	5846	903

ST	County	Elevation in Feet	Amenity Ranking	ST	County	Elevation in Feet	Amenity Ranking
ID	Franklin	5829	548	UT	Millard	5412	343
NV	Nye	5823	127	ID	Cassia	5375	522
NM	Grant	5823	50	CA	Lassen	5361	51
NV	Carson City	5780	27	NV	Washoe	5359	40
UT	Grand	5752	456	MT	Lewis & Clark	5337	287
CA	Sierra	5746	66	CO	Denver	5335	324
UT	Kane	5736	313	CA	Plumas	5309	44
AZ	Greenlee	5710	103	NM	Otero	5301	198
MT	Powell	5676	525	NV	Lincoln	5266	211
NV	Esmeralda	5670	192	CO	Pueblo	5212	451
UT	San Juan	5658	240	WY	Washakie	5211	779
CA	Tuolumne	5653	34	NV	Lyon	5207	74
UT	Weber	5649	224	NM	Guadalupe	5179	347
ID	Bannock	5633	542	ID	Power	5178	463
MT	Sweet Grass	5623	283	WY	Platte	5155	193
ID	Madison	5579	854	WY	Sheridan	5151	442
UT	Salt Lake	5577	187	OR	Lake	5132	188
MT	Carbon	5572	186	ID	Bingham	5125	496
NV	Storey	5565	113	CO	Lincoln	5122	791
WY	Johnson	5557	336	ID	Idaho	5119	285
ID	Boise	5531	258	CO	Adams	5088	374
ID	Oneida	5531	1325	NV	Humboldt	5085	207
UT	Juab	5528	497	UT	Washington	5072	365
CO	Arapahoe	5468	399	NM	Harding	5044	692
NM	Sierra	5445	41	MT	Judith Basin	5039	500
WY	Converse	5426	326	MT	Stillwater	5036	352
NM	Valencia	5424	306	MT	Broadwater	5015	205
NM	Union	5423	822				
WY	Big Horn	5422	372				

CHAPTER 5

Alphabetical Listing of 3,108 Lower Forty-Eight Counties

The pressure-sensitive adhesive used in 3M's famous Post-it Notes languished from 1968-1980. It can take a long time for a good idea to catch on. – Peggy Forney

The alphabetical listing of counties provides quick access to the specifics for any county. It also establishes a reference point for both the natural amenities and obesity rating sections. Here is some information that can help put the county data into context.

Below are the two counties with the lowest and highest obesity rates in the country. You will find that diabetes and leisure-time physical inactivity rates correlate significantly with obesity rates. In other words, a high obesity rate is associated with high diabetes and high leisure-time physical inactivity rates. Higher obesity rates are also correlated with lower longevity for both men and women.

COUNTY & STATE	% OBESITY	% DIABETES	% INACTIVE	MEN LONGEVITY	WOMEN LONGEVITY
Routt County, CO	13.5%	3.8%	11.1%	78.6 Years	83.3 Years
Green County, AL	47.9% *(355% higher)*	16.2% *(426% higher)*	37.3% *(336% higher)*	67.9 Years *(-10.7 Years)*	76.6 Years *(-6.7 Years)*

Take a look at the county you are currently residing in and you will likely see these correlations.

The blue book dataset headers are as follows:

ABBREVIATION	DESCRIPTION
ST	State
COUNTY	County
USDA	USDA numerical rating with +11.17 denoting the highest number of natural amenities and -6.40 denoting the lowest number of natural amenities[1]
AMEN	Numerical ranking of the USDA natural amenities data with +11.17 being #1 and -6.40 being #3,108. #1 denotes highest ranking and #3,108 denotes lowest ranking[1]
OBES	% obesity among adults ≥ 20[2]
DIAB	% diabetes among adults ≥ 20[2]
INACT	% leisure-time physical inactivity among adults ≥ 20[2]
M AGE	Longevity for men in years[3]
W AGE	Longevity for women in years[3]
ALT ft.	Mean county altitude in feet
ALT m.	Mean county altitude in meters

Alphabetical Listing of 3,108 Lower Forty-Eight Counties

ST	COUNTY	USDA	AMEN	OBES	DIAB	INACT	M AGE	W AGE	ALT ft	ALT m
AL	Autauga	0.78	920	33.9	11.7	31.9	72.9	78	365	111
AL	Baldwin	1.82	516	25.7	9.9	24.2	74.4	80.3	121	37
AL	Barbour	0.19	1314	37.1	13.2	33.8	71	76.9	374	114
AL	Bibb	-0.15	1559	34.1	11.2	36.8	69.8	77.1	413	126
AL	Blount	0.23	1273	32.1	11.5	35.1	72.5	78.8	788	240
AL	Bullock	-1.08	2177	39.2	15.6	30.9	68.4	75.3	415	126
AL	Butler	-1.16	2218	41.3	14.6	35.9	69.6	77.2	385	117
AL	Calhoun	0.22	1282	33.8	12.9	33.3	70.5	77.3	760	232
AL	Chambers	-0.34	1695	35.5	14.2	35	70.2	77.2	750	228
AL	Cherokee	0.64	986	31.1	11.2	34.6	71.3	77.9	756	231
AL	Chilton	0.38	1155	35.3	11.1	30.4	70.4	77.3	528	161
AL	Choctaw	0.92	850	38.8	14.3	34.1	70.4	77	197	60
AL	Clarke	1.26	703	35.7	12.9	37.1	72.1	77.6	228	69
AL	Clay	0.21	1292	34.8	12.7	36.2	71.8	78	1023	312
AL	Cleburne	0.21	1293	30.1	11.1	32.8	71.8	78	1050	320
AL	Coffee	-0.66	1918	32.2	12.5	28.2	73.4	79	328	100
AL	Colbert	0.70	957	33.4	11.7	33.7	71.9	78.3	589	180
AL	Conecuh	-1.00	2125	33.5	14.1	34.9	69.6	77.2	323	98
AL	Coosa	1.59	570	34	12.8	33.7	70.4	77.3	647	197
AL	Covington	-0.17	1569	37.2	10.9	36	71.4	77.9	299	91

HEALTHIEST PLACES TO LIVE

ST	COUNTY	USDA	AMEN	OBES	DIAB	INACT	M AGE	W AGE	ALT ft	ALT m
AL	Crenshaw	-0.91	2072	37.4	12.2	32.5	69.9	76.4	422	129
AL	Cullman	0.64	987	32.2	11.9	28.7	71.9	78.4	750	229
AL	Dale	-0.47	1798	35.6	12.6	31	72.9	79	314	96
AL	Dallas	-0.18	1581	41.9	14.2	33.3	68.5	75.3	195	59
AL	DeKalb	-1.60	2423	34	10.3	27	71.9	78.1	1216	371
AL	Elmore	2.11	449	31.3	11.8	31.5	73.1	78.8	382	117
AL	Escambia	-0.03	1461	35.9	12.1	37	71.5	77.6	242	74
AL	Etowah	0.96	829	32.5	11.8	33.3	70.5	77.2	766	233
AL	Fayette	-0.38	1733	36.9	12.2	31.8	70.5	78	487	148
AL	Franklin	0.16	1328	31.4	13.3	36.4	70.7	77.1	744	227
AL	Geneva	-0.51	1814	35.9	12	34.2	71.6	78.4	212	65
AL	Greene	-0.04	1469	47.9	16.2	37.3	67.9	76.6	167	51
AL	Hale	1.43	623	43.5	14	35.2	69.3	75.5	211	64
AL	Henry	0.07	1383	34	12.8	30.1	70.5	77.2	328	100
AL	Houston	-0.79	2000	33.3	11.2	32.5	73.3	79.5	219	67
AL	Jackson	1.25	708	30.8	12	29.3	71.2	77.6	1051	320
AL	Jefferson	0.51	1058	31.9	11.7	28.8	71	77.8	575	175
AL	Lamar	-0.85	2034	32.6	11.1	34.4	71.7	77.3	397	121
AL	Lauderdale	0.90	858	33	12.2	32	73.3	79.7	639	195
AL	Lawrence	0.54	1043	38	12.4	35.3	71.5	77.7	678	207
AL	Lee	-0.24	1626	29.8	11.3	27.9	73.9	78.6	615	187
AL	Limestone	-0.42	1767	31.3	10	30.9	73	79	690	210
AL	Lowndes	-0.41	1761	44.7	16.4	37.5	69.9	76.4	251	76
AL	Macon	-0.56	1850	41.7	14.2	31.1	68.4	75.3	328	100
AL	Madison	-1.25	2260	31.3	11.2	24.9	74.7	79.3	795	242
AL	Marengo	-0.72	1957	40.4	14.8	34.8	69.9	76.3	181	55
AL	Marion	-0.31	1678	33.2	10.6	34.5	71	77.7	635	193
AL	Marshall	0.37	1162	29.2	10.9	31.5	71.5	77.5	880	268
AL	Mobile	1.52	590	31.7	11.6	30.2	70.7	77.8	123	38
AL	Monroe	1.27	692	35.7	12.2	31.2	71.1	77.2	269	82
AL	Montgomery	-0.28	1650	34.1	13.5	29.5	71.7	78	270	82
AL	Morgan	1.09	778	33	10.2	26.6	72.9	78.9	703	214
AL	Perry	0.84	891	40.5	17.8	34.1	69.3	75.5	277	84
AL	Pickens	0.13	1347	36.9	13.9	32.5	70.3	76.7	273	83
AL	Pike	-0.93	2085	37	15	32.3	71.7	77.1	430	131
AL	Randolph	0.71	949	32.5	12.6	33.8	70.8	77.4	916	279
AL	Russell	-0.24	1627	39.5	12.5	36.5	69.3	76.3	339	103
AL	Shelby	1.12	763	27.6	8.3	23.5	75.6	80	578	176
AL	St. Clair	1.39	635	35.5	12.5	34.7	71.8	77.7	699	213
AL	Sumter	-0.48	1803	42.4	16.8	32.3	67.9	76.6	173	53
AL	Talladega	1.34	655	36.9	13.3	34.6	70.5	77.2	613	187
AL	Tallapoosa	2.19	432	37.7	12	30	71.7	78.2	631	192
AL	Tuscaloosa	0.50	1069	34.4	11.8	28.8	71.9	77.8	361	110
AL	Walker	0.51	1059	35	13	36.9	68.3	75.9	472	144
AL	Washington	-0.49	1806	36.3	11.4	32	72.9	78.5	148	45
AL	Wilcox	1.58	573	43.6	15.5	34.4	69.9	76.3	198	60
AL	Winston	0.88	867	36.5	10.3	32.4	70.9	77.6	722	220

ST	COUNTY	USDA	AMEN	OBES	DIAB	INACT	M AGE	W AGE	ALT ft	ALT m
AR	Arkansas	-0.87	2047	36.5	11.3	35.6	71.5	78.5	177	54
AR	Ashley	-1.12	2199	39.4	10.4	37.4	72.4	77.4	134	41
AR	Baxter	2.64	348	29.8	8	30.3	73.4	79.8	746	227
AR	Benton	2.39	389	28	7.2	27.8	76.8	81.8	1230	375
AR	Boone	1.98	478	29.7	9.9	30.6	74.1	79.6	1169	356
AR	Bradley	-1.06	2168	32.3	11.9	32	72	78.3	169	52
AR	Calhoun	-1.35	2299	34.5	10.5	35.2	70.8	77.4	171	52
AR	Carroll	1.75	535	26.6	9.1	26.8	74.3	79.4	1330	405
AR	Chicot	-0.45	1782	38.6	12.8	35.1	69.4	75.8	113	34
AR	Clark	1.15	748	34.1	10.7	30.5	72.9	78.5	317	97
AR	Clay	-2.30	2689	33.2	10.6	32.6	70.3	78.1	300	91
AR	Cleburne	2.19	433	27.4	10.4	30.4	74.4	79.5	714	218
AR	Cleveland	-1.59	2415	32.9	10.7	27.5	72	78.3	224	68
AR	Columbia	-1.63	2437	32.2	11.8	29	71.8	77.7	271	83
AR	Conway	-0.42	1768	33.2	10.3	29.1	72.5	78.1	492	150
AR	Craighead	-2.24	2665	33.1	10.9	32	72.3	78.5	257	78
AR	Crawford	1.44	618	33.3	8.2	29.4	72.7	78.6	930	284
AR	Crittenden	-1.05	2160	37.2	13.1	33.1	69.6	75.9	207	63
AR	Cross	-0.95	2102	34.5	10.6	35	70.7	77.2	234	71
AR	Dallas	-1.85	2522	34.2	10.7	32.8	70.8	77.4	276	84
AR	Desha	-1.04	2153	37.9	12.1	31.9	69.4	75.8	141	43
AR	Drew	-1.24	2255	35.9	11	32.8	71.8	77.4	190	58
AR	Faulkner	-0.08	1505	32.2	10.8	28.8	73.5	79.8	428	130
AR	Franklin	2.05	459	34.8	10	29.5	73.3	79.3	852	260
AR	Fulton	0.51	1060	31.7	9.3	28.1	72.5	78.7	737	225
AR	Garland	1.64	557	28.4	8.6	26.7	72.5	79.6	704	215
AR	Grant	-1.77	2497	35.7	9.2	33.1	73.7	79.6	252	77
AR	Greene	-2.00	2580	34.4	10	27	72.7	78.5	302	92
AR	Hempstead	-0.65	1911	36.4	12.4	31.6	71.5	77.2	343	105
AR	Hot Spring	0.49	1076	34.7	10.2	33.9	72.7	78.4	455	139
AR	Howard	0.99	816	34.7	11.6	32.8	72	78	584	178
AR	Independence	0.09	1370	30.1	10.1	32.3	73.5	78.9	433	132
AR	Izard	1.44	619	30	8.4	30.4	72.5	78.7	654	199
AR	Jackson	-1.85	2523	32	11	35.8	70.6	76.9	255	78
AR	Jefferson	-1.08	2178	38.2	12.9	34	70.4	77.2	216	66
AR	Johnson	2.37	393	35.6	9.8	30.7	72.5	78.7	1035	316
AR	Lafayette	-0.59	1874	31	10.5	31.8	70.2	77.1	252	77
AR	Lawrence	-0.10	1522	34.6	10.7	32.5	71.6	78.6	311	95
AR	Lee	-0.42	1769	36.7	12	37.1	69.5	76.3	194	59
AR	Lincoln	-1.24	2256	36.2	10.6	31.3	71.8	77.4	200	61
AR	Little River	-0.06	1489	33.1	10.4	31	72	78	315	96
AR	Logan	1.75	536	29.2	10.1	30.2	72.5	78.7	666	203
AR	Lonoke	-0.79	2001	33.8	11	30.8	73.3	79	233	71
AR	Madison	-0.43	1774	30.9	9.8	28.2	73	79.4	1651	503
AR	Marion	2.74	336	33.3	10.4	25.9	75.1	79.4	849	259
AR	Miller	-0.30	1664	37.9	12.3	35	73.3	79	261	80
AR	Mississippi	-1.76	2491	38.8	12.1	42	68.7	76.2	234	71

40

ST	COUNTY	USDA	AMEN	OBES	DIAB	INACT	M AGE	W AGE	ALT ft	ALT m
AR	Monroe	-1.13	2206	36.8	11	35.2	69.5	76.3	171	52
AR	Montgomery	1.32	666	28.7	9.1	27	73.2	78.7	906	276
AR	Nevada	-2.12	2622	35.6	12	33.6	70.2	77.1	292	89
AR	Newton	-0.26	1641	35.9	11	31.5	73.1	79.2	1557	475
AR	Ouachita	-0.88	2055	37.4	11.6	34.2	71.1	76.9	185	56
AR	Perry	0.89	861	32.8	10	33.1	72.5	78.1	557	170
AR	Phillips	-0.68	1927	39.7	13.2	37.8	66.8	75	174	53
AR	Pike	1.15	749	31.4	9.7	27.6	73.1	79.3	586	179
AR	Poinsett	-2.26	2676	36.9	10.4	37.3	69.3	76.6	231	71
AR	Polk	1.08	780	38.5	9.4	30.9	73.1	79.3	1180	360
AR	Pope	2.29	414	32	9	25.3	75.1	79	857	261
AR	Prairie	-0.86	2041	32.5	9.5	30.2	70.9	77.3	200	61
AR	Pulaski	0.85	887	32.1	10	28.6	72.1	78.9	335	102
AR	Randolph	-0.32	1685	35.7	11.1	31.7	72.6	79.1	407	124
AR	Saline	0.49	1077	31.1	10	25.2	74.7	79.8	537	164
AR	Scott	1.02	804	32.3	9.4	32	73.2	78.7	933	284
AR	Searcy	1.26	704	31.7	10.1	31.9	73.1	79.2	1137	346
AR	Sebastian	1.10	775	30	9.7	33.9	73.6	79.3	633	193
AR	Sevier	-0.13	1547	32.2	12	32.7	71.8	77.9	435	132
AR	Sharp	0.49	1078	29.2	8.9	32.1	72.7	79.4	560	171
AR	St. Francis	-1.28	2271	37.8	12.1	39.8	69.4	75.3	215	65
AR	Stone	1.55	582	32.6	9.3	33.8	73.5	79.7	885	270
AR	Union	-0.50	1811	31	10.1	27.3	71.2	77.6	170	52
AR	Van Buren	2.41	387	31.9	9.1	33	73.5	79.7	978	298
AR	Washington	1.22	720	29.6	9.1	24.9	74.9	80.1	1399	426
AR	White	-0.84	2025	31.5	9.4	27.8	73.2	78.8	352	107
AR	Woodruff	-1.47	2360	34.2	10.6	33.9	70.9	77.3	198	60
AR	Yell	1.63	561	36.3	12.2	28.6	71.6	78.3	608	185
AZ	Apache	3.45	249	33.1	13.1	27.5	70.8	80	6554	1998
AZ	Cochise	7.13	32	23.8	7.2	22.3	75.8	81.1	4635	1413
AZ	Coconino	4.93	134	24.9	7.5	17	75.8	80.8	5914	1803
AZ	Gila	7.50	24	26.5	8.7	23.1	72.9	79.6	4662	1421
AZ	Graham	5.20	98	32.5	9.6	27.3	74.6	79.5	4541	1384
AZ	Greenlee	5.18	103	35.4	8.7	25	74.6	79.5	5710	1740
AZ	La Paz	4.24	182	32.6	9.2	31.2	73.9	81	1370	418
AZ	Maricopa	4.87	139	23.6	7.6	19.3	76.8	81.6	1677	511
AZ	Mohave	5.84	68	27.9	9.5	28	72	78.5	3769	1149
AZ	Navajo	1.91	494	31.6	12.3	24.9	71.4	79.5	6016	1834
AZ	Pima	4.04	196	25.9	7.1	19.3	75.8	81.7	2647	807
AZ	Pinal	3.36	263	29.8	9	23.6	75.3	80.7	2340	713
AZ	Santa Cruz	5.95	63	21.8	6.1	16.7	74.3	81	4548	1386
AZ	Yavapai	5.21	97	22	6.6	19.1	75.8	81.6	4508	1374
AZ	Yuma	4.24	183	30.2	8.7	23.2	78	83.8	878	268
CA	Alameda	5.13	110	20.1	7.3	16.6	77.7	82.3	864	263
CA	Alpine	7.41	26	24.9	7.9	19.4	77	80.7	7732	2357
CA	Amador	7.23	29	24.8	8	16.6	76.3	81.1	2655	809
CA	Butte	5.11	112	24.8	8	16.3	74	80	1558	475

ST	COUNTY	USDA	AMEN	OBES	DIAB	INACT	M AGE	W AGE	ALT ft	ALT m
CA	Calaveras	8.27	14	25.6	6.7	19.3	76.6	81.6	2430	741
CA	Colusa	4.34	173	24.4	7.4	17.2	74.2	80.3	767	234
CA	Contra Costa	8.36	13	24.2	6.9	17.3	78.3	82.4	486	148
CA	Del Norte	10.75	5	27.2	7.6	18.1	72.8	79.8	2189	667
CA	El Dorado	6.10	55	20.4	6.5	14.1	77.2	81.5	4256	1297
CA	Fresno	6.03	60	29.2	9.3	21	75.2	80.2	3364	1025
CA	Glenn	4.38	169	26.9	7.3	18.5	73.6	79.2	1263	385
CA	Humboldt	11.15	2	25.9	8.1	18.9	73.9	79.1	1754	535
CA	Imperial	6.45	48	24.6	7.3	22.6	75.1	81.7	415	126
CA	Inyo	7.08	35	23.1	6.9	16.7	75.5	81.1	4163	1269
CA	Kern	4.84	142	28.6	8.1	23.7	73.5	78.7	2377	724
CA	Kings	3.48	247	27.5	7.6	22.4	74.6	79.6	343	105
CA	Lake	6.55	43	26.5	7.8	16.6	73.2	78.4	2327	709
CA	Lassen	6.35	51	26.4	7.6	18.9	75.5	79.8	5361	1634
CA	Los Angeles	10.33	7	21.4	7.7	18.9	77.4	82.5	2265	691
CA	Madera	6.00	61	29.9	8.5	20.4	74.6	80.2	3089	942
CA	Marin	8.14	18	15	5.4	12.1	80.8	84.5	426	130
CA	Mariposa	8.25	15	24.1	7.2	19.4	76.3	81.1	3637	1108
CA	Mendocino	10.93	4	22.6	6.3	17	75.6	80.8	1827	557
CA	Merced	4.51	162	31.8	7.6	20.3	75	79.9	368	112
CA	Modoc	4.99	121	24.7	6.7	18.9	75.5	79.8	4979	1517
CA	Mono	8.21	16	20.3	6.5	13.6	77	80.7	7760	2365
CA	Monterey	9.24	9	22.3	7.3	16	78	82.6	1464	446
CA	Napa	7.53	23	22.1	6.2	15.1	77.2	81.9	935	285
CA	Nevada	7.26	28	20.1	5.5	12.9	78	81.8	4139	1262
CA	Orange	8.74	10	20.5	7.1	16.4	79.3	83.6	725	221
CA	Placer	6.00	62	20.3	6.5	13.8	79	82.8	3812	1162
CA	Plumas	6.55	44	23.9	6.6	18.4	76.3	81.5	5309	1618
CA	Riverside	6.64	42	27.5	8.9	21.5	75.8	81.3	1857	566
CA	Sacramento	3.65	230	28	8.3	19	75.6	81	103	32
CA	San Benito	5.20	99	23.9	7	16.1	77.7	82	1939	591
CA	San Bernardino	3.57	241	27.8	8.1	21.7	74.3	79.5	2666	813
CA	San Diego	9.78	8	22.8	7.3	17.4	77.6	82.4	1975	602
CA	San Francisco	10.52	6	17.2	7.3	17	77.6	83.8	236	72
CA	San Joaquin	4.77	145	29.6	8.5	21.4	74.9	80.1	158	48
CA	San Luis Obispo	7.87	21	21.5	5.9	14.2	77.9	82.2	1552	473
CA	San Mateo	8.19	17	19.8	6.5	16.1	79.8	84.5	669	204
CA	Santa Barbara	10.97	3	19.9	6.6	15.8	78.3	83.1	1823	556
CA	Santa Clara	5.95	64	21.1	7.4	16.6	80.6	83.9	1226	374
CA	Santa Cruz	8.49	12	19.5	6.1	12.4	78.1	82.6	939	286
CA	Shasta	5.69	75	28	7.1	18.9	73.9	79.1	2997	913
CA	Sierra	5.90	66	23.4	6.9	17.7	76.3	81.5	5746	1751
CA	Siskiyou	3.36	264	25	7	18.7	74.6	80.7	4254	1297
CA	Solano	5.88	67	26.7	9.7	21.2	76.1	81	167	51
CA	Sonoma	7.93	20	22.7	6.1	14.2	77.8	82.1	729	222
CA	Stanislaus	7.21	30	30.2	8.2	23.9	74.8	79.4	491	150
CA	Sutter	1.72	541	26.4	7.8	21.9	75	80.4	77	23

ST	COUNTY	USDA	AMEN	OBES	DIAB	INACT	M AGE	W AGE	ALT ft	ALT m
CA	Tehama	3.24	278	25.2	8.3	16.7	74.1	79.1	2144	653
CA	Trinity	4.07	194	23.6	7.3	20.6	74.6	80.7	3805	1160
CA	Tulare	5.65	76	31.1	7.9	24.5	74.1	79.4	4352	1326
CA	Tuolumne	7.10	34	23.1	6	18.1	77	80.7	5653	1723
CA	Ventura	11.17	1	22.9	6.8	16.8	78.1	82.6	2690	820
CA	Yolo	5.10	114	26.1	7.8	16.5	76.9	81.5	340	104
CA	Yuba	4.97	126	31	7.3	24.8	72.1	78.9	1073	327
CO	Adams	2.48	373	24.6	6.9	21.3	77.6	81.4	5088	1551
CO	Alamosa	1.59	571	20.4	6.2	19.9	74.5	80.1	7744	2360
CO	Arapahoe	2.35	398	19.4	5.8	17.2	78.4	82.3	5468	1667
CO	Archuleta	5.58	80	16.5	5	16.7	76.8	81.4	8265	2519
CO	Baca	0.48	1084	22.7	5.7	22.3	74.2	79.3	4292	1308
CO	Bent	2.45	379	24.5	6	22.6	74.2	79.3	4130	1259
CO	Boulder	5.82	71	14.5	4.6	11.3	77.6	81.4	7381	2250
CO	Chaffee	6.46	47	15.9	4.6	15.6	77.1	81.1	9959	3035
CO	Cheyenne	-0.04	1470	20.9	5.4	19.6	74.4	80.6	4350	1326
CO	Clear Creek	6.96	37	17.7	5.1	17.3	78.2	82	10296	3138
CO	Conejos	4.98	123	17.2	4.7	18.9	76.8	81.4	8951	2728
CO	Costilla	4.96	130	20.4	5.7	18.8	74.5	80.1	8861	2701
CO	Crowley	2.60	359	22.5	6.4	22.9	74.1	80	4539	1383
CO	Custer	5.61	78	20.2	5.4	20.5	74.9	79.9	9062	2762
CO	Delta	3.64	232	20.3	5.6	22.7	75.9	81.5	6982	2128
CO	Denver	2.88	323	18.2	6.1	16.3	74.4	80.9	5335	1626
CO	Dolores	4.38	170	20.3	5.2	20.8	75.6	80.9	8330	2539
CO	Douglas	5.15	104	15.7	4.6	11.1	80.3	83.5	6876	2096
CO	Eagle	4.57	156	13.9	4.2	11.8	79.1	83.1	9074	2766
CO	El Paso	5.15	105	21	6	18.2	76.6	81.1	6423	1958
CO	Elbert	0.90	859	21.2	4.5	18.9	77.9	81.9	5965	1818
CO	Fremont	4.82	143	22.2	6.8	19.6	74.9	79.9	7525	2294
CO	Garfield	3.81	214	17.3	5.4	15.5	76.7	81.5	7893	2406
CO	Gilpin	6.97	36	19.2	5.4	18.7	77.1	81.8	9303	2836
CO	Grand	7.47	25	18.3	5.2	16.9	78.2	82	9259	2822
CO	Gunnison	4.94	132	15.7	4.8	15.3	80	84.2	9548	2910
CO	Hinsdale	6.90	38	18.9	5.3	18.3	75.7	81.2	10935	3333
CO	Huerfano	5.20	100	20.1	5.5	23.1	74.5	80.1	7507	2288
CO	Jackson	6.45	49	20.5	5.4	17.9	78.6	83.3	8919	2719
CO	Jefferson	5.61	79	18.7	5.2	15.7	77.6	81.4	7056	2151
CO	Kiowa	2.31	409	23.9	5.5	19.8	74.4	80.6	4157	1267
CO	Kit Carson	-0.01	1442	27	5.5	26.4	75.2	79.9	4418	1347
CO	La Plata	5.83	69	15.9	4.6	15.5	77.9	82.2	7988	2435
CO	Lake	8.52	11	17.7	5.1	18.9	77.1	81.6	10931	3332
CO	Larimer	5.62	77	18.5	5	14.2	79.2	82.7	7725	2355
CO	Las Animas	3.60	238	21.9	6.2	23.3	75	80.5	5947	1813
CO	Lincoln	1.05	789	21.6	6.4	23.1	74.4	80.6	5122	1561
CO	Logan	1.29	682	23.1	5.5	22.1	75.8	80.2	4193	1278
CO	Mesa	2.26	420	22.2	5.4	17.8	75.9	81.2	6846	2087
CO	Mineral	5.79	72	18.7	5.2	17.2	75.7	81.2	10492	3198

ST	COUNTY	USDA	AMEN	OBES	DIAB	INACT	M AGE	W AGE	ALT ft	ALT m
CO	Moffat	4.14	190	23.2	6	26.1	74.8	80.3	6733	2052
CO	Montezuma	4.41	167	18.9	5.7	19.8	75.6	80.9	6813	2077
CO	Montrose	2.94	315	18.6	4.9	18.9	75.3	81	6943	2116
CO	Morgan	1.43	624	25.9	6.6	23	75	80.7	4492	1369
CO	Otero	2.24	425	25.5	6.4	22.1	74.4	80.6	4448	1356
CO	Ouray	6.08	57	17	5.4	15	75.7	81.2	8980	2737
CO	Park	7.11	33	17.7	5	19.2	77.1	81.6	9672	2948
CO	Phillips	-0.71	1946	22.1	5.8	18.5	75.8	80.2	3819	1164
CO	Pitkin	6.14	54	14.2	4.7	12.7	80	84.2	10010	3051
CO	Prowers	1.13	757	22.3	6.1	26.9	74.2	79.3	3801	1159
CO	Pueblo	2.11	450	23.6	6.9	19.3	74.1	80	5212	1589
CO	Rio Blanco	3.59	240	20	5.4	18.9	74.8	80.3	7231	2204
CO	Rio Grande	5.26	92	21.1	6	22.5	75.7	81.2	9029	2752
CO	Routt	5.29	90	13.5	3.8	11.1	78.6	83.3	8197	2499
CO	Saguache	4.91	137	20.7	4.8	18.2	74.9	79.9	9206	2806
CO	San Juan	7.16	31	18.8	5.3	18.4	75.6	80.9	11344	3458
CO	San Miguel	5.14	108	16.4	5.4	13.7	75.6	80.9	7943	2421
CO	Sedgwick	0.92	851	24.3	5.2	19.4	75.8	80.2	3761	1146
CO	Summit	8.08	19	15.1	4.7	12.3	79.3	83	10481	3195
CO	Teller	6.29	52	17.8	6	18.7	77.9	81.8	9181	2798
CO	Washington	0.58	1027	21.1	5.6	24.3	75	80.7	4604	1403
CO	Weld	1.70	543	25	6.2	18.5	77.6	81.4	4964	1513
CO	Yuma	0.30	1213	23.7	5.3	21.1	75.2	79.9	3934	1199
CT	Fairfield	2.25	421	18	5.8	19.2	78.9	83.3	378	115
CT	Hartford	1.05	790	23.8	7.3	22.5	76.6	81.7	316	96
CT	Litchfield	1.04	796	19.7	6.1	18.5	77.3	82.5	914	279
CT	Middlesex	2.32	407	22.9	6.3	20.2	77.8	82.5	286	87
CT	New Haven	2.52	369	26.7	8.2	26	76.3	81.3	319	97
CT	New London	2.43	384	23.3	7.4	22.1	76.4	81.5	248	76
CT	Tolland	1.48	602	22.2	6.9	19.1	78.3	82.5	581	177
CT	Windham	1.28	687	29.7	8.3	25.2	75.4	80.7	471	143
DC	Dist of Columbia	-0.76	1976	21.6	8.5	19.9	71.6	78.5	139	42
DE	Kent	-0.07	1498	32.5	11	27.9	73.5	79.5	33	10
DE	New Castle	0.01	1427	26.8	7.2	21.9	75.2	80.1	90	27
DE	Sussex	0.05	1401	29.2	9.3	24.8	74.8	80.8	31	9
FL	Alachua	2.44	383	25.1	8.3	22.6	75.1	79.8	103	31
FL	Baker	0.65	980	34.8	12.7	32.6	68.1	77.7	126	38
FL	Bay	2.15	442	26.8	8.9	23.5	73.7	79.2	55	17
FL	Bradford	1.34	656	35.1	12.1	29.8	71.8	78.9	144	44
FL	Brevard	3.93	204	28.8	9.7	23.7	75.9	81.2	16	5
FL	Broward	4.98	124	25.3	8.3	22.5	76.5	82	11	3
FL	Calhoun	1.12	764	34.4	11.6	29.7	72	77.7	97	29
FL	Charlotte	5.10	115	27.2	8.7	19.4	76.2	83.1	27	8
FL	Citrus	3.43	253	29.8	9.6	25.1	73.1	80.8	53	16
FL	Clay	2.01	466	29.2	10	24.1	74.8	79.1	89	27
FL	Collier	5.00	120	22.1	7.2	16.2	80.2	86	11	3
FL	Columbia	0.59	1023	33.8	10.9	28.4	71.8	77.8	109	33

44

HEALTHIEST PLACES TO LIVE

ST	COUNTY	USDA	AMEN	OBES	DIAB	INACT	M AGE	W AGE	ALT ft	ALT m
FL	DeSoto	2.74	337	34.6	11.2	30.7	74.2	80.1	55	17
FL	Dixie	2.42	385	34.9	10.6	33.2	71.3	78.8	27	8
FL	Duval	2.31	410	27.8	11	26.2	72.5	78	36	11
FL	Escambia	2.34	400	29.4	10.5	25.5	73.6	79	150	46
FL	Flagler	2.70	339	29	9	22.4	76.7	83.1	21	6
FL	Franklin	2.66	345	27.5	9.1	28.9	72.4	78.5	13	4
FL	Gadsden	1.65	556	35.7	12.6	31.1	70.1	77.9	202	62
FL	Gilchrist	1.21	728	32.8	10	28	71.3	78.8	58	18
FL	Glades	5.15	106	35.9	10.2	33	74.2	80.1	29	9
FL	Gulf	2.25	422	29.8	10.3	27.1	72	77.7	17	5
FL	Hamilton	0.58	1028	38.3	13.3	33.3	70.2	76.5	108	33
FL	Hardee	2.25	423	37.6	12.2	31.2	73.2	78.9	87	26
FL	Hendry	4.22	185	34.6	10.7	31.2	71.8	77.8	21	6
FL	Hernando	3.71	222	29.2	8.6	24.8	74.3	81.1	73	22
FL	Highlands	4.14	191	30.2	9.8	26.6	75.5	81.6	74	23
FL	Hillsborough	4.32	175	26	9.6	24.1	74.7	80.4	63	19
FL	Holmes	0.89	862	30.4	12.9	32.7	71.8	78	131	40
FL	Indian River	4.72	147	22.2	8.4	22.6	77	82.6	25	8
FL	Jackson	1.76	529	33	12.3	31	72.5	77.9	124	38
FL	Jefferson	2.00	469	34.2	11.6	27.9	72.5	78.3	88	27
FL	Lafayette	0.84	892	32.9	11.5	29.9	72.4	78.2	65	20
FL	Lake	3.40	256	27.1	9.1	22.2	76.8	82.9	83	25
FL	Lee	5.23	94	26.4	8.6	22.3	76.4	83.1	15	5
FL	Leon	1.75	537	28.1	9.8	21.2	76.1	80.4	102	31
FL	Levy	2.47	375	34.2	10.6	31.4	71.5	78.7	40	12
FL	Liberty	0.36	1173	35.8	11.5	31.7	72.4	78.5	75	23
FL	Madison	1.30	676	36.3	12.2	31.1	70.2	76.5	104	32
FL	Manatee	4.66	152	25.9	8.9	24	75.9	82.8	55	17
FL	Marion	2.59	361	32.7	9.9	26.9	73.9	80.9	81	25
FL	Martin	5.34	88	21.7	6.2	18.9	77.7	83.4	21	6
FL	Miami-Dade	5.48	84	23.9	8.6	23.6	76.6	82.8	5	1
FL	Monroe	6.05	59	19.4	6.1	18.1	76	81.8	3	1
FL	Nassau	2.04	461	28.5	8.6	23.6	74.6	79.4	39	12
FL	Okaloosa	2.01	467	29.4	8.9	22.2	75.6	80.2	172	52
FL	Okeechobee	4.70	149	31.7	9.4	31	72.2	78.7	44	13
FL	Orange	2.96	313	26.6	9.6	24.1	75.5	80.9	77	23
FL	Osceola	4.50	163	29.2	9.3	26	76	80.8	60	18
FL	Palm Beach	5.14	109	22.2	8	21.6	77.1	83.5	15	5
FL	Pasco	3.37	261	28.9	8.8	27.4	73.7	80.6	72	22
FL	Pinellas	5.05	117	24	8.2	19.5	74.7	81.4	21	6
FL	Polk	3.98	201	33.5	10.9	25.3	74.3	80	117	36
FL	Putnam	2.35	399	35.6	11.8	30.9	70.9	78	54	16
FL	Santa Rosa	1.94	487	28	10	24.6	75.6	79.8	146	45
FL	Sarasota	4.78	144	21.3	7.3	18.1	77.8	83.8	21	6
FL	Seminole	3.14	289	25	10.1	20.2	77.1	81.5	37	11
FL	St. Johns	2.98	310	21.5	7.4	17.7	77.6	82.8	22	7
FL	St. Lucie	5.03	118	26.9	10.9	24.3	75.1	81.5	23	7

ST	COUNTY	USDA	AMEN	OBES	DIAB	INACT	M AGE	W AGE	ALT ft	ALT m
FL	Sumter	2.84	326	29.4	9.4	19.5	74.4	80.2	74	23
FL	Suwannee	0.70	958	30.7	9.8	29.1	72.4	78.2	96	29
FL	Taylor	2.32	408	35.4	11	30.7	72.5	78.3	41	12
FL	Union	1.60	568	35.7	12.9	31.7	68.1	77.7	124	38
FL	Volusia	3.45	250	25.9	9.6	24.6	74.3	80.6	28	9
FL	Wakulla	1.95	483	34.8	10.5	27.3	74.5	79.8	33	10
FL	Walton	2.18	435	26.4	9.4	25.7	73.7	79.7	165	50
FL	Washington	1.95	484	35.6	12.3	29.6	71.3	77.6	103	32
GA	Appling	0.06	1395	32.5	11.1	31.4	70.8	76.9	174	53
GA	Atkinson	0.24	1261	29.1	10.1	29.5	69.4	76.5	212	65
GA	Bacon	-0.47	1799	31	10	33.8	68.8	76.4	181	55
GA	Baker	-0.07	1499	32.6	13	27.5	70.1	77.2	176	54
GA	Baldwin	2.09	453	31.2	11.6	27.8	72.1	77.7	388	118
GA	Banks	-1.21	2239	27.3	9.8	24.2	72.9	79	862	263
GA	Barrow	-0.70	1940	28.7	10.9	28	72.5	78.6	863	263
GA	Bartow	1.17	741	25.3	9.3	24.8	71.9	78.2	856	261
GA	Ben Hill	-0.10	1523	32.6	12	29.9	70.1	76	297	90
GA	Berrien	0.32	1202	30.4	10.5	29.1	71.1	77.6	256	78
GA	Bibb	1.81	520	30	11.8	28.2	70	76.9	383	117
GA	Bleckley	0.15	1334	28.7	10.6	27.2	70.5	77.1	328	100
GA	Brantley	0.05	1402	28.9	9.5	28	70.6	77.2	66	20
GA	Brooks	0.35	1183	30.8	12.6	30.3	70.1	76.7	191	58
GA	Bryan	0.70	959	28	9.6	24.6	73.7	78.9	43	13
GA	Bulloch	0.19	1315	31.1	12.2	26.1	73.2	78.9	158	48
GA	Burke	-0.77	1987	37	11.4	30.7	68.3	75	255	78
GA	Butts	1.86	508	30.8	11.8	25.7	71.9	76.9	630	192
GA	Calhoun	0.21	1294	33.8	12.6	27.4	67.6	74.7	238	73
GA	Camden	1.88	501	29.1	11.2	24.1	74.2	79.5	15	5
GA	Candler	0.39	1145	31	10.3	27.5	70.1	77.7	214	65
GA	Carroll	-0.11	1532	30.7	12.7	24.7	72.6	77.8	1035	315
GA	Catoosa	-0.54	1836	32.8	10	29	73.3	79.2	857	261
GA	Charlton	-0.36	1718	30.8	10.8	29.8	70.6	77.2	96	29
GA	Chatham	1.76	530	29	10.9	23.4	73	78.4	11	3
GA	Chattahoochee	-0.35	1708	32.7	12	27.2	71.9	78.2	409	125
GA	Chattooga	-1.08	2179	30.7	10.1	27.6	70.1	76.9	899	274
GA	Cherokee	1.93	488	27.2	7.8	22.3	76	79.7	1072	327
GA	Clarke	-0.71	1947	28.1	11	20.3	74.3	79.6	722	220
GA	Clay	1.34	657	33	14.2	28.8	69.6	75.8	300	91
GA	Clayton	-0.32	1686	34.7	12.4	29.9	73.5	78.8	886	270
GA	Clinch	0.31	1207	32.7	11.1	29.9	72.2	77.9	150	46
GA	Cobb	-0.17	1570	23.3	9.1	21.3	77.6	81.3	981	299
GA	Coffee	-0.49	1807	29.5	11.3	32.2	70.2	78	254	77
GA	Colquitt	0.26	1245	31.4	11	28.2	70.9	77.2	282	86
GA	Columbia	0.79	915	25.4	9.3	22.2	75.4	80.2	357	109
GA	Cook	0.70	960	32.9	11.5	27.8	70	76.4	246	75
GA	Coweta	-0.28	1651	29.3	9.9	23.7	74.1	79.1	839	256
GA	Crawford	0.97	824	29.7	10.5	27.5	70.6	76.6	473	144

HEALTHIEST PLACES TO LIVE

ST	COUNTY	USDA	AMEN	OBES	DIAB	INACT	M AGE	W AGE	ALT ft	ALT m
GA	Crisp	0.36	1174	34.1	11.4	31.3	69.8	76.6	326	99
GA	Dade	-0.39	1743	27.9	10	23.2	71.7	78.3	1293	394
GA	Dawson	2.48	374	26.6	9.2	22.9	74.6	80.2	1469	448
GA	Decatur	1.04	797	33.7	12.5	31.8	70.7	77.8	168	51
GA	DeKalb	-0.30	1665	26.1	9.9	21.2	75.9	81.4	915	279
GA	Dodge	-0.08	1506	35.8	12.6	30.1	70.7	76.4	300	92
GA	Dooly	-0.12	1538	34	11.5	29.4	69.2	76.2	333	101
GA	Dougherty	-0.31	1679	34.7	13	27.5	70.8	77.6	203	62
GA	Douglas	-0.45	1783	30.7	10.3	25.8	73.4	77.5	987	301
GA	Early	0.16	1329	30.1	12.2	29.5	69.6	75.8	225	69
GA	Echols	0.73	939	28.9	10.2	24.9	72.2	77.9	142	43
GA	Effingham	-0.10	1524	31.4	10.5	25.7	74.4	78.8	70	21
GA	Elbert	-0.34	1696	36.3	12.2	30	71.7	78.1	553	169
GA	Emanuel	-0.16	1564	30.9	11.2	26.8	69.3	75.6	260	79
GA	Evans	0.28	1229	31.8	12.2	28.6	70.1	77.7	141	43
GA	Fannin	2.78	334	29	9.9	23.5	72.9	79.3	2109	643
GA	Fayette	-0.24	1628	23.6	9.8	20.3	77.8	82	865	264
GA	Floyd	0.33	1197	28.9	9.2	28.7	72.1	78.2	755	230
GA	Forsyth	0.99	817	23	9.2	20.2	77.2	81.8	1156	352
GA	Franklin	-0.50	1812	28.1	9.5	24.7	72	78.9	760	232
GA	Fulton	-0.24	1629	23.8	9.2	19.8	75	80.2	940	287
GA	Gilmer	2.33	403	30.3	10.2	24.4	72.6	78.5	1839	560
GA	Glascock	-0.78	1995	27.4	10.2	28	68.4	75.4	445	136
GA	Glynn	2.06	456	27	9.3	24.6	73	79	13	4
GA	Gordon	-0.52	1822	31.2	9.7	28.4	72	78.5	762	232
GA	Grady	0.16	1330	32.9	11.5	29.5	70.8	78	229	70
GA	Greene	2.34	401	32.4	11.6	25.8	73.2	78.5	568	173
GA	Gwinnett	-0.35	1709	25.2	8.7	20.7	77.2	80.9	997	304
GA	Habersham	1.22	721	26.7	9	25.5	74.6	80	1527	465
GA	Hall	0.96	830	27.9	10.5	21.9	74.7	79.7	1136	346
GA	Hancock	1.52	591	36.8	14.5	28.5	68.4	75.4	486	148
GA	Haralson	-0.39	1744	30.7	10.4	27.8	71.4	77.7	1166	355
GA	Harris	0.18	1318	27	10.5	20	74.9	80.1	696	212
GA	Hart	0.62	1006	30.4	9.6	24.4	72	78.4	742	226
GA	Heard	0.22	1283	28.1	9.9	27.3	71.4	77.1	794	242
GA	Henry	-0.53	1833	27.8	10.6	23.5	74	78.7	784	239
GA	Houston	-0.04	1471	28.7	10.5	25.6	74.2	79.6	347	106
GA	Irwin	0.23	1274	31.1	10.9	25.4	70.8	76.6	314	96
GA	Jackson	-1.20	2232	25.6	10.2	25.5	72.2	78.6	827	252
GA	Jasper	1.46	608	28.7	10.8	27.6	73	78.7	545	166
GA	Jeff Davis	-0.60	1878	26.9	10.1	25.8	68.8	76.4	219	67
GA	Jefferson	-0.46	1790	37.3	12.4	29.7	67.9	75.2	335	102
GA	Jenkins	-0.22	1611	32.4	11.5	26.7	70.1	76.4	208	63
GA	Johnson	-0.01	1443	34.8	12.8	29.4	70.6	76.1	332	101
GA	Jones	0.98	822	29.3	10.4	29.4	73.1	79.3	468	143
GA	Lamar	-0.57	1857	29.8	10.8	26.8	72.1	77.9	746	227
GA	Lanier	0.94	840	31	11.7	29.4	69.4	76.5	200	61

ST	COUNTY	USDA	AMEN	OBES	DIAB	INACT	M AGE	W AGE	ALT ft	ALT m
GA	Laurens	0.01	1428	35.9	11.3	28.4	71.4	77.2	284	87
GA	Lee	0.22	1284	27.6	9.7	24.3	74.9	80	271	83
GA	Liberty	1.46	609	31.8	13.1	27	73	78.1	35	11
GA	Lincoln	1.13	758	32.6	11.4	28.7	70.8	76.8	394	120
GA	Long	-0.04	1472	30.1	11.2	25.3	70.6	77.8	63	19
GA	Lowndes	0.27	1237	33.9	11.9	27.6	72.2	77.9	192	59
GA	Lumpkin	1.28	688	27.5	8.6	20.3	73.6	79	1658	505
GA	Macon	-0.54	1837	33.2	13.7	26.6	69.2	76.2	375	114
GA	Madison	-1.05	2161	30.5	10.1	24	72.5	78.7	740	225
GA	Marion	-0.86	2042	31.1	11	26.4	71.9	78.2	563	172
GA	McDuffie	1.96	481	29.9	11.6	26.9	70.1	76.3	441	134
GA	McIntosh	2.00	470	31.3	11.4	28.8	70.6	77.8	14	4
GA	Meriwether	-0.59	1875	31.4	11.9	26.5	69.4	76	827	252
GA	Miller	-1.12	2200	32.8	12.5	32.1	70.1	77.2	167	51
GA	Mitchell	-0.45	1784	34.1	11.6	30.2	69.8	76.7	217	66
GA	Monroe	1.13	759	30.6	10.6	26	73.1	78.1	542	165
GA	Montgomery	0.07	1384	31.2	10.5	26.7	71.3	76.5	227	69
GA	Morgan	0.37	1163	29	11.1	24.5	73.2	78.5	609	186
GA	Murray	1.16	745	29.3	10.4	31.4	70.8	77.8	1107	338
GA	Muscogee	0.08	1376	35	12.4	27.8	70.9	77.5	389	119
GA	Newton	1.45	612	31.1	10.8	26	72.6	78.1	700	213
GA	Oconee	-1.04	2154	25.6	8.4	21.5	76.8	81.3	700	213
GA	Oglethorpe	-1.15	2212	30.5	10.1	23.7	71.7	78.1	598	182
GA	Paulding	0.44	1113	26	10.9	25.7	74.1	78.4	1026	313
GA	Peach	-0.64	1904	30.2	12.4	28.5	70.6	76.3	435	133
GA	Pickens	1.56	579	26.4	10	22.5	74.5	79.7	1417	432
GA	Pierce	-0.63	1893	28.8	10.6	27.6	70.3	77.5	103	32
GA	Pike	-0.63	1894	29.7	10.4	25.4	72.1	77.9	825	251
GA	Polk	0.21	1295	29.1	11.1	26.4	70.4	76.9	914	279
GA	Pulaski	0.28	1230	30.2	10.7	30.4	70.9	77.1	278	85
GA	Putnam	2.34	402	29.3	11.3	24.2	73	78.7	490	149
GA	Quitman	1.05	791	32.8	12.3	30.7	69.6	75.8	331	101
GA	Rabun	3.11	294	27.1	9.4	23.1	75.1	81	2289	698
GA	Randolph	-0.49	1808	36.1	13.4	31.9	67.6	74.7	386	118
GA	Richmond	0.02	1417	32.4	11.2	27.3	69.7	77.2	290	89
GA	Rockdale	0.14	1338	32.1	10.9	27.2	74.4	78.9	785	239
GA	Schley	-1.42	2331	30.4	11.3	27.3	70.9	77	483	147
GA	Screven	-0.02	1452	30.7	11.9	29.5	70.1	76.4	149	45
GA	Seminole	0.87	875	32.9	11.7	25.8	70.1	77.2	137	42
GA	Spalding	-0.33	1690	31.6	10.9	27.6	71.2	77	818	249
GA	Stephens	0.53	1048	32.7	10.4	27.1	71.7	78.1	910	277
GA	Stewart	0.01	1429	35.3	13.7	29	69.6	75.8	417	127
GA	Sumter	0.23	1275	34.7	13	29.7	70.9	77	385	117
GA	Talbot	1.10	776	34.7	13	28.6	69.4	76	620	189
GA	Taliaferro	-0.13	1548	34.8	12.7	30.1	70.8	76.8	535	163
GA	Tattnall	0.54	1044	28.9	10.9	28.1	70.6	77.1	162	49
GA	Taylor	-0.62	1890	33.8	11.9	29.1	70.6	76.6	503	153

HEALTHIEST PLACES TO LIVE

ST	COUNTY	USDA	AMEN	OBES	DIAB	INACT	M AGE	W AGE	ALT ft	ALT m
GA	Telfair	-0.36	1719	29.6	11.5	27	70.1	76	205	62
GA	Terrell	-0.21	1603	37.3	12.5	29.7	67.6	74.7	336	102
GA	Thomas	0.29	1220	34.1	12.2	28.4	72	78.8	210	64
GA	Tift	0.33	1198	33.2	12.1	28.9	72.1	78.2	328	100
GA	Toombs	0.24	1262	31.5	11.8	31.6	70.6	77.5	197	60
GA	Towns	3.18	283	27.4	9.4	26.2	75.1	81	2551	778
GA	Treutlen	0.02	1418	34.9	10.7	28.3	71.3	76.5	269	82
GA	Troup	0.93	847	32.7	11.9	28.9	71.4	77.1	725	221
GA	Turner	0.11	1358	34.1	12.4	32.4	70.8	76.6	356	109
GA	Twiggs	-0.11	1533	32	12.2	29.4	70.5	77.1	390	119
GA	Union	2.94	316	27.8	9.7	23	74.9	80.1	2362	720
GA	Upson	1.37	645	30.3	11.3	26.7	70.5	76.3	660	201
GA	Walker	-0.40	1751	30.5	10	34.9	71.3	78	1078	329
GA	Walton	-0.94	2090	28.2	10.3	30.5	74.4	79.6	809	247
GA	Ware	-0.17	1571	31.2	12.1	33.7	69.7	76.6	139	42
GA	Warren	1.04	798	35	12.3	27.3	68.4	75.4	502	153
GA	Washington	-0.21	1604	34.5	12.7	27.3	70.1	77	371	113
GA	Wayne	-0.12	1539	32.2	9.6	31.3	70.9	77.3	85	26
GA	Webster	-0.55	1839	31.6	12.3	27.1	69.6	75.8	455	139
GA	Wheeler	0.07	1385	30.1	10.9	26.3	71.3	76.5	179	55
GA	White	1.55	583	29.3	9.2	23	74.6	79.7	1737	529
GA	Whitfield	-0.36	1720	29	10.7	27.9	72.5	78.6	842	257
GA	Wilcox	-0.29	1660	32.9	11	31.9	70.9	77.1	302	92
GA	Wilkes	0.65	981	31	12.3	28.4	70.8	76.8	500	153
GA	Wilkinson	1.54	587	32	11.8	27.2	70.6	76.1	345	105
GA	Worth	0.06	1396	29.5	10.2	26.4	71.8	78.3	331	101
IA	Adair	-1.59	2416	30.7	8	28.7	76.1	82.6	1276	389
IA	Adams	-1.00	2126	32.5	7	24.1	76.4	80.9	1214	370
IA	Allamakee	-0.27	1646	28.9	7.7	22.1	76	80.2	974	297
IA	Appanoose	-0.51	1815	30	7.1	28.8	75	80.2	952	290
IA	Audubon	-1.94	2560	33.1	7.8	26.5	76.1	82.6	1380	421
IA	Benton	-3.66	3030	30.3	7	25	77.7	82	893	272
IA	Black Hawk	-3.07	2917	28.8	8.5	23	76.8	80.8	921	281
IA	Boone	-3.35	2974	33.7	6.8	26.4	76.4	81.5	1058	322
IA	Bremer	-3.16	2936	27.4	7.1	22.7	77.6	82.2	1022	312
IA	Buchanan	-3.24	2954	29.3	7.8	25.7	76.2	81.3	987	301
IA	Buena Vista	-2.44	2756	28.5	7.1	26.4	76.7	81.2	1376	419
IA	Butler	-3.94	3058	25.4	6.1	25.9	76.3	81	998	304
IA	Calhoun	-2.73	2846	30.7	7.9	27.7	76.3	81.2	1198	365
IA	Carroll	-1.70	2470	30.8	6.2	27.9	76.7	82	1311	400
IA	Cass	-1.79	2501	35.7	6.5	25.3	77	81.6	1270	387
IA	Cedar	-3.28	2960	32.9	7.1	24	76.9	82.2	798	243
IA	Cerro Gordo	-2.96	2898	26.5	8	23.5	75.7	81.5	1183	361
IA	Cherokee	-2.66	2828	26	6.8	21.3	75.9	81.8	1365	416
IA	Chickasaw	-3.65	3028	31.1	7.1	26.4	76.3	81	1137	346
IA	Clarke	-2.42	2746	29.5	6.7	28	75.5	80.8	1095	334
IA	Clay	-2.52	2789	30.5	6.8	26.5	77	81.6	1391	424

ST	COUNTY	USDA	AMEN	OBES	DIAB	INACT	M AGE	W AGE	ALT ft	ALT m
IA	Clayton	-1.01	2134	29.2	6.5	28.3	76.1	81.5	968	295
IA	Clinton	-2.35	2707	29.8	7.3	28.7	75.5	80.7	726	221
IA	Crawford	-1.89	2539	31.4	7	30.8	75.4	81.7	1361	415
IA	Dallas	-2.56	2800	30	8.1	23.9	77	81.9	992	302
IA	Davis	-1.96	2567	30.7	7.2	27.9	74.7	80.9	841	256
IA	Decatur	-2.04	2592	29.4	6.6	25.3	75.5	80.8	1054	321
IA	Delaware	-3.45	2995	32.4	6.9	27.4	77.4	81.7	1016	310
IA	Des Moines	-2.04	2593	33.8	8.5	28.5	75.9	81.6	691	210
IA	Dickinson	-1.51	2380	26.6	6.8	20.9	78	82.1	1470	448
IA	Dubuque	-0.79	2002	26.8	7	20.1	76.9	81.5	957	292
IA	Emmet	-2.10	2614	31.4	7.4	27.2	75.7	81.2	1304	397
IA	Fayette	-4.09	3077	33.5	6.4	24.1	76.1	80.8	1100	335
IA	Floyd	-4.03	3072	29.5	7.3	24.6	76.5	81.1	1072	327
IA	Franklin	-4.18	3082	32.6	7.8	26.5	76.6	81.4	1174	358
IA	Fremont	-0.81	2012	32.2	7.1	29.8	76.2	81.1	1028	313
IA	Greene	-2.37	2723	29.1	6.8	26.3	76.2	82	1106	337
IA	Grundy	-4.86	3097	31.2	7.4	23.4	77.1	81.4	1036	316
IA	Guthrie	-1.19	2229	30.3	6.6	25.8	76.2	82	1206	368
IA	Hamilton	-3.74	3042	31.6	7.2	23.6	76.7	82.4	1127	344
IA	Hancock	-4.06	3076	28.6	7.1	23.8	76.6	81.4	1233	376
IA	Hardin	-3.63	3027	33.4	7	29.6	76	81.1	1113	339
IA	Harrison	-1.06	2169	30.9	7.2	27.2	75	80.4	1171	357
IA	Henry	-2.95	2894	30.1	8	24.2	76	81.4	690	210
IA	Howard	-4.16	3080	28.3	6.8	22	76.6	81.4	1271	387
IA	Humboldt	-4.05	3073	30.6	7.4	24.7	75.9	81.1	1140	347
IA	Ida	-2.14	2631	27.3	6.5	24.2	75.1	80.4	1357	414
IA	Iowa	-3.84	3051	28.7	6.9	29.1	76.6	81.8	811	247
IA	Jackson	-0.85	2035	31.2	6.6	23.5	76	80.8	794	242
IA	Jasper	-3.19	2943	35.1	8.3	23.5	76.9	80.9	902	275
IA	Jefferson	-3.35	2975	29	7.9	22.1	76.9	80.9	741	226
IA	Johnson	-2.64	2823	23.6	6.5	19.3	79.3	82.5	745	227
IA	Jones	-3.45	2996	30	7.4	24.7	76.1	81.4	879	268
IA	Keokuk	-3.95	3059	33.5	6.6	24.3	76.6	81.8	784	239
IA	Kossuth	-4.47	3092	28.9	6.7	32.2	77.1	82.7	1182	360
IA	Lee	-1.95	2564	30.6	7.3	26.7	74.5	80.1	646	197
IA	Linn	-2.83	2865	28.1	7.8	23.4	77.6	81.5	851	259
IA	Louisa	-1.83	2516	33.8	7	26.8	76.4	82	623	190
IA	Lucas	-2.61	2814	31.3	6.7	28.3	75	80.2	979	298
IA	Lyon	-4.49	3093	26.5	6.5	26.6	75.8	81.2	1417	432
IA	Madison	-2.15	2634	28.5	7.4	20.6	76.5	81.5	1072	327
IA	Mahaska	-1.82	2512	28	7.4	29.4	76.3	81.6	808	246
IA	Marion	-2.28	2684	31.5	7.2	23.7	75.7	81.1	832	254
IA	Marshall	-3.70	3034	31.6	7.3	24.2	74.4	81.7	985	300
IA	Mills	-1.00	2127	25.7	6.8	23.5	75.9	80.4	1089	332
IA	Mitchell	-4.10	3078	26	6.4	26.9	76.6	81.4	1196	365
IA	Monona	-1.03	2147	27.2	7	29.7	75.1	80.4	1153	352
IA	Monroe	-2.36	2714	32.5	7.2	34.4	74.7	80.9	887	270

ST	COUNTY	USDA	AMEN	OBES	DIAB	INACT	M AGE	W AGE	ALT ft	ALT m
IA	Montgomery	-1.67	2450	30.5	7.7	24.4	76.2	81.1	1161	354
IA	Muscatine	-2.37	2724	31.6	6.7	23.8	75.7	80.7	670	204
IA	O'Brien	-4.23	3086	30.1	7.5	24.2	75.9	81.8	1455	443
IA	Osceola	-3.19	2944	30.9	6.5	23.9	75.8	81.2	1542	470
IA	Page	-1.83	2517	32.6	8.5	28.2	76.3	80.7	1107	337
IA	Palo Alto	-2.29	2686	28.5	7.4	24.9	75.7	81.2	1285	392
IA	Plymouth	-2.69	2836	30.3	7.3	28.7	76.4	81.8	1329	405
IA	Pocahontas	-2.95	2895	29.6	8	24.5	75.9	81.1	1243	379
IA	Polk	-2.13	2628	27.5	7.7	23.9	76.4	81.2	904	276
IA	Pottawattamie	-1.03	2148	29.9	7.3	26.7	74.9	80	1188	362
IA	Poweshiek	-3.42	2987	30.5	7.5	24.8	77.4	80.8	920	280
IA	Ringgold	-1.90	2544	29.4	6.9	26.1	76.4	80.9	1174	358
IA	Sac	-1.45	2350	29.1	7.1	24.9	76.3	81.2	1331	406
IA	Scott	-2.39	2732	27.2	7.6	20.8	76	80.9	707	216
IA	Shelby	-2.01	2582	32.1	7.6	24.1	77	81.6	1335	407
IA	Sioux	-3.70	3035	26.3	5.7	23.3	77.5	82.8	1367	417
IA	Story	-3.54	3008	26	6.5	21.1	78.5	83.1	1006	307
IA	Tama	-3.34	2972	25.7	7.8	28.5	77.1	81.4	951	290
IA	Taylor	-1.44	2344	30.2	7.2	23.5	76.4	80.9	1204	367
IA	Union	-1.83	2518	30.2	7.2	27.6	76.5	81.5	1219	371
IA	Van Buren	-1.07	2175	32.3	7.4	24.3	76.9	80.9	705	215
IA	Wapello	-1.40	2321	29.1	8.7	25.5	75.1	80.8	782	238
IA	Warren	-2.16	2638	35	7.6	26.6	77.1	81.8	906	276
IA	Washington	-3.28	2961	30.6	7	22.9	76.4	82	727	222
IA	Wayne	-1.90	2545	33.5	6.7	25.1	74.7	80.9	1042	318
IA	Webster	-3.20	2947	30	8.6	30.4	75.1	80.2	1131	345
IA	Winnebago	-3.81	3048	26.1	7.4	22.7	76.5	81.8	1264	385
IA	Winneshiek	-4.44	3091	24.5	7.2	21.6	77.6	82.9	1142	348
IA	Woodbury	-1.51	2381	30.5	8.4	29.1	75.4	80.5	1230	375
IA	Worth	-3.51	3006	28.7	7.5	24.2	76.5	81.8	1232	375
IA	Wright	-3.56	3011	30	7	28	76	81.9	1179	359
ID	Ada	1.87	504	23.2	7	15.1	77.8	81.9	3074	937
ID	Adams	3.83	212	27.3	7.6	22	76.7	81	4804	1464
ID	Bannock	1.73	540	29.6	8.8	20.3	75.9	80.3	5633	1717
ID	Bear Lake	3.62	235	25	7.5	28.9	76.2	80.9	6769	2063
ID	Benewah	3.10	295	29.1	8.7	28.1	74.6	80.2	3123	952
ID	Bingham	1.91	495	33.5	10.8	22.8	75.4	80.4	5125	1562
ID	Blaine	2.94	317	17.2	5.3	13.3	79.3	83.6	6103	1860
ID	Boise	3.40	257	27.9	7.3	19	75.8	80.4	5531	1686
ID	Bonner	4.57	157	22.2	6.6	19	76.1	80.7	3168	966
ID	Bonneville	2.00	471	26.6	8.3	20.4	76.4	80	6090	1856
ID	Boundary	2.61	357	23.2	7.1	25.9	76.1	80.7	4068	1240
ID	Butte	0.07	1386	29	8	23.2	76.2	80.4	5977	1822
ID	Camas	2.70	340	25.9	7.6	20.9	74.3	80	6320	1926
ID	Canyon	1.82	517	29.4	8.5	22.6	75.1	80.3	2490	759
ID	Caribou	3.08	297	23.9	7	26.2	76.2	80.9	6494	1979
ID	Cassia	1.81	521	28.6	8.5	22.8	75.6	80.5	5375	1638

ST	COUNTY	USDA	AMEN	OBES	DIAB	INACT	M AGE	W AGE	ALT ft	ALT m
ID	Clark	-0.06	1490	28.2	8.1	22.8	76.2	80.4	6414	1955
ID	Clearwater	2.33	404	31.6	7.6	24.9	75.8	80.6	3881	1183
ID	Custer	0.86	879	27.2	7.3	22.7	75.8	80.4	7615	2321
ID	Elmore	2.94	318	28.5	8.5	23.9	75.5	79.9	4737	1444
ID	Franklin	1.68	546	30	8.2	23.3	76.2	80.9	5829	1777
ID	Fremont	2.95	314	23.4	7.9	22.3	76.2	80.4	6163	1879
ID	Gem	2.45	380	30.5	7.1	25.2	75.8	80.4	3598	1097
ID	Gooding	0.76	926	28.9	7.8	26.2	74.3	80	3867	1179
ID	Idaho	3.17	284	29.3	7.6	24	75.8	80.6	5119	1560
ID	Jefferson	1.40	631	25.3	8.4	23.8	75.4	80.4	4879	1487
ID	Jerome	0.63	998	31.6	8.2	19.5	74.7	80.3	3996	1218
ID	Kootenai	3.50	245	25.4	7.5	19.6	77.5	81.8	2940	896
ID	Latah	1.13	760	26.3	7.8	17.7	77.6	81.6	2944	897
ID	Lemhi	0.43	1121	23	7.3	16.4	76.2	80.4	6928	2112
ID	Lewis	0.99	818	30.5	8	24.1	75.8	80.6	3403	1037
ID	Lincoln	-0.41	1762	24.7	7.4	23.2	74.3	80	4370	1332
ID	Madison	0.92	852	27.4	8	22.9	76.7	80.4	5579	1700
ID	Minidoka	1.42	627	30.1	9.5	25.6	74.2	79.6	4374	1333
ID	Nez Perce	1.41	629	30.5	9.6	22.8	76.1	80.7	2558	780
ID	Oneida	0.17	1322	28.7	7.1	25.7	75.6	80.5	5531	1686
ID	Owyhee	2.10	452	29.9	8.7	28.4	75.5	79.9	4773	1455
ID	Payette	1.79	523	26.6	8.1	24.6	75	79.6	2596	791
ID	Power	2.04	462	30	7.5	24.1	75.6	80.5	5178	1578
ID	Shoshone	3.64	233	29.6	7.8	26.9	74.6	80.2	4239	1292
ID	Teton	1.90	497	24.7	7.7	17.4	76.7	80.4	6512	1985
ID	Twin Falls	0.96	831	26.1	8.2	23.1	75.4	79.9	4795	1461
ID	Valley	4.59	154	27	6.8	23.3	76.7	81	6466	1971
ID	Washington	2.17	440	27.7	8.7	24.9	76.7	81	3698	1127
IL	Adams	-2.10	2615	30.7	8.7	32.8	74.4	80.7	648	197
IL	Alexander	0.95	836	31	9.3	29.8	69.9	77	392	119
IL	Bond	-2.01	2583	29.1	8.6	30.8	74.1	79.5	537	164
IL	Boone	-3.32	2969	29	7.3	26	76.5	80.6	864	263
IL	Brown	-2.39	2733	29.7	8.5	28.2	74.4	79.5	625	191
IL	Bureau	-3.05	2913	27.8	7.5	28.1	75.9	80.7	708	216
IL	Calhoun	-0.75	1970	27.9	8.1	32.3	74.5	79.5	557	170
IL	Carroll	-0.08	1507	26.7	8.6	30.3	75.6	81.1	765	233
IL	Cass	-1.94	2561	29.3	8.2	29.1	74.8	80	533	162
IL	Champaign	-4.55	3094	26.6	7.7	25.6	76.6	80.8	714	218
IL	Christian	-2.19	2648	29.1	8.3	25.9	73.6	80.2	617	188
IL	Clark	-2.35	2708	30.3	8.1	30.3	74.5	80.5	590	180
IL	Clay	-3.01	2907	28.3	7.6	29.9	74.4	80	487	148
IL	Clinton	-0.72	1958	28.2	8	27.3	74.9	81.2	454	138
IL	Coles	-2.99	2906	29.2	7.3	24.8	74.7	80.1	677	206
IL	Cook	-1.04	2155	26	8.8	23.6	75.1	80.7	659	201
IL	Crawford	-2.44	2757	30.4	7.9	31.1	74.9	79.6	503	153
IL	Cumberland	-2.80	2860	27.8	8.2	29.9	75.3	80.2	602	184
IL	De Witt	-2.52	2790	28.5	7.5	27.9	73.9	79.6	723	220

HEALTHIEST PLACES TO LIVE

ST	COUNTY	USDA	AMEN	OBES	DIAB	INACT	M AGE	W AGE	ALT ft	ALT m
IL	DeKalb	-3.58	3017	29.7	7.9	25.4	77	81	832	254
IL	Douglas	-3.50	3004	29.6	7.1	27.8	74.6	80.3	659	201
IL	DuPage	-2.33	2699	24.2	6.8	18.9	79	82.4	733	223
IL	Edgar	-3.65	3029	30.3	8.1	28.4	73.8	79.7	666	203
IL	Edwards	-2.90	2886	26.6	7.5	26.5	75.2	80.1	440	134
IL	Effingham	-2.81	2862	27.7	7.6	28.3	75.3	80.7	575	175
IL	Fayette	-1.97	2570	30	7.7	30.9	73.6	79.2	550	168
IL	Ford	-4.02	3070	31.8	7.9	29.4	74.6	79.5	748	228
IL	Franklin	-1.19	2230	29.6	8.8	28.9	72.2	78.6	435	133
IL	Fulton	-1.77	2498	30.3	7.3	29.9	73.9	79.8	604	184
IL	Gallatin	-0.19	1584	28.2	7.7	27	73	79.5	391	119
IL	Greene	-2.24	2666	31.6	8.5	31	74.5	79.5	545	166
IL	Grundy	-2.11	2618	31.3	7.5	34.8	75.8	80.5	584	178
IL	Hamilton	-2.97	2902	29.7	7.8	30.4	73	79.5	441	134
IL	Hancock	-1.63	2438	27.9	8	29	76	81.2	632	193
IL	Hardin	0.07	1387	30.1	8	26	73	79.5	482	147
IL	Henderson	-1.29	2277	30.5	8	26.2	75.9	80.9	630	192
IL	Henry	-3.43	2991	27.1	7.8	29.4	75.9	81	704	215
IL	Iroquois	-4.00	3068	31.3	7.8	30.4	74.6	79.5	665	203
IL	Jackson	0.71	950	27.5	8.3	27.7	75.3	80.1	449	137
IL	Jasper	-2.25	2669	28.8	7.5	30.7	75.3	80.2	528	161
IL	Jefferson	-1.74	2482	32.4	9	29.4	74.3	79.7	489	149
IL	Jersey	-1.68	2457	27.1	7.4	27.2	75.3	79.8	575	175
IL	Jo Daviess	-0.40	1752	28.9	7.5	22.9	76.5	81.6	838	255
IL	Johnson	0.28	1231	28.9	8.2	29.5	72.8	78.8	506	154
IL	Kane	-2.77	2852	27.5	8.1	23.6	77.4	81	816	249
IL	Kankakee	-3.30	2964	30.9	8.2	27.9	73.3	79	646	197
IL	Kendall	-2.85	2874	25.3	6.6	24.8	77.4	81.9	654	199
IL	Knox	-2.43	2751	32.9	8	31	74.2	79.3	714	218
IL	La Salle	-2.75	2850	29.6	8.1	25.7	74.4	80.1	658	201
IL	Lake	-0.30	1666	24	7.1	18.9	78.5	81.7	740	226
IL	Lawrence	-2.34	2703	29.2	7.8	28.8	73.7	79.3	454	138
IL	Lee	-2.93	2889	26.4	8.5	27.2	74.8	79.9	789	240
IL	Livingston	-3.95	3060	29	8.3	30.9	74	79.3	683	208
IL	Logan	-3.89	3053	34.6	8.3	28.9	74	79.8	599	183
IL	Macon	-2.79	2856	32.3	7.9	27	74	80.1	665	203
IL	Macoupin	-2.36	2715	28.7	8.2	25.4	74.6	80.2	630	192
IL	Madison	-1.69	2465	29.7	9.6	27.3	74.5	79.5	512	156
IL	Marion	-2.18	2644	29.3	6.7	29.3	73.6	79.5	535	163
IL	Marshall	-1.89	2540	26.1	7.7	28.5	74.9	80.3	656	200
IL	Mason	-1.86	2528	30.5	7.6	28.6	74.4	79.5	502	153
IL	Massac	-1.69	2466	31.4	8.8	29.5	72.8	78.8	394	120
IL	McDonough	-3.19	2945	29.5	7.4	27.4	76.1	80.5	667	203
IL	McHenry	-2.40	2736	23.8	6.4	23.5	77.7	81.6	873	266
IL	McLean	-3.57	3013	30.2	7.6	24.7	76.6	80.9	767	234
IL	Menard	-3.04	2909	25.9	7.5	29	74.8	80	570	174
IL	Mercer	-2.47	2767	30.4	7.5	25	75.9	80.9	677	206

53

ST	COUNTY	USDA	AMEN	OBES	DIAB	INACT	M AGE	W AGE	ALT ft	ALT m
IL	Monroe	-0.06	1491	27.9	7.8	29.2	76.8	80.7	510	156
IL	Montgomery	-2.18	2645	24.5	8.3	27.4	74.1	79.8	640	195
IL	Morgan	-2.25	2670	29.2	7.4	28.6	74.6	79.5	613	187
IL	Moultrie	-1.96	2568	28.3	8.2	28.5	75.1	81	662	202
IL	Ogle	-2.82	2864	27.6	7.4	28	75.8	80.5	812	247
IL	Peoria	-2.41	2741	28.6	9.6	25.6	74.5	79.9	651	198
IL	Perry	-1.20	2233	29.3	8.3	29.8	73.4	79.1	462	141
IL	Piatt	-4.21	3084	28.4	7.9	30.2	75.1	81	695	212
IL	Pike	-1.88	2534	28.2	7.6	26	75	80.5	601	183
IL	Pope	-0.22	1612	29.8	7.9	28	72.4	78.7	507	155
IL	Pulaski	-1.43	2338	31.4	9.8	29.3	69.9	77	367	112
IL	Putnam	-1.52	2384	28.1	7.9	27	75.9	80.7	591	180
IL	Randolph	0.63	999	29.2	7.4	25.3	73.8	79.2	464	141
IL	Richland	-2.20	2651	29.9	8.2	29.2	74.4	80	474	145
IL	Rock Island	-1.87	2531	27.2	7.6	26.4	75.7	81	654	199
IL	Saline	-0.41	1763	29.2	8.3	31.6	72.4	78.7	421	128
IL	Sangamon	-2.47	2768	28.8	8.6	25.6	74.8	80	597	182
IL	Schuyler	-2.08	2610	27	7.4	29.9	74.4	79.5	584	178
IL	Scott	-2.47	2769	28.5	7.9	28.9	75	80.5	530	162
IL	Shelby	-2.34	2704	27.4	7.6	30.6	75.9	80.5	635	194
IL	St. Clair	-1.81	2507	29.7	8.8	28.7	72.2	78.5	466	142
IL	Stark	-3.87	3052	29.4	7.6	28.1	74.9	80.3	721	220
IL	Stephenson	-3.75	3045	29.9	8	27.9	75.5	80.8	871	265
IL	Tazewell	-2.55	2797	26.7	6.6	26.6	75.4	80.3	614	187
IL	Union	0.57	1034	30.4	7.7	31.5	72.9	79.7	503	153
IL	Vermilion	-3.21	2950	28.5	9	30.1	73.1	78.7	683	208
IL	Wabash	-1.68	2458	28.4	7.9	28.8	75.2	80.1	430	131
IL	Warren	-3.17	2940	29.1	8.1	26.8	75.1	79.6	715	218
IL	Washington	-2.23	2660	30.2	7.6	27.3	75.3	80.6	482	147
IL	Wayne	-2.61	2815	29.1	7.3	26	74.6	80.3	435	132
IL	White	-1.82	2513	28.9	8.1	30.7	73.5	79.5	403	123
IL	Whiteside	-2.32	2695	27.4	7.8	29.2	75.2	80.2	657	200
IL	Will	-2.41	2742	30.3	8.6	25	77	80.9	661	202
IL	Williamson	1.05	792	30.4	7.4	31.1	73.2	79.2	466	142
IL	Winnebago	-2.50	2783	28.6	9.1	26.2	75.1	80.8	803	245
IL	Woodford	-2.26	2677	28.7	7.4	23.5	76.6	81.4	706	215
IN	Adams	-3.55	3010	33.3	7.9	24.6	75.9	80.8	810	247
IN	Allen	-2.97	2903	32.8	9.9	25.3	75.4	80.6	793	242
IN	Bartholomew	-2.38	2728	30.5	9.8	25.9	75.3	80.4	677	206
IN	Benton	-4.71	3095	32.3	9.8	33	74.8	80.6	757	231
IN	Blackford	-3.27	2959	33	10	28.7	74.2	79.5	868	265
IN	Boone	-3.68	3032	29.8	8.5	29.8	76.6	80.9	918	280
IN	Brown	-0.29	1661	29	9.6	24.8	75.8	81	756	230
IN	Carroll	-2.83	2866	31.7	9.2	26	75.3	80.8	680	207
IN	Cass	-3.04	2910	34	9.3	27.9	74.5	79.4	731	223
IN	Clark	-2.49	2780	30.7	8.7	31.3	73.3	78.8	606	185
IN	Clay	-2.56	2801	35.7	9.2	28.6	73.7	78.7	610	186

HEALTHIEST PLACES TO LIVE

ST	COUNTY	USDA	AMEN	OBES	DIAB	INACT	M AGE	W AGE	ALT ft	ALT m
IN	Clinton	-4.37	3090	28.4	11.9	26.3	74.6	79.9	844	257
IN	Crawford	-0.20	1594	36	9.8	30.2	73.5	78.9	638	195
IN	Daviess	-1.70	2471	32.3	9.7	26.3	74.2	79.8	494	150
IN	Dearborn	-2.04	2594	32.7	9.5	28	75.3	80.6	796	243
IN	Decatur	-3.09	2922	30.4	9.4	24.5	74.3	80.2	885	270
IN	DeKalb	-2.81	2863	31	8.8	26.3	75.4	80.4	884	269
IN	Delaware	-2.60	2809	32.7	9.4	29.3	73.6	78.9	938	286
IN	Dubois	-0.34	1697	31.5	8.3	24	75.5	80.9	534	163
IN	Elkhart	-2.72	2843	28.3	9	25.7	75.6	80.3	817	249
IN	Fayette	-3.35	2976	34	9.2	30.4	72.9	79.2	974	297
IN	Floyd	-1.04	2156	30.9	8.7	24.1	74.9	79.3	709	216
IN	Fountain	-2.68	2833	28.9	9.5	28.7	74.3	79.5	649	198
IN	Franklin	-1.45	2351	27.9	11	25.5	74.7	80.7	902	275
IN	Fulton	-3.13	2932	31.2	9	25.9	73.3	79.3	791	241
IN	Gibson	-1.56	2404	28	8.6	26.5	74.8	80	439	134
IN	Grant	-3.54	3009	29.6	10.2	31.4	73	79.2	842	257
IN	Greene	-0.77	1988	30.7	10.9	27.8	74.2	79.4	591	180
IN	Hamilton	-2.53	2792	21.9	8.1	19.4	78.6	82.7	851	259
IN	Hancock	-3.58	3018	27.1	8.7	23.6	76.2	80.4	868	264
IN	Harrison	-0.78	1996	29.6	9.5	28.4	75.1	80.2	673	205
IN	Hendricks	-3.61	3022	33.1	8.9	23.4	76.9	80.8	888	271
IN	Henry	-2.61	2816	30.8	9.1	30.1	73.2	79.3	1051	320
IN	Howard	-3.61	3023	34.1	9.7	31	73.8	79.3	814	248
IN	Huntington	-2.34	2705	34.8	10.3	29.8	75.7	81	804	245
IN	Jackson	-0.57	1858	30.6	8.9	32.4	74.7	79.4	626	191
IN	Jasper	-3.57	3014	32.1	9.9	29.1	74.9	80.6	681	208
IN	Jay	-3.98	3064	34.3	9.6	31.2	74.2	79.5	905	276
IN	Jefferson	-0.89	2061	30.4	8.8	30	74.4	79.9	738	225
IN	Jennings	-2.48	2772	29.2	9	28.1	73.2	79.2	699	213
IN	Johnson	-1.16	2219	29	9.9	27.6	76	80.3	778	237
IN	Knox	-1.98	2576	31.9	8.9	32.9	73.5	79.9	462	141
IN	Kosciusko	-2.25	2671	32.4	9.2	26.3	75.2	80.8	853	260
IN	LaGrange	-2.36	2716	29.5	8.8	24.3	74.1	79.7	907	276
IN	Lake	-1.14	2210	33.9	11	29.8	72.6	78.6	656	200
IN	LaPorte	-1.87	2532	30.9	9.7	25.9	73.7	80.1	729	222
IN	Lawrence	-0.35	1710	28.1	11.2	28.8	74	79.5	653	199
IN	Madison	-3.47	2998	36.6	11	32.8	74.1	79.1	864	263
IN	Marion	-2.51	2787	30.1	10.5	26.1	72.6	78.7	794	242
IN	Marshall	-2.41	2743	28.7	8.4	28.6	75	81.1	803	245
IN	Martin	-0.19	1585	29.2	8.6	30	74.2	79.8	571	174
IN	Miami	-2.83	2867	31.8	10.3	30.2	74.2	79.9	775	236
IN	Monroe	0.29	1221	25.8	9.6	22.3	76.6	81.6	733	224
IN	Montgomery	-3.35	2977	31	9.4	30.1	74.9	80.3	803	245
IN	Morgan	-0.88	2056	30.1	9.2	27.2	74.6	79.2	729	222
IN	Newton	-3.42	2988	30.3	9.8	28.6	74	79.3	671	205
IN	Noble	-1.93	2557	30.6	9.4	27.2	74.4	79.9	929	283
IN	Ohio	-0.49	1809	29.4	9.5	28.2	74.7	79.5	712	217

ST	COUNTY	USDA	AMEN	OBES	DIAB	INACT	M AGE	W AGE	ALT ft	ALT m
IN	Orange	0.21	1296	32.7	10.4	35.4	73.5	78.9	675	206
IN	Owen	-0.76	1977	35	9.7	29.5	73.6	79	672	205
IN	Parke	-2.30	2690	28.3	9.8	32.5	74.5	80.1	637	194
IN	Perry	-0.38	1734	32.4	8.6	29	74	79.5	548	167
IN	Pike	-1.75	2487	30.5	9.2	28.1	74.8	80	479	146
IN	Porter	-0.54	1838	29.6	9.1	25.8	76.2	80.5	693	211
IN	Posey	-1.53	2392	30.2	9.3	26.7	75.1	80.9	402	123
IN	Pulaski	-3.48	3000	33.7	9.7	26.9	73.3	79.3	698	213
IN	Putnam	-2.71	2842	31.1	10.1	29.8	75.8	79.7	795	242
IN	Randolph	-3.72	3038	34.5	10.2	36.5	74.2	79.5	1083	330
IN	Ripley	-2.40	2737	30.6	8	29.5	74.9	79.8	933	284
IN	Rush	-3.97	3063	32	9.9	30.2	74.5	80.1	951	290
IN	Scott	-1.92	2552	28.9	10.8	31.5	72	77.9	626	191
IN	Shelby	-3.76	3046	35.1	10	32.4	74.4	79.6	771	235
IN	Spencer	-2.20	2652	30.4	9.4	25.2	75.3	80.3	434	132
IN	St. Joseph	-2.51	2788	29.2	8.9	26.7	74.4	80.8	770	235
IN	Starke	-2.85	2875	32.1	9.9	33.8	72.1	77.8	700	213
IN	Steuben	-1.61	2427	31.9	10.9	27.3	75.2	80.5	999	305
IN	Sullivan	-2.07	2605	31.2	8.8	32.1	73.1	79	507	154
IN	Switzerland	-0.20	1595	27.5	9.7	27.1	74.7	79.5	749	228
IN	Tippecanoe	-2.79	2857	28.1	9.4	24.2	75.6	80.7	676	206
IN	Tipton	-5.40	3106	30.4	9.3	28.2	75.7	80.7	872	266
IN	Union	-1.51	2382	32.2	9.5	25.3	74.7	80.7	973	296
IN	Vanderburgh	-2.48	2773	28.8	9.3	27.1	73.8	79.4	424	129
IN	Vermillion	-2.30	2691	30.4	10.9	26.8	73.8	79.2	599	182
IN	Vigo	-2.12	2623	32.6	8.7	27.8	73.6	79.2	540	165
IN	Wabash	-2.05	2598	35.7	9.3	25.2	74.9	80.5	779	237
IN	Warren	-3.25	2956	29.4	10.2	29.9	74.8	80.6	701	214
IN	Warrick	-1.81	2508	31.4	9.5	22.8	76.2	79.7	437	133
IN	Washington	-2.13	2629	29.7	9.1	32.5	73.7	79	761	232
IN	Wayne	-2.54	2794	27.8	7.6	27.6	73.4	79.6	1048	319
IN	Wells	-3.73	3041	31.5	8.7	25.9	75.7	81.4	820	250
IN	White	-2.73	2847	33.3	8.6	27.6	74.5	80.7	693	211
IN	Whitley	-2.56	2802	32.3	7.7	20.1	75.2	80.6	871	265
KS	Allen	-1.43	2339	34.5	9	26.2	74.7	79.4	1018	310
KS	Anderson	-2.42	2747	32.1	7.4	25.8	75.2	80.6	1049	320
KS	Atchison	-0.76	1978	33.4	7.8	29.5	75.2	79.9	1033	315
KS	Barber	-1.28	2272	34.5	8.9	32.4	75.3	80.1	1639	500
KS	Barton	-0.88	2057	34.5	9.4	26.4	75.6	81.9	1891	576
KS	Bourbon	-1.85	2524	34.8	7.9	26.1	74.6	79.4	919	280
KS	Brown	-2.64	2824	36.7	9.2	28.9	75.1	80.9	1091	333
KS	Butler	0.58	1029	32.5	8.3	23.5	75.8	80.3	1396	425
KS	Chase	-0.88	2058	31.8	8.1	22.5	74.7	80.4	1361	415
KS	Chautauqua	0.23	1276	29.5	7.7	24.7	73	79.9	958	292
KS	Cherokee	-0.98	2115	35.7	9.1	25.5	73.2	78.9	867	264
KS	Cheyenne	-0.14	1554	32.8	7.6	20.4	76	80.6	3450	1052
KS	Clark	0.22	1285	32.4	7.9	27.8	75.4	80	2162	659

HEALTHIEST PLACES TO LIVE

ST	COUNTY	USDA	AMEN	OBES	DIAB	INACT	M AGE	W AGE	ALT ft	ALT m
KS	Clay	-0.80	2007	30.9	8.1	26.9	75.8	81.2	1291	394
KS	Cloud	-1.49	2367	31.3	9.7	23	75.8	81.2	1444	440
KS	Coffey	-0.95	2103	34.9	9.2	23.4	75.2	80.6	1106	337
KS	Comanche	-1.26	2266	29.3	7.7	28.8	75.4	80	1937	590
KS	Cowley	-1.25	2261	32.9	8.5	28.4	73.1	79.9	1249	381
KS	Crawford	-1.00	2128	34.8	9.4	27.7	73.9	79.6	938	286
KS	Decatur	-0.83	2023	32	9.5	26.1	76	80.6	2648	807
KS	Dickinson	-0.96	2106	31.3	8.3	25.9	75.1	81.2	1272	388
KS	Doniphan	-2.07	2606	35.6	8.5	27.6	75.2	79.9	985	300
KS	Douglas	0.36	1175	26.5	7	19.6	78.1	81.9	966	295
KS	Edwards	-3.01	2908	34.6	8.5	26.7	74.9	80.1	2173	662
KS	Elk	0.13	1348	32.3	9.8	26.5	73	79.9	1109	338
KS	Ellis	-2.31	2693	31.1	7.5	24.3	76.6	81.6	2039	621
KS	Ellsworth	-0.19	1586	35.5	8.7	24.2	75.2	80.7	1675	511
KS	Finney	-0.35	1711	32.8	9.1	25.8	75.3	80.2	2834	864
KS	Ford	-0.84	2026	32.8	9.2	28.6	75.4	80	2492	759
KS	Franklin	-1.97	2571	33.5	9.2	27.1	75.7	79.6	986	300
KS	Geary	0.39	1146	29.3	9.1	29.9	74.4	80.2	1272	388
KS	Gove	-1.79	2502	31.1	9	27.7	76.3	81.5	2676	816
KS	Graham	-1.28	2273	32.2	8.2	23.6	76.3	81.5	2345	715
KS	Grant	-0.97	2110	33.4	8.5	20.1	74.6	79.4	3056	931
KS	Gray	-0.96	2107	29.5	8.7	25.8	75.3	80.2	2738	834
KS	Greeley	-1.80	2505	34.1	8.5	28.6	75.9	81.2	3661	1116
KS	Greenwood	0.66	978	34.3	7.8	30.4	74.7	80.4	1175	358
KS	Hamilton	-0.59	1876	31.7	7.8	25.9	75.9	81.2	3446	1050
KS	Harper	-1.26	2267	28.5	8.8	31.5	75.3	80.1	1374	419
KS	Harvey	-1.71	2474	29.2	7.5	23.6	76	80.9	1445	440
KS	Haskell	-0.61	1883	30.4	9.3	27.2	75.3	80.2	2917	889
KS	Hodgeman	-0.94	2091	32.9	9	27.1	75.2	80.6	2386	727
KS	Jackson	-2.85	2876	31.5	8.2	26.3	75.8	80.8	1115	340
KS	Jefferson	-1.06	2170	37.5	9.4	22.8	75.4	80	1026	313
KS	Jewell	-0.20	1596	34.2	8.6	24.7	75.7	82	1664	507
KS	Johnson	-1.69	2467	23.6	6.4	17.5	78.9	82.6	991	302
KS	Kearny	-0.36	1721	31.2	8.7	24.9	74.6	79.4	3161	963
KS	Kingman	-0.77	1989	31	8.5	29.7	75.3	80.1	1575	480
KS	Kiowa	-2.08	2611	31.2	7.8	24.4	75.4	80	2185	666
KS	Labette	-1.05	2162	32.2	9.3	31.4	73.8	79	867	264
KS	Lane	-0.90	2068	34.3	8.3	24.8	75.9	81.2	2757	840
KS	Leavenworth	-0.35	1712	31.2	9.1	24.8	75.2	80	938	286
KS	Lincoln	-1.33	2291	28.3	7.6	24.2	75.2	80.7	1515	462
KS	Linn	-1.53	2393	34.8	8.8	28.8	74.7	79.4	931	284
KS	Logan	-1.43	2340	32.4	8.9	29.4	76.3	81.5	3090	942
KS	Lyon	-0.48	1804	30.5	8.1	24.7	75.5	79.5	1207	368
KS	Marion	-0.81	2013	31.4	8	27.7	75.1	81.2	1426	435
KS	Marshall	-1.38	2312	34.5	8.1	25.3	76.3	81.7	1305	398
KS	McPherson	-1.81	2509	31.2	8.4	24	76.7	81.3	1501	458
KS	Meade	-0.16	1565	30.9	8.4	23.9	75.4	80	2527	770

ST	COUNTY	USDA	AMEN	OBES	DIAB	INACT	M AGE	W AGE	ALT ft	ALT m
KS	Miami	-1.15	2213	29.5	8.1	25.2	75.9	80.2	985	300
KS	Mitchell	0.32	1203	28	8.5	24.3	75.5	80.1	1509	460
KS	Montgomery	-0.81	2014	30.9	9.1	30.3	73	79.9	826	252
KS	Morris	-0.40	1753	33.6	8.9	24.7	74.7	80.4	1410	430
KS	Morton	-1.59	2417	33.1	8.1	29.8	74.6	79.4	3429	1045
KS	Nemaha	-3.62	3025	28.2	8.7	25.4	75.1	80.9	1257	383
KS	Neosho	-1.01	2135	36.3	10	30	74	79.6	945	288
KS	Ness	-1.54	2398	29.1	8.2	24.8	75.2	80.6	2379	725
KS	Norton	1.57	576	30.4	8.2	24.8	76.3	81.5	2342	714
KS	Osage	-1.17	2223	35.3	9.2	27.3	75.3	80.4	1095	334
KS	Osborne	-1.07	2176	32.9	9	25.3	75.7	82	1751	534
KS	Ottawa	-1.67	2451	32	7.7	31.2	75.5	80.1	1345	410
KS	Pawnee	-2.07	2607	34	8.8	28.7	75.2	80.6	2089	637
KS	Phillips	0.15	1335	34.3	8.3	24.6	76.3	81.5	2024	617
KS	Pottawatomie	-0.09	1517	30.8	8.7	24.2	75.8	80.8	1223	373
KS	Pratt	-1.42	2332	32	7.5	29.2	75.4	80.6	1923	586
KS	Rawlins	-1.50	2376	33.3	7.8	26.3	76	80.6	3060	933
KS	Reno	-0.42	1770	33.1	9.4	22.2	75.4	80.6	1602	488
KS	Republic	-1.61	2428	32.7	8.3	26.5	76.3	81.7	1537	468
KS	Rice	-1.62	2434	37.4	9	23.8	74.9	80.1	1694	516
KS	Riley	-0.11	1534	26.5	8	19.6	78.1	81.9	1244	379
KS	Rooks	-0.94	2092	30.3	8.7	25.8	75.7	82	2013	614
KS	Rush	-2.57	2804	29	7.6	25.7	75.2	80.6	2082	635
KS	Russell	0.12	1351	32.5	8	27.3	75.2	80.7	1751	534
KS	Saline	-1.03	2149	34.2	8	24.2	75.5	80.1	1332	406
KS	Scott	-1.50	2377	29.1	7.2	23.1	75.9	81.2	2984	910
KS	Sedgwick	-0.70	1941	29.3	9.1	23.1	74.3	79.8	1361	415
KS	Seward	-0.21	1605	35.8	7.7	29.6	73.3	79.2	2809	856
KS	Shawnee	-1.76	2492	32.8	8.9	23.4	74.6	80.4	1007	307
KS	Sheridan	-1.21	2240	29.9	7.7	25.7	76.3	81.5	2727	831
KS	Sherman	-1.34	2293	32.2	9.7	26.9	76	80.6	3657	1115
KS	Smith	-0.94	2093	31.7	7.3	30.9	75.7	82	1830	558
KS	Stafford	-1.52	2385	33.6	8.7	31.1	74.9	80.1	1901	579
KS	Stanton	-1.59	2418	31.2	8.5	25.5	75.9	81.2	3367	1026
KS	Stevens	-1.18	2227	29.9	9.7	26.4	74.6	79.4	3101	945
KS	Sumner	-1.15	2214	34	9.1	27.3	75	79.7	1225	373
KS	Thomas	-1.58	2411	31.4	8.1	20.8	76	80.6	3170	966
KS	Trego	0.81	907	33.1	7.6	28.7	76.3	81.5	2346	715
KS	Wabaunsee	0.40	1138	31.7	7.7	24.8	75.3	80.4	1253	382
KS	Wallace	-1.45	2352	32	8	27.6	75.9	81.2	3620	1103
KS	Washington	-2.95	2896	33.3	8.2	22.5	76.3	81.7	1393	425
KS	Wichita	-1.80	2506	31.9	8.8	28.7	75.9	81.2	3295	1004
KS	Wilson	-1.75	2488	34.9	9	25.3	74	79.6	919	280
KS	Woodson	-0.36	1722	31.4	9.1	31.1	74	79.6	1037	316
KS	Wyandotte	-0.17	1572	37.9	11.7	32.5	71.1	77.5	882	269
KY	Adair	0.24	1263	36.5	12.1	37.5	72.6	78.1	848	258
KY	Allen	-1.50	2378	33.5	10.6	28.6	71.5	77.9	689	210

HEALTHIEST PLACES TO LIVE

ST	COUNTY	USDA	AMEN	OBES	DIAB	INACT	M AGE	W AGE	ALT ft	ALT m
KY	Anderson	-0.45	1785	35.3	11	34.5	75	79	776	237
KY	Ballard	-0.55	1840	32.4	10.5	32.4	73.6	79.1	367	112
KY	Barren	-1.47	2361	29.2	11.8	30.4	73.4	78.6	725	221
KY	Bath	0.32	1204	33	12.1	34.6	71	77.5	844	257
KY	Bell	0.12	1352	35.9	13.9	32.3	69.3	75.9	1659	506
KY	Boone	0.29	1222	30.8	9.4	28.3	75.4	79.6	751	229
KY	Bourbon	-3.18	2941	35	11.8	35.3	74	79.2	891	271
KY	Boyd	0.28	1232	35.9	13.1	32.6	72.5	78.2	727	221
KY	Boyle	-0.23	1618	31.3	11.1	29.9	73.9	79	958	292
KY	Bracken	0.50	1070	33.3	11.1	30.3	72.3	78.5	798	243
KY	Breathitt	-1.36	2302	39.6	14.7	33.7	68.2	76.1	1045	318
KY	Breckinridge	0.35	1184	33.4	11.2	31.3	72.8	78.9	618	188
KY	Bullitt	-0.87	2048	33.8	10.9	33.8	75.4	80.2	577	176
KY	Butler	-0.06	1492	33.2	11.5	30.6	72.8	77.8	515	157
KY	Caldwell	-0.52	1823	35	10.4	31.7	73	79.3	507	155
KY	Calloway	-0.58	1868	29.4	10.8	24	74.7	79.7	493	150
KY	Campbell	0.39	1147	27.9	9.6	26.3	73.7	79.6	679	207
KY	Carlisle	-1.03	2150	32.6	11.1	29.5	73.6	79.1	383	117
KY	Carroll	0.37	1164	31.9	10.5	34.4	72.8	78.6	645	196
KY	Carter	0.12	1353	34.5	11.4	42.8	70.8	77.5	860	262
KY	Casey	-1.97	2572	36.5	12.2	35.6	71.1	78.2	1008	307
KY	Christian	-0.63	1895	31.3	11.1	33.2	72.7	78.6	568	173
KY	Clark	-0.51	1816	28.8	10.5	29.5	74.1	78.8	900	274
KY	Clay	-1.46	2357	32.4	13.2	35.4	69.2	76.1	1178	359
KY	Clinton	0.62	1007	32.8	10.2	36.1	70.2	77.3	961	293
KY	Crittenden	0.46	1097	33	9.9	37.8	72.3	77.9	477	145
KY	Cumberland	0.65	982	33.7	11	32.1	70.2	77.3	762	232
KY	Daviess	-1.20	2234	30.5	10.1	27.8	74.3	79.7	429	131
KY	Edmonson	0.62	1008	33.5	12.5	28.1	72.8	77.8	627	191
KY	Elliott	0.29	1223	37.6	10.6	37.5	70.2	77.3	914	279
KY	Estill	0.55	1040	34.6	11.7	36.8	70.3	76.9	900	274
KY	Fayette	-2.39	2734	30.7	9.7	24.7	75.4	80.3	944	288
KY	Fleming	-0.86	2043	34.7	10.6	34.6	71	77.5	862	263
KY	Floyd	0.04	1409	36.8	14.6	39.9	69.7	76.2	1031	314
KY	Franklin	-0.34	1698	33	10.1	31.1	74.3	78.7	730	223
KY	Fulton	-0.46	1791	32.8	11	36	72.6	78.2	331	101
KY	Gallatin	0.63	1000	32.8	11.1	37.2	72.6	78.7	644	196
KY	Garrard	-1.23	2250	33.3	11.1	35.2	74.5	78.8	918	280
KY	Grant	-0.93	2086	37.6	10.4	36.7	72.6	78.7	809	247
KY	Graves	-2.48	2774	33.8	10.5	31	72.6	78.2	465	142
KY	Grayson	0.21	1297	30.9	11.7	32.8	71.9	77.8	638	194
KY	Green	-3.72	3039	32	11.4	36.2	71.9	77.9	711	217
KY	Greenup	0.62	1009	35.3	13.3	31.7	73.3	78.5	758	231
KY	Hancock	0.48	1085	34.5	9.7	30.8	72.8	78.9	504	154
KY	Hardin	-0.69	1934	30.9	11.5	29.7	75.2	80.2	718	219
KY	Harlan	0.37	1165	32.3	13.8	34.8	68.4	76.2	2095	638
KY	Harrison	-1.72	2477	30	11.6	33.5	72.5	78	808	246

ST	COUNTY	USDA	AMEN	OBES	DIAB	INACT	M AGE	W AGE	ALT ft	ALT m
KY	Hart	-0.07	1500	34	10	35.6	72.4	78.2	707	216
KY	Henderson	-0.72	1959	33.5	10.4	26.9	73.6	78.7	399	122
KY	Henry	-0.46	1792	35.1	11.4	32.4	73	78.9	775	236
KY	Hickman	-0.84	2027	33.7	11.4	32.2	72.6	78.2	375	114
KY	Hopkins	-0.21	1606	35.4	10.7	33.4	72.3	78.1	445	136
KY	Jackson	-0.82	2019	33.4	11.3	36	70.3	76.9	1216	371
KY	Jefferson	0.32	1205	33.6	10.5	28.5	73.4	79.2	556	169
KY	Jessamine	-1.99	2578	30.4	11.4	30.6	74.3	79.5	886	270
KY	Johnson	0.64	988	38.2	11.7	34.5	69.7	77.4	891	272
KY	Kenton	-1.62	2435	30.2	10.1	27.1	73.5	78.6	767	234
KY	Knott	0.07	1388	33.7	13.2	36.5	69.7	77.6	1332	406
KY	Knox	-1.49	2368	35.6	13.2	35.6	69.9	76.4	1238	377
KY	Larue	-1.22	2246	33	11.6	30.9	72.4	78.2	781	238
KY	Laurel	1.25	709	37	12.9	35.7	72	77.7	1138	347
KY	Lawrence	-0.19	1587	36.1	12	35.7	70.2	77.3	812	247
KY	Lee	0.53	1049	33.4	11.1	35.5	68.2	76.2	946	288
KY	Leslie	-0.41	1764	36.2	14	37.5	69.2	76.1	1419	433
KY	Letcher	-0.74	1966	38.9	15.2	36.1	69.4	76.8	1717	523
KY	Lewis	0.78	921	35	12.2	34.8	69.8	77.2	867	264
KY	Lincoln	-1.25	2262	40.1	11.7	37.8	71.7	78.2	1060	323
KY	Livingston	0.75	933	33.8	12.5	34.6	73.8	79.6	428	130
KY	Logan	-0.75	1971	34.1	10.3	33.5	72.5	78.1	597	182
KY	Lyon	1.51	595	34.3	10.1	29.8	72.3	77.9	433	132
KY	Madison	-0.10	1525	30.2	9.7	30.3	73.8	79.5	888	271
KY	Magoffin	-1.67	2452	32.1	11.8	41.1	70.8	76.9	1076	328
KY	Marion	-1.32	2288	33.8	10.6	34.7	73.3	79.6	790	241
KY	Marshall	-0.24	1630	37.1	9.5	25.8	73.8	79.6	414	126
KY	Martin	-0.92	2080	38.6	12.6	38.1	69.7	77.4	943	288
KY	Mason	0.40	1139	31.5	10.5	29.8	72.9	79.1	831	253
KY	McCracken	-0.87	2049	30.1	9.6	28.4	73.6	79.1	375	114
KY	McCreary	0.73	940	32.3	12.4	40.8	69	76.2	1159	353
KY	McLean	-1.52	2386	31.3	11.2	34.1	72.4	78.9	416	127
KY	Meade	0.76	927	35.6	11.6	31.8	74.4	79.6	640	195
KY	Menifee	0.46	1098	35.9	11.9	31.6	70.8	77.6	1059	323
KY	Mercer	-0.03	1462	33.8	10.5	33.8	73.2	79.1	846	258
KY	Metcalfe	-3.16	2937	35.3	10.9	33.7	71.9	77.9	850	259
KY	Monroe	-0.10	1526	35.5	10.5	32.4	71.5	77.9	833	254
KY	Montgomery	-1.12	2201	31.7	10.2	31.6	72.3	79.1	929	283
KY	Morgan	0.39	1148	35.1	12.6	34.4	70.8	76.9	976	297
KY	Muhlenberg	0.21	1298	31.8	9.9	31.9	71.6	77.8	481	146
KY	Nelson	-0.63	1896	30	10.3	28.5	73.9	80.4	639	195
KY	Nicholas	-1.43	2341	33.6	11.4	34.9	72.5	78	851	259
KY	Ohio	-0.21	1607	32.6	12.2	35.3	72.8	78.3	489	149
KY	Oldham	-0.85	2036	29.2	9.3	27.5	76.4	80.7	694	211
KY	Owen	-0.64	1905	33.8	11.4	36.3	72.8	78.6	762	232
KY	Owsley	-1.67	2453	32.7	11	33.6	68.2	76.1	1025	313
KY	Pendleton	-0.74	1967	35.9	10.1	31.6	72.3	78.5	729	222

ST	COUNTY	USDA	AMEN	OBES	DIAB	INACT	M AGE	W AGE	ALT ft	ALT m
KY	Perry	-0.19	1588	38.8	13.1	39.2	68.4	76.6	1261	384
KY	Pike	-0.18	1582	36.9	13.9	38.1	68.7	76.3	1297	395
KY	Powell	-1.28	2274	35.4	12.8	40.4	70.8	77.6	915	279
KY	Pulaski	0.61	1015	30.5	10.2	32.2	72.5	78.9	1012	308
KY	Robertson	-1.91	2549	32	10.8	33.9	72.3	78.5	782	238
KY	Rockcastle	-0.35	1713	36.5	10.7	37.3	71.1	77.2	1154	352
KY	Rowan	0.97	825	35.4	10.3	30.6	72.4	79	992	302
KY	Russell	1.33	661	33.8	11	32.6	72.5	78.5	902	275
KY	Scott	-1.89	2541	32.5	10.1	31.7	74.9	80.4	871	265
KY	Shelby	-0.71	1948	34.3	10.9	28	75.4	80.2	783	239
KY	Simpson	-3.98	3065	32.3	11.5	35.4	73.1	79.3	668	204
KY	Spencer	0.39	1149	36.2	10.3	29.9	75	79	654	199
KY	Taylor	0.45	1102	33.2	10.5	26.8	73.2	78.7	837	255
KY	Todd	-0.98	2116	32.3	10.2	35.9	72.5	78.1	623	190
KY	Trigg	0.99	819	34.2	9.7	33.5	73	79.3	484	147
KY	Trimble	0.31	1208	33.6	11	34.1	73	78.9	728	222
KY	Union	0.72	943	35.8	10.4	33.2	72.8	78.8	401	122
KY	Warren	-0.68	1928	29.2	9.5	28.7	73.9	80	574	175
KY	Washington	-0.58	1869	31.6	11.2	29.4	73.3	79.6	757	231
KY	Wayne	0.89	863	33.3	11.3	40.6	71.6	77.8	1049	320
KY	Webster	-2.30	2692	36.9	11.6	33.8	72.4	78.9	436	133
KY	Whitley	1.15	750	33.1	12.9	34.1	70.7	77	1194	364
KY	Wolfe	-1.00	2129	31.8	10.6	33	68.2	76.2	1063	324
KY	Woodford	-2.04	2595	31.5	9.6	27.3	75.5	80.1	811	247
LA	Acadia	-1.56	2405	32.5	8.9	31.6	70	76.7	27	8
LA	Allen	-2.38	2729	38.4	12.2	33.8	73.1	78.7	77	24
LA	Ascension	-1.22	2247	31.8	9.7	28.5	73.3	78.9	9	3
LA	Assumption	-0.22	1613	32.8	10.9	30	71.1	77.8	5	2
LA	Avoyelles	-0.50	1813	36.9	11.2	36.1	69.4	76.3	47	14
LA	Beauregard	-1.45	2353	32.6	10.8	30.2	72.2	77.7	114	35
LA	Bienville	-0.03	1463	39.1	11.2	29	70	76.1	241	73
LA	Bossier	0.25	1252	31	11.7	26.4	73.4	79.1	209	64
LA	Caddo	0.65	983	32.1	11.5	30.4	70.8	77.6	212	65
LA	Calcasieu	-0.67	1923	34.5	11.6	29.4	71.2	78.1	17	5
LA	Caldwell	0.35	1185	37.5	11.1	31.4	70.1	76.8	119	36
LA	Cameron	0.77	924	32.1	10.2	25	72.6	78	3	1
LA	Catahoula	0.08	1377	34	11.3	33.6	70.1	76.8	67	21
LA	Claiborne	0.08	1378	34.2	12.3	32.7	71.1	76.7	265	81
LA	Concordia	-0.18	1583	33.1	10.7	32.2	69.9	76.7	44	14
LA	De Soto	0.37	1166	36.6	11.8	30.9	70.5	77.3	240	73
LA	E Baton Rouge	-0.73	1963	31.5	11.1	25.9	72.3	78	59	18
LA	East Carroll	-1.24	2257	36.2	13.4	32.8	70.1	76.2	87	26
LA	East Feliciana	-1.46	2358	34.9	11.9	27.6	69.9	76.7	197	60
LA	Evangeline	-0.56	1851	33	10.5	30	69.8	75.5	69	21
LA	Franklin	-1.35	2300	36.2	10.6	36	70	76.6	66	20
LA	Grant	-0.20	1597	31.6	10.8	32.1	71.3	78.1	139	42
LA	Iberia	0.48	1086	33.7	11.3	31	72	78	7	2

ST	COUNTY	USDA	AMEN	OBES	DIAB	INACT	M AGE	W AGE	ALT ft	ALT m
LA	Iberville	-0.56	1852	36.8	12.2	32.6	69.4	76.3	8	3
LA	Jackson	0.20	1303	30.6	9.3	32.4	71.5	77.1	230	70
LA	Jefferson	0.18	1319	31.9	11.1	28.6	72.4	79.5	4	1
LA	Jefferson Davis	-1.04	2157	33.2	12	31	72.6	78	22	7
LA	La Salle	-0.02	1453	32.7	10.9	30.9	71.8	77.4	126	38
LA	Lafayette	-2.47	2770	29.1	7.8	25.1	73.3	78.7	29	9
LA	Lafourche	0.11	1359	35.7	12	31	73.1	79.3	4	1
LA	Lincoln	-0.99	2122	34.4	10.8	30.8	74	78.9	229	70
LA	Livingston	0.07	1389	30.8	9.7	30	72.3	78.6	32	10
LA	Madison	-0.68	1929	36.7	12.6	34.5	69.3	75.3	72	22
LA	Morehouse	-1.85	2525	37.8	11.6	35.7	69.5	75.6	90	28
LA	Natchitoches	0.39	1150	35.7	11.6	33.1	70.9	77.2	166	51
LA	Orleans	0.14	1339	29.7	11.7	28.8	68.4	79.5	3	1
LA	Ouachita	0.51	1061	31.8	12.3	29.5	72.1	77.8	102	31
LA	Plaquemines	0.30	1214	34	12.3	30.9	72.8	79.1	4	1
LA	Pointe Coupee	0.17	1323	31.9	10.9	29.9	71.7	78.1	24	7
LA	Rapides	-0.21	1608	32.6	12.4	30.5	72	77.5	119	36
LA	Red River	1.11	768	34.8	11.3	32.4	70	76.1	161	49
LA	Richland	-1.75	2489	36.3	10.4	29.1	69.3	75.3	71	22
LA	Sabine	1.63	562	36.2	12.5	31.6	72.8	78.9	254	77
LA	St. Bernard	0.37	1167	32.3	10.8	31.7	70.6	76.1	3	1
LA	St. Charles	-0.10	1527	32.2	10.1	28.8	73.6	79.3	4	1
LA	St. Helena	-2.02	2589	36.4	13	33.9	69.9	76.7	210	64
LA	St. James	-1.12	2202	35.7	11.5	32.6	71.3	78.3	6	2
LA	St. John Baptist	-0.34	1699	38.5	11.5	32	71.3	76.8	4	1
LA	St. Landry	-0.71	1949	38.1	12.6	32.5	70.7	77.2	34	10
LA	St. Martin	-0.34	1700	35.5	11.7	29.7	71.6	77.5	8	2
LA	St. Mary	0.85	888	37.9	11.6	32.2	70.3	78	4	1
LA	St. Tammany	0.76	928	27.2	8.9	23.9	74.1	79.6	48	14
LA	Tangipahoa	-0.28	1652	35.3	10.6	31.4	70.2	76	118	36
LA	Tensas	-0.47	1800	35.4	12.4	33.3	69.9	76.7	61	18
LA	Terrebonne	0.50	1071	38.9	12.4	32.5	71.8	78.6	3	1
LA	Union	0.22	1286	35.7	12.2	34.7	71.7	77.6	148	45
LA	Vermilion	0.44	1114	33.3	10.4	27.6	71.9	78.5	6	2
LA	Vernon	0.20	1304	36.4	11.3	28.9	73.8	79.3	251	77
LA	Washington	-1.57	2409	34.3	13.5	34.7	68.8	75.7	204	62
LA	Webster	0.71	951	35.7	11.7	30.8	70.7	77.1	228	70
LA	W Baton Rouge	-0.01	1444	31.8	11.5	29.3	71.7	77.2	15	5
LA	W Carroll	-2.79	2858	31.5	11.2	32.1	70.1	76.2	95	29
LA	W Feliciana	-0.27	1647	32.3	12	29.8	71.7	77.2	137	42
LA	Winn	-0.04	1473	32.6	10.3	36.8	69.7	76.8	165	50
MA	Barnstable	1.52	592	18.1	6.1	16.6	78.1	82.9	55	17
MA	Berkshire	0.81	908	23.5	7.5	21.1	76.9	81.1	1404	428
MA	Bristol	0.54	1045	28.8	9.9	28.1	75.8	81.4	100	30
MA	Dukes	2.89	321	18.2	7.8	18.1	78.2	82.9	58	18
MA	Essex	1.43	625	23.2	8.3	21.7	77.4	81.7	86	26
MA	Franklin	0.00	1440	24.2	6.7	18.7	77.1	81.3	853	260

HEALTHIEST PLACES TO LIVE

ST	COUNTY	USDA	AMEN	OBES	DIAB	INACT	M AGE	W AGE	ALT ft	ALT m
MA	Hampden	-0.08	1508	28.4	9.3	25.7	75.2	80.5	629	192
MA	Hampshire	-0.01	1445	22.1	6.6	16.9	77.5	81.6	739	225
MA	Middlesex	-1.12	2203	23	7.6	20.8	78.8	82.9	226	69
MA	Nantucket	2.89	322	22.6	7.6	19.8	78.1	82.9	26	8
MA	Norfolk	-0.64	1906	20	6.4	19.4	78.2	82.6	191	58
MA	Plymouth	1.09	779	22.8	7.4	20.5	76.3	81.3	80	24
MA	Suffolk	0.83	896	22.1	8.6	22.1	75.8	81.9	57	17
MA	Worcester	0.24	1264	25.2	8	22.6	76.4	81.2	709	216
MD	Allegany	1.26	705	30.7	12.3	31	74	79.7	1252	382
MD	Anne Arundel	0.71	952	27.4	8.5	20.1	75.7	80.2	88	27
MD	Baltimore	-0.37	1729	31	11.7	30.6	66.7	75.6	436	133
MD	Baltimore City	-0.37	1730	27.2	8.6	27.1	75.1	80.3	202	62
MD	Calvert	0.65	984	27.8	8.8	23.1	75	79.7	79	24
MD	Caroline	-1.68	2459	32.1	11.1	29.2	73.2	78.7	40	12
MD	Carroll	-1.34	2294	27.5	8	20.8	76.6	80.5	646	197
MD	Cecil	0.10	1366	31.2	8.9	27.9	73.8	79.4	181	55
MD	Charles	0.55	1041	32.3	10	24.7	74.7	79.2	113	34
MD	Dorchester	0.20	1305	35.6	11.1	29.8	72.5	78.7	12	4
MD	Frederick	0.10	1367	26.2	8.2	21.8	76.8	81.2	599	183
MD	Garrett	0.35	1186	30	10.1	29.5	75	80.2	2460	750
MD	Harford	0.04	1410	27.8	8.3	24.5	75.6	80.6	320	98
MD	Howard	-1.42	2333	24.4	7.3	17.6	79.8	82.6	442	135
MD	Kent	-0.23	1619	28.1	8.8	25.8	74.5	80.6	39	12
MD	Montgomery	-0.57	1859	18.1	6.5	16.6	80.7	84.5	404	123
MD	Prince George's	-0.61	1884	33.8	11	24.9	73.5	79.2	147	45
MD	Queen Anne's	-0.08	1509	26.8	7.8	23.4	76.1	81.8	42	13
MD	Somerset	-0.04	1474	39.7	11.4	32	72	77.4	11	3
MD	St. Mary's	0.53	1050	28.6	9.6	23.4	75.5	80.3	75	23
MD	Talbot	0.10	1368	26.3	7.5	20.9	76.4	81.7	26	8
MD	Washington	0.85	889	29.9	9.8	27.7	74.6	79.7	639	195
MD	Wicomico	-0.70	1942	33.3	10.4	27.5	73	78.9	31	9
MD	Worcester	0.34	1191	30.2	8.3	23.2	75.3	80.7	23	7
ME	Androscoggin	-0.32	1687	32.1	8.7	26.5	75.2	79.9	345	105
ME	Aroostook	-0.14	1555	31.8	10.5	32.4	74.6	80.1	855	261
ME	Cumberland	1.05	793	21.6	6.8	16.3	77.1	81.7	282	86
ME	Franklin	0.17	1324	28.7	7.1	21.4	76.1	80.3	1552	473
ME	Hancock	1.87	505	25.1	7.2	19.6	76	81.3	293	89
ME	Kennebec	-0.14	1556	30.1	8.2	22.5	75.7	80.4	287	87
ME	Knox	2.06	457	25.8	7.6	20.7	76.7	81.4	235	72
ME	Lincoln	1.55	584	23.8	6.7	19.4	77.3	81	158	48
ME	Oxford	1.28	689	27.4	8.3	24.1	74.5	80	1175	358
ME	Penobscot	-0.52	1824	31	9.7	25.5	75	80.1	440	134
ME	Piscataquis	1.20	732	33.7	8.6	23.5	74.3	80.5	1073	327
ME	Sagadahoc	1.05	794	25.7	7.6	19.8	76.5	80.5	139	42
ME	Somerset	0.47	1093	35.1	9.8	26.4	74.8	79.8	1180	360
ME	Waldo	0.20	1306	27.8	8.1	22.2	75.4	80.8	357	109
ME	Washington	2.69	341	30.9	9.5	29.8	73.1	80.1	277	84

PEGGY FORNEY

ST	COUNTY	USDA	AMEN	OBES	DIAB	INACT	M AGE	W AGE	ALT ft	ALT m
ME	York	0.86	880	25.7	7.2	20.4	77	81.5	309	94
MI	Alcona	0.35	1187	30.5	9.3	24	75.2	79.6	853	260
MI	Alger	-0.91	2073	30.6	8.7	24	74.7	80	858	262
MI	Allegan	-0.52	1825	31.4	8.5	23.3	76	80.9	711	217
MI	Alpena	0.07	1390	31.2	8	21	75.4	81.2	745	227
MI	Antrim	0.58	1030	30.6	8.1	22.6	76.2	80.9	895	273
MI	Arenac	-1.04	2158	35.2	8.6	24	74.1	79.6	683	208
MI	Baraga	-0.55	1841	32.4	10.4	23.1	75.1	80.9	1336	407
MI	Barry	-2.15	2635	35.2	8.3	25.7	75.4	80.7	878	268
MI	Bay	-1.53	2394	34.5	9.2	24.7	74.7	80.4	632	193
MI	Benzie	0.75	934	29.5	8.8	23	75.7	80.9	777	237
MI	Berrien	-0.30	1667	32.9	9.4	27.6	74.8	79.8	680	207
MI	Branch	-2.45	2760	32.9	9.2	28.9	74.7	79.6	949	289
MI	Calhoun	-2.73	2848	35.5	10.3	27.3	73.1	79.1	938	286
MI	Cass	-2.14	2632	30.6	8.5	27.4	74.6	79.6	846	258
MI	Charlevoix	0.94	841	28	8.9	21.2	76.8	81.4	798	243
MI	Cheboygan	0.08	1379	39.1	9.1	26.7	75.8	80.6	744	227
MI	Chippewa	-1.40	2322	31.4	10	22.9	75.9	80.7	722	220
MI	Clare	-2.36	2717	30.3	8.9	30.4	72.7	79	1069	326
MI	Clinton	-3.49	3003	31.2	9	24.9	77	81.5	768	234
MI	Crawford	-2.37	2725	30.1	8.3	23.4	74.1	79.2	1218	371
MI	Delta	-1.94	2562	30.1	8.7	24.3	76.5	80.9	733	224
MI	Dickinson	-3.58	3019	27.4	8.4	22.4	76.5	81.9	1186	362
MI	Eaton	-3.14	2935	31.1	8.5	22.4	76	80.4	892	272
MI	Emmet	0.93	848	31.7	7.9	21.5	77.7	81.6	794	242
MI	Genesee	-1.90	2546	35.9	10.6	29.7	73.2	78.6	787	240
MI	Gladwin	-2.23	2661	34	8.8	26.7	74.2	79.6	792	242
MI	Gogebic	-1.69	2468	30.9	8.4	24.7	75	80.7	1481	451
MI	Grand Traverse	0.37	1168	30.2	7.5	19.5	77.7	82	905	276
MI	Gratiot	-3.92	3056	37.7	9.1	27.9	75.2	79.6	735	224
MI	Hillsdale	-2.40	2738	28	9.1	25.8	75.2	80.5	1057	322
MI	Houghton	-0.58	1870	26.2	8.8	26.2	75.2	80.1	1026	313
MI	Huron	-0.74	1968	30.9	7.8	22.6	75.1	80	682	208
MI	Ingham	-3.38	2983	30.9	8.3	22.4	76.1	80.4	914	279
MI	Ionia	-3.07	2918	33.2	9.8	23.4	75.1	80	799	244
MI	Iosco	-0.17	1573	34.3	8.3	22.9	73.5	79.5	737	225
MI	Iron	-2.88	2881	30.2	9.2	23	75.1	80.9	1538	469
MI	Isabella	-3.10	2928	32.8	8.5	24.2	75.5	80.4	859	262
MI	Jackson	-2.45	2761	36.4	9.4	27	74.4	79.3	983	300
MI	Kalamazoo	-2.10	2616	28.4	9.3	22.3	75.7	80.8	880	268
MI	Kalkaska	-1.11	2192	30.4	10	25	74.8	80	1121	342
MI	Kent	-2.28	2685	30.1	8.9	21.3	76.5	81	796	243
MI	Keweenaw	0.44	1115	31.9	8.9	25.1	75.2	80.1	847	258
MI	Lake	-1.68	2460	32.4	10	24.5	74.1	78.9	969	295
MI	Lapeer	-2.12	2624	33.3	8.3	25.8	76.1	80.1	862	263
MI	Leelanau	0.73	941	31.3	8.5	26.6	78.6	82.8	731	223
MI	Lenawee	-2.31	2694	33.4	8.5	23.8	76.2	79.8	828	252

64

ST	COUNTY	USDA	AMEN	OBES	DIAB	INACT	M AGE	W AGE	ALT ft	ALT m
MI	Livingston	-1.82	2514	26.2	7.6	19	77.2	81.2	935	285
MI	Luce	-1.21	2241	31.8	9.1	26.6	75	80.3	780	238
MI	Mackinac	-0.95	2104	33.8	9	25.3	75	80.3	733	223
MI	Macomb	-1.24	2258	30.8	9.4	24.6	75.6	80.5	680	207
MI	Manistee	0.89	864	27.5	8.5	27.2	75.3	80.8	790	241
MI	Marquette	-1.09	2186	29.8	7.9	20.9	76.3	80.4	1246	380
MI	Mason	0.60	1021	32	8.6	26.7	75.5	80.5	693	211
MI	Mecosta	-1.94	2563	32.6	9.6	25.5	75.3	80.6	1002	306
MI	Menominee	-1.61	2429	30.9	8.3	25.6	76.2	81	799	243
MI	Midland	-3.09	2923	31	8.1	21.6	77.1	81.2	669	204
MI	Missaukee	-1.95	2565	33.4	9.7	25.1	75.1	79	1213	370
MI	Monroe	-1.43	2342	34.7	10.1	27	74.6	79.7	635	194
MI	Montcalm	-2.48	2775	33.6	9	22.6	74.4	79	883	269
MI	Montmorency	-0.92	2081	31.9	8.9	24.4	74.7	80.4	960	293
MI	Muskegon	-0.40	1754	34.7	9.9	25.8	74.3	79.3	667	203
MI	Newaygo	-1.30	2280	34.5	11.5	25.2	75	79.8	885	270
MI	Oakland	-1.78	2499	27	8.7	20.3	77.3	81.5	935	285
MI	Oceana	0.26	1246	35.2	9.6	24.9	75.4	80.9	763	233
MI	Ogemaw	-1.89	2542	34	9	29.2	73.1	78.6	1033	315
MI	Ontonagon	-0.72	1960	32.5	9.3	20.9	75	80.7	1110	338
MI	Osceola	-2.35	2709	33.2	9.1	26.6	74.1	78.9	1194	364
MI	Oscoda	-1.37	2307	31.6	9.8	26.7	75.2	79.6	1136	346
MI	Otsego	-0.89	2062	30.4	8.5	23.6	76	80.4	1219	371
MI	Ottawa	-0.04	1475	25.2	8.2	21.3	78.8	82.4	655	200
MI	Presque Isle	0.18	1320	32.8	9.1	23.3	74.7	80.4	746	228
MI	Roscommon	-1.20	2235	36.1	9.7	30.3	73.8	79.9	1169	356
MI	Saginaw	-3.33	2970	39.9	9.8	30.2	73.5	79.1	624	190
MI	Sanilac	-1.23	2251	35.4	8.8	27.8	75.2	79.5	765	233
MI	Schoolcraft	-1.05	2163	30	9.3	24.8	74.7	80	745	227
MI	Shiawassee	-3.48	3001	31.7	9.5	25.6	75.2	80.5	787	240
MI	St. Clair	-1.25	2263	30.6	9.3	24	75.5	79.8	697	213
MI	St. Joseph	-2.40	2739	32	9.5	25.5	73.5	79.8	848	258
MI	Tuscola	-1.63	2439	30.6	9	26.4	74.7	79.7	709	216
MI	Van Buren	-0.61	1885	30.1	9.2	27.3	73.9	79.6	737	225
MI	Washtenaw	-2.19	2649	24.4	8.5	19.4	77.9	81.7	881	268
MI	Wayne	-1.73	2479	34	11.6	27.6	71.9	78	642	196
MI	Wexford	-0.76	1979	33.3	8.4	27.3	74.9	79.9	1181	360
MN	Aitkin	-1.74	2483	27.9	7.6	20.2	76.2	81.6	1274	388
MN	Anoka	-2.41	2744	30	7.7	20.8	78.3	82.4	909	277
MN	Becker	-2.34	2706	28.5	7.5	21.1	75.7	81.2	1454	443
MN	Beltrami	-2.89	2884	30.2	7.4	21.3	74.6	81	1261	384
MN	Benton	-3.43	2992	27.3	8.4	21.6	75.4	80.2	1123	342
MN	Big Stone	-2.77	2853	27.7	6.7	20.2	76.5	82.2	1096	334
MN	Blue Earth	-2.48	2776	27.4	7.2	25	77.4	81.6	997	304
MN	Brown	-3.07	2919	30.6	7.4	22.1	77.4	82	1019	310
MN	Carlton	-2.15	2636	27.9	8.1	19.1	74.9	81	1195	364
MN	Carver	-2.70	2839	25.9	6.6	16.9	78.6	83	971	296

ST	COUNTY	USDA	AMEN	OBES	DIAB	INACT	M AGE	W AGE	ALT ft	ALT m
MN	Cass	-2.38	2730	27.5	6.8	21	75.3	81.1	1345	410
MN	Chippewa	-3.42	2989	31.6	7.3	20.7	76.8	81.7	1036	316
MN	Chisago	-2.23	2662	26.7	7.9	18.8	76.7	81	907	276
MN	Clay	-4.17	3081	29.9	7.9	22.3	77.3	82.6	1022	312
MN	Clearwater	-2.96	2899	30.4	7.5	21	74.9	81	1427	435
MN	Cook	2.99	309	26.9	7.3	18.3	76.3	81.7	1617	493
MN	Cottonwood	-2.35	2710	27.4	7.7	25.2	76.3	81.8	1364	416
MN	Crow Wing	-2.14	2633	24.8	6.4	17.3	77.3	81.8	1256	383
MN	Dakota	-3.05	2914	26	6.3	16.9	78.7	81.7	922	281
MN	Dodge	-5.08	3101	31.3	7.2	19.6	77.5	82.3	1259	384
MN	Douglas	-2.23	2663	27.8	6.8	19	78	82.8	1385	422
MN	Faribault	-2.91	2887	28.5	7.2	22.8	76	81.8	1114	340
MN	Fillmore	-2.93	2890	28.4	6.7	21.7	76.4	82	1194	364
MN	Freeborn	-2.38	2731	28.7	7	21.5	76.6	81.7	1257	383
MN	Goodhue	-1.38	2313	27.5	7.4	18.1	77.7	82	1048	319
MN	Grant	-2.69	2837	26.9	6.8	20.8	76.5	82.4	1143	348
MN	Hennepin	-2.15	2637	21	6	16.3	78.1	82.4	924	282
MN	Houston	-1.52	2387	26.5	7.1	19.1	76.9	81.8	974	297
MN	Hubbard	-3.24	2955	24.9	6.9	18.7	76	81.5	1453	443
MN	Isanti	-2.66	2829	28.6	7.6	18.7	76.7	81.7	956	291
MN	Itasca	-2.36	2718	26	7	18	76	81.1	1363	416
MN	Jackson	-2.05	2599	30.3	6.6	22.2	77.5	82.9	1435	437
MN	Kanabec	-3.04	2911	28.2	7.4	21.3	76.2	80.7	1087	331
MN	Kandiyohi	-2.60	2810	28.7	6.5	22.8	77.2	82.5	1176	358
MN	Kittson	-4.90	3098	28.8	7.6	22.3	75.3	82.4	904	276
MN	Koochiching	-4.20	3083	29.4	8.1	19.8	75.3	81.1	1215	370
MN	Lac qui Parle	-3.43	2993	29.4	7.7	19.8	76.5	82.2	1068	326
MN	Lake	0.24	1265	29.2	7.4	22.2	76.3	81.7	1560	475
MN	Lk of the Woods	-3.09	2924	27.8	7.1	21.6	75.3	81.1	1134	345
MN	Le Sueur	-2.17	2641	29	6.9	21	77.6	81.9	1016	310
MN	Lincoln	-2.16	2639	27.5	6.6	21.6	75.1	81.8	1689	515
MN	Lyon	-2.70	2840	29.3	7.1	22.5	76.9	81.6	1306	398
MN	Mahnomen	-3.09	2925	31.6	9.1	27	74.9	81	1365	416
MN	Marshall	-4.05	3074	26.1	6.9	20.7	75.3	82.4	1025	312
MN	Martin	-2.48	2777	26.9	6.6	20.4	76.5	82.8	1205	367
MN	McLeod	-2.93	2891	28.6	6.9	18.6	77.3	82.4	1057	322
MN	Meeker	-2.65	2827	25.7	8.2	23.6	76.4	80.8	1139	347
MN	Mille Lacs	-1.74	2484	26.5	7.1	22.6	75.1	80.6	1185	361
MN	Morrison	-3.09	2926	28.3	6.8	20.6	75	81.1	1221	372
MN	Mower	-5.18	3103	28.5	7.2	21.8	77.6	82.6	1309	399
MN	Murray	-2.21	2654	30.6	7	18.9	75.8	82.1	1611	491
MN	Nicollet	-2.58	2805	27.8	7.5	17	78	82.1	987	301
MN	Nobles	-2.48	2778	26.8	8.2	22.1	77.5	82.9	1607	490
MN	Norman	-5.37	3105	30.4	8.1	21.2	75.7	81.2	984	300
MN	Olmsted	-3.96	3062	28	7	17.4	78.3	83.7	1172	357
MN	Otter Tail	-2.41	2745	30.2	6.7	22.7	76.5	82.4	1355	413
MN	Pennington	-4.97	3099	28.1	8.6	23.1	74.9	81	1121	342

HEALTHIEST PLACES TO LIVE

ST	COUNTY	USDA	AMEN	OBES	DIAB	INACT	M AGE	W AGE	ALT ft	ALT m
MN	Pine	-2.77	2854	27.1	7	19.7	75.3	80.1	1079	329
MN	Pipestone	-4.13	3079	27.8	7.4	19.2	75.1	81.8	1714	522
MN	Polk	-3.76	3047	30.5	7.7	26	75.3	81.4	1012	308
MN	Pope	-2.45	2762	28	7.1	23.4	77.8	81.9	1281	391
MN	Ramsey	-2.08	2612	24.1	7	15	77.4	82.5	918	280
MN	Red Lake	-6.40	3108	31.8	7.2	19.8	75.3	81.4	1089	332
MN	Redwood	-3.67	3031	29.2	6.9	21	76	81.1	1073	327
MN	Renville	-3.90	3054	32	7.4	23	76.2	80.9	1066	325
MN	Rice	-2.20	2653	24	7.3	17.2	77.3	82	1095	334
MN	Rock	-4.25	3087	24.3	6.7	22.2	75.8	82.1	1547	471
MN	Roseau	-4.30	3088	31.6	6.7	22.2	75.9	81.3	1092	333
MN	Scott	-2.95	2897	24.6	6.2	17.4	78.3	82.4	928	283
MN	Sherburne	-2.88	2882	30.4	7.9	22.4	77.3	80.8	979	298
MN	Sibley	-3.10	2929	29.8	6.9	23.1	76.6	81.5	1012	308
MN	St. Louis	-0.66	1919	27.5	6.9	17.5	75.8	80.9	1378	420
MN	Stearns	-2.87	2880	28.4	7.6	19	78.8	83.9	1197	365
MN	Steele	-3.05	2915	29.5	6.6	21.2	77.7	82.5	1215	370
MN	Stevens	-3.31	2967	27.4	7.1	21.3	77.8	81.9	1133	345
MN	Swift	-3.74	3043	28.7	8.2	26.5	76.8	81.7	1076	328
MN	Todd	-2.84	2872	30	7.4	25.8	75.7	81.1	1335	407
MN	Traverse	-3.57	3015	28.2	7.2	21.8	76.5	82.2	1041	317
MN	Wabasha	-1.13	2207	24	6.3	22.3	77.1	81.8	985	300
MN	Wadena	-3.74	3044	30.7	7.8	21.7	76	81.5	1358	414
MN	Waseca	-2.36	2719	30.3	7.7	23	77.5	81.3	1124	343
MN	Washington	-0.63	1897	25.4	6.8	16.6	78.8	82	918	280
MN	Watonwan	-2.85	2877	27.8	7.2	21.7	76.3	81.8	1106	337
MN	Wilkin	-6.10	3107	28.6	7.2	25	76.5	82.4	993	303
MN	Winona	-1.61	2430	30.5	7.2	19.5	77.3	82.2	1063	324
MN	Wright	-2.50	2784	24.4	6.2	17.9	77.8	82.1	1005	306
MN	Yellow Medicine	-3.98	3066	25	7	19.5	76	81.1	1127	343
MO	Adair	-1.11	2193	28.4	9.3	31.5	74.8	80.2	896	273
MO	Andrew	-1.01	2136	31.1	8.5	24.3	74.8	79.6	979	298
MO	Atchison	-0.76	1980	29.7	8.5	27	76.2	80.7	998	304
MO	Audrain	-2.43	2752	31.1	8.4	31.1	73.6	79.3	790	241
MO	Barry	1.95	485	30.2	8.7	31.6	72.7	79.2	1319	402
MO	Barton	-1.93	2558	32.5	9.6	27.7	73.9	80	944	288
MO	Bates	-1.65	2444	30.1	8.9	27.4	73.8	79.5	848	259
MO	Benton	1.47	605	33	9.4	29.7	73	78.8	856	261
MO	Bollinger	0.49	1079	35.1	8.9	31.5	72.7	78.7	596	182
MO	Boone	-0.02	1454	27.4	7.5	21.6	76.5	80.5	765	233
MO	Buchanan	-0.47	1801	37.4	10.3	30.1	73.8	79.6	923	281
MO	Butler	-0.84	2028	32.6	8.6	31.7	70.7	77.8	372	113
MO	Caldwell	-2.83	2868	34.7	9.2	30.2	74.5	80.4	895	273
MO	Callaway	-0.06	1493	35.4	10.4	28.7	73.9	80.1	765	233
MO	Camden	1.68	547	27.1	8.3	30.7	75	81	864	263
MO	Cape Irardeau	0.91	854	27.4	9	27.2	75	80.2	462	141
MO	Carroll	-0.14	1557	31.7	7.9	25.6	74.5	80.4	737	225

ST	COUNTY	USDA	AMEN	OBES	DIAB	INACT	M AGE	W AGE	ALT ft	ALT m
MO	Carter	1.23	717	30.5	9.3	29.7	70.4	77.3	726	221
MO	Cass	-1.68	2461	33.1	9.8	27.1	75	79.4	921	281
MO	Cedar	1.24	715	31.3	9.1	27.8	73.9	80	907	276
MO	Chariton	0.06	1397	31.2	9.7	28.8	75.2	79.9	695	212
MO	Christian	0.08	1380	27.1	7.7	26.2	75.1	80.1	1246	380
MO	Clark	-0.52	1826	32.5	8.6	30.6	74	80.2	644	196
MO	Clay	0.15	1336	27.6	8.5	26.5	76.1	80.3	883	269
MO	Clinton	-1.49	2369	31	9.9	29	74.2	80.1	981	299
MO	Cole	0.96	832	27.9	8.8	26.1	75.7	80.5	696	212
MO	Cooper	-0.08	1510	30.4	9.1	25.7	74.4	79.9	743	227
MO	Crawford	-0.28	1653	32.3	8	28.4	73.1	79.2	928	283
MO	Dade	0.95	837	29.5	8.8	26.4	73.7	79	1024	312
MO	Dallas	-0.20	1598	32	8.1	28.6	73.1	78.7	1093	333
MO	Daviess	-2.06	2601	32.2	9.1	27.4	74.9	80.2	870	265
MO	DeKalb	-2.33	2700	31.9	8.4	29.8	74.8	79.6	967	295
MO	Dent	0.61	1016	31.7	8.6	29.6	72.8	78.6	1189	362
MO	Douglas	-0.88	2059	31.7	9.3	28.1	72.5	79.3	1142	348
MO	Dunklin	-2.10	2617	34.9	10.6	40.7	69.8	76.6	267	81
MO	Franklin	0.38	1156	30.7	8.3	26.7	74.2	79.4	667	203
MO	Gasconade	0.47	1094	32.4	8.5	31.1	73.7	79.1	774	236
MO	Gentry	-1.76	2493	31.2	9.5	28.2	74.9	80.2	951	290
MO	Greene	0.62	1010	30.2	8.5	25.2	74.7	80.7	1226	374
MO	Grundy	-0.57	1860	28.9	8	26.2	73.9	80	835	254
MO	Harrison	-1.19	2231	32.5	9	30.3	74.9	80.2	974	297
MO	Henry	-0.46	1793	32.2	9	30	73.7	78.9	796	242
MO	Hickory	1.22	722	32.7	8.6	26.4	72.8	79	947	289
MO	Holt	-0.15	1560	30.6	8.8	26.9	76.2	80.7	939	286
MO	Howard	0.29	1224	31.1	8.4	31.5	75.2	79.9	712	217
MO	Howell	0.31	1209	30.6	10.1	29	72.2	79	1058	322
MO	Iron	0.81	909	33.6	9.1	28	70.4	77.3	1078	328
MO	Jackson	-1.49	2370	32.5	8.9	25.4	73.2	79.2	894	272
MO	Jasper	-2.26	2678	33.1	8.2	26.5	73.1	78.9	991	302
MO	Jefferson	0.96	833	34.9	10.1	30.9	74.1	78.4	614	187
MO	Johnson	-2.00	2581	33.5	10.1	29.5	74.6	80.1	830	253
MO	Knox	-1.47	2362	31.9	8.6	29.4	73.8	79.8	774	236
MO	Laclede	-0.11	1535	31.9	8.8	33.8	73.4	78.8	1138	347
MO	Lafayette	-1.70	2472	30.8	8.4	26.8	73.9	79.9	804	245
MO	Lawrence	-2.46	2765	29.8	8.4	28.5	73.3	79.4	1239	378
MO	Lewis	-0.40	1755	33.9	8.6	29	74	80.2	631	192
MO	Lincoln	0.37	1169	35.4	10.1	26.8	73.7	79	607	185
MO	Linn	-1.26	2268	37.5	8.8	32.9	74.2	80.2	815	248
MO	Livingston	-2.04	2596	28.4	9.3	32.5	74.2	80.2	770	235
MO	Macon	-0.55	1842	30.6	8.8	29.1	73.8	79.8	830	253
MO	Madison	1.01	809	34.7	9.4	28.6	72.7	78.7	809	247
MO	Maries	0.20	1307	31.1	9.2	29.4	74.3	79.8	885	270
MO	Marion	-1.48	2365	29	7.9	30.2	74	79.2	621	189
MO	McDonald	-0.20	1599	31.8	8.6	31.2	71.9	77.8	1100	335

HEALTHIEST PLACES TO LIVE

ST	COUNTY	USDA	AMEN	OBES	DIAB	INACT	M AGE	W AGE	ALT ft	ALT m
MO	Mercer	-1.24	2259	31.9	8.7	33	74.8	80.2	965	294
MO	Miller	0.83	897	30.2	8.4	30	73.6	78.9	787	240
MO	Mississippi	-1.39	2317	31.4	9.7	37.3	69.9	76.9	305	93
MO	Moniteau	0.39	1151	29.6	9.2	32	74.4	79.9	802	244
MO	Monroe	-0.94	2094	31	9.6	27.1	74.4	80.1	722	220
MO	Montgomery	-0.31	1680	31.6	9.3	28.5	73.7	79.1	732	223
MO	Morgan	1.22	723	29.1	8.6	35	73.5	79.6	884	269
MO	New Madrid	-1.52	2388	31.8	10	30.3	69.9	76.9	283	86
MO	Newton	-0.36	1723	32.3	10.2	30.5	74.7	80	1135	346
MO	Nodaway	-2.85	2878	30.7	8.2	30.5	76.2	80.7	1049	320
MO	Oregon	-0.76	1981	32.7	9.6	32.7	71.9	78.7	767	234
MO	Osage	0.42	1125	29.7	8.7	26.8	74.3	79.8	715	218
MO	Ozark	1.60	569	27.7	8.2	29	72.5	79.3	904	276
MO	Pemiscot	-1.16	2220	38.2	10	35.8	68.5	76.5	261	79
MO	Perry	2.29	415	33.6	9.4	25.8	74.8	80	553	169
MO	Pettis	-2.05	2600	29.5	8.4	31.8	74.7	79.7	825	251
MO	Phelps	-0.16	1566	31.3	8.4	27.5	74.4	79.2	990	302
MO	Pike	0.46	1099	32.7	10.2	31.5	73.8	78.8	668	204
MO	Platte	0.12	1354	28	8.8	28.1	76.8	81.5	889	271
MO	Polk	-0.62	1891	33.2	10	27.2	73.7	79	1050	320
MO	Pulaski	0.54	1046	32.4	9.5	27.5	74.6	79.5	984	300
MO	Putnam	-0.90	2069	29.4	7.7	28.5	74.8	80.2	964	294
MO	Ralls	-1.20	2236	30.5	8.5	27.9	74.4	80.1	679	207
MO	Randolph	-0.22	1614	34.8	10.3	31.6	73.7	79.9	794	242
MO	Ray	-0.72	1961	31.7	9.4	30.9	74.8	79.6	849	259
MO	Reynolds	1.41	630	33.4	9.2	32.8	70.4	77.3	950	290
MO	Ripley	0.48	1087	31.6	8.9	34.4	70.7	77.8	519	158
MO	Saline	-1.00	2130	31.3	9.4	28.7	74	78.6	720	219
MO	Schuyler	-1.90	2547	32	9.1	28.4	74.8	80.2	892	272
MO	Scotland	-1.56	2406	34.4	7.9	27.9	74	80.2	759	231
MO	Scott	-1.44	2345	34.4	10	32.7	73	79	345	105
MO	Shannon	-0.23	1620	34.7	10.1	30.9	71.9	78.7	981	299
MO	Shelby	-2.29	2687	32.9	10	28.4	73.8	79.8	764	233
MO	St. Charles	0.86	881	29.3	8	24.4	77.5	81.1	531	162
MO	St. Clair	1.11	769	31.7	9	30.7	72.8	79	816	249
MO	St. Francois	1.70	544	31.4	9.4	27.2	72.1	77.6	922	281
MO	St. Louis	0.64	989	28.8	8	23.8	76.1	80.8	542	165
MO	St. Louis City	-0.48	1805	33.7	11.8	27.6	69.6	77.7	477	145
MO	Ste. Genevieve	2.06	458	30.6	9.1	33	74.8	80.2	679	207
MO	Stoddard	-2.43	2753	29	8.7	39.4	71.8	78.2	343	105
MO	Stone	2.24	426	30.4	8.9	26.7	75.1	81.2	1138	347
MO	Sullivan	-1.58	2412	28.7	9.3	29.1	73.9	80	927	282
MO	Taney	1.63	563	32.4	8.8	29.3	74.5	79.9	966	295
MO	Texas	0.45	1103	35.6	8.2	31.9	72	78.5	1253	382
MO	Vernon	-1.60	2424	34	9.4	30.5	73.2	78.6	824	251
MO	Warren	0.14	1340	31.7	8.9	28.2	75.3	80.2	706	215
MO	Washington	0.86	882	29.7	9	27.8	70.4	77.3	933	284

ST	COUNTY	USDA	AMEN	OBES	DIAB	INACT	M AGE	W AGE	ALT ft	ALT m
MO	Wayne	2.18	436	29.5	9.2	30.1	71.8	78.2	578	176
MO	Webster	-0.45	1786	31.8	8.6	25.3	73.5	79.7	1411	430
MO	Worth	-1.56	2407	30.4	8.6	28.3	74.9	80.2	1035	315
MO	Wright	0.87	876	33.5	8	34	72.1	78.8	1320	402
MS	Adams	0.12	1355	37.8	12.5	38.8	70.8	77.6	170	52
MS	Alcorn	-1.30	2281	32.8	10.7	33.8	71.9	77.9	490	149
MS	Amite	-1.01	2137	37.8	11.9	32.3	69.3	76.1	351	107
MS	Attala	0.02	1419	38.6	12.7	35.2	68.2	77.3	403	123
MS	Benton	-1.04	2159	36.4	11.8	33.3	70.6	77.9	503	153
MS	Bolivar	-0.57	1861	39.2	13.3	31.4	67.9	75.2	136	42
MS	Calhoun	0.23	1277	33	12.2	36	70.6	77.9	346	105
MS	Carroll	-1.02	2144	34.7	10.9	31.6	70.7	77.9	312	95
MS	Chickasaw	-0.98	2117	35.3	11.7	33.1	69.8	77.5	335	102
MS	Choctaw	-0.16	1567	34.3	12	29	71.1	77.3	475	145
MS	Claiborne	-0.35	1714	41.6	14.5	39.9	67.8	74.5	177	54
MS	Clarke	0.42	1126	33.8	10.9	37.7	71.2	77.6	325	99
MS	Clay	-0.36	1724	38.1	12.9	36.8	71	77.8	242	74
MS	Coahoma	-0.65	1912	44.3	14.7	36.1	66.8	75	158	48
MS	Copiah	-1.08	2180	36	12.2	37.1	69.6	76.7	325	99
MS	Covington	-1.11	2194	40.7	12	30.8	69.2	77	323	98
MS	DeSoto	-0.24	1631	32.4	10	30.3	73.9	78.8	293	89
MS	Forrest	-0.03	1464	36.4	12	32.7	71.9	77.5	217	66
MS	Franklin	-1.29	2278	39	12.6	37.9	70.8	77.6	322	98
MS	George	-0.81	2015	37.9	10.1	33	70.4	77	134	41
MS	Greene	0.02	1420	39.7	12.1	32.7	70.7	76.6	170	52
MS	Grenada	1.78	526	37.6	12.3	35	68.8	76.7	253	77
MS	Hancock	0.25	1253	35.4	10.9	28.9	73.9	79.7	59	18
MS	Harrison	1.00	813	36	11.3	29.5	71	78.6	77	23
MS	Hinds	-1.21	2242	36	12.4	35.2	71.1	79	259	79
MS	Holmes	-0.92	2082	40.8	14.1	35.3	65.9	73.5	246	75
MS	Humphreys	-1.17	2224	41.4	13.6	33.4	66.5	74.1	101	31
MS	Issaquena	-0.89	2063	37.8	13.2	33.8	69.9	75.9	90	27
MS	Itawamba	1.01	810	35.1	12.2	35.6	71.6	77.3	394	120
MS	Jackson	0.85	890	32.8	11.3	28.7	72.1	77.7	45	14
MS	Jasper	-1.11	2195	39.5	14.4	35.5	70.5	77.2	404	123
MS	Jefferson	-0.71	1950	44.9	15.3	37.2	67.8	74.5	256	78
MS	Jefferson Davis	-1.10	2189	35.2	11.5	31	69.9	76.9	390	119
MS	Jones	-0.38	1735	37.6	12.3	32	71.8	77.9	247	75
MS	Kemper	-0.60	1879	38.1	14.3	32.9	68.9	76.5	344	105
MS	Lafayette	0.50	1072	32.3	10.3	28.9	72.5	79.4	389	119
MS	Lamar	-0.26	1642	31.4	9.2	28.8	74	78.9	307	93
MS	Lauderdale	1.31	670	35.4	13.2	29.8	70	77.1	383	117
MS	Lawrence	-0.08	1511	36.5	14.2	34	69.9	76.9	311	95
MS	Leake	0.72	944	35.9	13	38.7	68.4	76.2	406	124
MS	Lee	-0.86	2044	33.6	11.7	30.5	70.9	77	335	102
MS	Leflore	-1.41	2325	39	13.8	35.2	68.5	75.5	122	37
MS	Lincoln	-0.99	2123	36.1	11.8	34.1	71.8	77.9	418	127

HEALTHIEST PLACES TO LIVE

ST	COUNTY	USDA	AMEN	OBES	DIAB	INACT	M AGE	W AGE	ALT ft	ALT m
MS	Lowndes	-0.07	1501	37.3	13	33.5	72.5	78.4	222	68
MS	Madison	-0.01	1446	28.5	10.8	25.9	69.9	75.9	283	86
MS	Marion	0.04	1411	36.3	12	28.9	68.7	76.2	246	75
MS	Marshall	-1.00	2131	38.8	14.7	37.5	68.5	76	438	134
MS	Monroe	0.86	883	35.5	12.1	35.7	71.2	78.3	283	86
MS	Montgomery	0.05	1403	36.4	13.7	36.1	70.7	77.9	379	115
MS	Neshoba	0.61	1017	35	13.6	33.7	71.1	77.3	455	139
MS	Newton	0.34	1192	33.4	11.4	33	71.8	77.9	426	130
MS	Noxubee	0.39	1152	39.9	13.7	33.4	68.9	76.5	230	70
MS	Oktibbeha	-0.62	1892	31.6	11.4	26.9	73.9	79.3	301	92
MS	Panola	-0.06	1494	35.9	12.6	36.7	68.8	75.7	287	88
MS	Pearl River	-0.91	2074	32.9	11.6	28.8	71.8	78	184	56
MS	Perry	-0.28	1654	35.5	12.4	35.8	70.7	76.6	175	53
MS	Pike	-0.29	1662	39.9	13.7	35.2	69.9	76.5	347	106
MS	Pontotoc	-0.45	1787	33.8	10.7	34.3	72.1	79.4	409	125
MS	Prentiss	-0.79	2003	34.1	11.6	32.1	71.3	78.9	445	136
MS	Quitman	-1.97	2573	40.1	15.1	34.8	66	74.1	156	48
MS	Rankin	0.16	1331	34.7	10.7	27.9	74.8	80.9	360	110
MS	Scott	-1.15	2215	38	13.6	35	69.3	77.8	422	128
MS	Sharkey	-1.34	2295	40.2	13.3	35.2	66.5	74.1	92	28
MS	Simpson	-0.80	2008	34.9	11.7	32.2	70.3	76.4	384	117
MS	Smith	-1.23	2252	34.3	11.3	35	69.6	77	384	117
MS	Stone	-1.13	2208	34	11.4	30.6	70.4	77	177	54
MS	Sunflower	-1.47	2363	41.4	14.4	34.6	67.1	73.6	122	37
MS	Tallahatchie	-0.92	2083	37.6	12.8	33.5	68.6	76.3	187	57
MS	Tate	-0.70	1943	35.5	12.4	32.2	72	77.2	302	92
MS	Tippah	-1.17	2225	35.2	11.7	39.4	70.6	77.9	517	158
MS	Tishomingo	1.66	553	29	10.3	29.5	70.8	77.8	527	161
MS	Tunica	-0.40	1756	40.2	14.2	39.1	66	74.1	181	55
MS	Union	-0.85	2037	34.4	10.8	31.9	72.3	78.4	422	128
MS	Walthall	-0.87	2050	39.6	12.4	34.9	69.9	76.9	355	108
MS	Warren	-0.14	1558	39.1	12	30.9	71.1	77.3	156	48
MS	Washington	-1.03	2151	38.2	11.6	36.1	68.1	75.3	109	33
MS	Wayne	-0.79	2004	35.5	10.2	32	71.1	77.2	253	77
MS	Webster	-0.32	1688	33.9	11.5	34	71.1	77.3	418	127
MS	Wilkinson	-0.09	1518	39.7	14.9	35.3	69.3	76.1	214	65
MS	Winston	0.49	1080	36.8	14.2	34.1	70.4	78.6	456	139
MS	Yalobusha	0.53	1051	38.8	13.4	34.5	68.6	76.3	327	100
MS	Yazoo	-0.91	2075	35.5	12.8	35.2	69.9	75.9	210	64
MT	Beaverhead	3.50	246	23	7.1	20	76.6	79.8	7078	2157
MT	Big Horn	1.38	640	36.3	11.8	27.1	74.6	80.3	3982	1214
MT	Blaine	0.19	1316	35.3	10.9	32.4	74.4	80.2	3070	936
MT	Broadwater	3.93	205	25.8	6.2	23.2	75.9	80.9	5015	1529
MT	Carbon	4.22	186	27	6.1	24.8	74.6	80.3	5572	1698
MT	Carter	-0.58	1871	23.9	6	30.7	75	80.7	3426	1044
MT	Cascade	2.20	431	25.5	7.6	23.4	75.6	81.2	4273	1302
MT	Chouteau	-0.98	2118	29.7	7.9	27.7	74.4	80.2	3231	985

71

ST	COUNTY	USDA	AMEN	OBES	DIAB	INACT	M AGE	W AGE	ALT ft	ALT m
MT	Custer	-1.06	2171	23.3	7.1	24	75	80.7	2845	867
MT	Daniels	-3.82	3050	22.9	6.5	23.6	73.6	79.5	2635	803
MT	Dawson	-1.01	2138	27.8	6.7	29.7	75.3	80.5	2575	785
MT	Deer Lodge	1.51	596	27	6.7	22.9	76.6	79.8	6664	2031
MT	Fallon	-1.33	2292	25	6.3	30.8	75.7	81	3018	920
MT	Fergus	2.63	350	23.7	6	22.7	75.3	80.8	3779	1152
MT	Flathead	2.80	332	21.8	5.6	19.2	75.5	80.5	4908	1496
MT	Gallatin	3.86	210	17.4	4.4	17.3	78.3	82.4	6274	1912
MT	Garfield	0.65	985	25.8	6.2	26.8	75.7	81	2810	856
MT	Glacier	4.69	150	30.9	11.5	30.8	74.4	80.2	4812	1467
MT	Golden Valley	0.06	1398	27.2	6.5	24.2	75.8	80.9	4220	1286
MT	Granite	2.27	418	22.7	5.8	24.3	75.5	80.5	6118	1865
MT	Hill	-1.22	2248	32.4	7.3	28.8	74.6	80.7	2969	905
MT	Jefferson	2.27	419	20.9	6.6	19.9	75.9	80.9	5869	1789
MT	Judith Basin	1.89	499	24.7	5.8	28	75.6	81.2	5039	1536
MT	Lake	3.82	213	27.8	7	21.9	75.9	80.6	3973	1211
MT	Lewis and Clark	3.16	286	23.2	6.2	19	76.7	80.5	5337	1627
MT	Liberty	0.45	1104	26.2	5.9	32.5	74.6	80.7	3372	1028
MT	Lincoln	2.33	405	25.4	7.2	23.2	74.7	79.8	4259	1298
MT	Madison	3.22	280	24.2	6	26.3	74.6	79.8	6657	2029
MT	McCone	0.52	1053	26	6	26.2	75.7	81	2483	757
MT	Meagher	2.83	328	25	6.5	27.3	75.9	80.9	5861	1786
MT	Mineral	1.80	522	28.4	6.9	28.3	76.7	81	4712	1436
MT	Missoula	1.74	539	20.5	5.3	16.7	76.7	81	4954	1510
MT	Musselshell	1.22	724	21.5	6.6	26.7	75.8	80.9	3510	1070
MT	Park	3.61	237	21.2	5.2	21.4	78.3	82.4	6960	2122
MT	Petroleum	1.86	509	23.7	6.6	24.5	76.1	81	2958	901
MT	Phillips	0.29	1225	26.4	6.2	30.4	75.3	80.8	2666	813
MT	Pondera	3.45	251	29	7	28.2	74.4	80.2	4062	1238
MT	Powder River	-1.02	2145	24	6.4	29.1	75	80.7	3503	1068
MT	Powell	1.79	524	24.4	7	25.5	75.5	80.5	5676	1730
MT	Prairie	-0.39	1745	27.5	6.6	27.8	75.7	81	2724	830
MT	Ravalli	1.59	572	20.8	5.3	20	77.1	81.3	5918	1804
MT	Richland	-0.22	1615	30.9	6	28.9	75.3	80.5	2283	696
MT	Roosevelt	-2.45	2763	34.8	12.1	32.4	73.6	79.5	2288	697
MT	Rosebud	-0.34	1701	35.1	9.1	29.3	76.1	81	3092	943
MT	Sanders	2.33	406	23.1	7.1	25.5	74.7	79.8	4102	1250
MT	Sheridan	-2.12	2625	27.4	6	28.5	73.6	79.5	2233	681
MT	Silver Bow	2.15	443	25.2	7.1	24.6	74.6	79.8	6456	1968
MT	Stillwater	2.63	351	26.6	6.3	22.3	75.8	80.9	5036	1535
MT	Sweet Grass	3.19	282	20.8	6.2	27.9	75.8	80.9	5623	1714
MT	Teton	3.88	206	24.8	6.2	25.1	74.4	80.2	4502	1372
MT	Toole	0.97	826	28.6	7.6	26.6	74.6	80.7	3508	1069
MT	Treasure	-0.02	1455	24.6	6.2	26.8	76.1	81	3032	924
MT	Valley	-0.03	1465	27.2	7.8	28.7	75.7	81	2581	787
MT	Wheatland	3.07	298	25.4	6.6	29.9	75.8	80.9	4859	1481
MT	Wibaux	-0.81	2016	26.1	6.5	29.9	75.7	81	2715	828

HEALTHIEST PLACES TO LIVE

ST	COUNTY	USDA	AMEN	OBES	DIAB	INACT	M AGE	W AGE	ALT ft	ALT m
MT	Yellowstone	1.08	781	27.6	7.3	23.5	76.1	81	3482	1061
NC	Alamance	-0.96	2108	33.6	10.1	27.7	74.2	79.4	643	196
NC	Alexander	1.17	742	28.3	8.9	24	73.9	78.9	1197	365
NC	Alleghany	1.47	606	25.5	8.6	28.2	73.7	79.2	2868	874
NC	Anson	0.06	1399	35.5	12.3	29.5	70.9	77.1	336	102
NC	Ashe	2.28	417	23.3	7.4	24.7	73.7	79.2	3198	975
NC	Avery	1.95	486	30.2	9.1	20.7	73.1	79.5	3536	1078
NC	Beaufort	0.02	1421	36.2	10.4	28.4	73	78.5	23	7
NC	Bertie	-0.30	1668	37.7	13	29.9	68.8	76.2	38	12
NC	Bladen	-0.31	1681	37.1	12.2	30	69.3	76.7	86	26
NC	Brunswick	1.12	765	29.9	8.6	25.6	74.4	80	40	12
NC	Buncombe	2.18	437	24	7.9	19.6	74.6	80.5	2684	818
NC	Burke	1.82	518	28.5	10.1	27.2	73.3	79.3	1492	455
NC	Cabarrus	-1.08	2181	30.7	9.4	23.1	74.2	79	644	196
NC	Caldwell	1.51	597	30.6	9.1	26.7	72.9	78.7	1503	458
NC	Camden	0.42	1127	32	9.8	25.4	72.9	78.2	10	3
NC	Carteret	1.22	725	28.5	8.4	27.2	74.6	79.8	13	4
NC	Caswell	0.45	1105	30.9	12.1	27.9	71.7	78.1	577	176
NC	Catawba	1.32	667	26.4	8.2	26.1	74	79.1	981	299
NC	Chatham	0.41	1134	24.8	8	21.7	75.4	80.5	424	129
NC	Cherokee	3.00	308	27.4	9.7	25.5	73.4	79.7	2133	650
NC	Chowan	0.51	1062	30.4	10.8	28.1	73	78.8	18	5
NC	Clay	3.05	300	25.8	8.1	22.3	73.4	79.7	2683	818
NC	Cleveland	0.76	929	32.5	11.6	29.2	71.8	78.2	889	271
NC	Columbus	-0.39	1746	33.9	11.3	27.8	69.4	76.8	70	21
NC	Craven	0.19	1317	33.9	10.5	26.3	74.4	79.2	27	8
NC	Cumberland	-0.71	1951	33.1	12.4	29.8	72.6	78.4	147	45
NC	Currituck	0.88	868	32.3	9.1	23.5	73.7	79.6	6	2
NC	Dare	1.63	564	28.5	8.4	23.7	75.9	80.4	4	1
NC	Davidson	-0.09	1519	29.3	8.9	29.1	73	78.8	761	232
NC	Davie	-0.46	1794	28.5	8.9	27.7	74.7	80.2	749	228
NC	Duplin	-1.51	2383	34.5	11.5	33.1	71.3	78.3	89	27
NC	Durham	-0.26	1643	30.1	9.4	20.8	74.4	80.1	369	112
NC	Edgecombe	-2.13	2630	39.7	12.1	30.4	68.9	75.6	71	22
NC	Forsyth	-1.06	2172	25.5	8.8	21	74.5	79.5	848	258
NC	Franklin	-1.43	2343	34.2	9.8	28.1	72.4	78.8	314	96
NC	Gaston	0.42	1128	26.2	9	28.4	71.9	78.1	763	233
NC	Gates	-1.00	2132	34.7	11.2	29.4	72.9	78.2	28	9
NC	Graham	3.14	290	28.2	10.1	25.9	72	78.6	2801	854
NC	Granville	-0.94	2095	31.9	10.9	26.6	71.8	78.4	424	129
NC	Greene	-2.33	2701	33.3	11.3	29.2	70.4	76.7	79	24
NC	Guilford	-0.85	2038	28	9.8	23	74.9	80.5	787	240
NC	Halifax	-1.30	2282	38.7	12.6	33.3	69.5	76.9	153	47
NC	Harnett	-0.52	1827	31.6	9.5	27.6	72.6	78.2	247	75
NC	Haywood	2.23	427	28.8	8.5	22.7	74	80.2	3581	1092
NC	Henderson	1.99	475	24.3	7.9	22.1	75.6	80.8	2413	736
NC	Hertford	-1.25	2264	35.5	12	33.6	69.8	75.8	40	12

ST	COUNTY	USDA	AMEN	OBES	DIAB	INACT	M AGE	W AGE	ALT ft	ALT m
NC	Hoke	-1.26	2269	33.2	12.7	29.4	71	76.9	278	85
NC	Hyde	1.48	603	32.2	11.3	30.1	71.6	77.6	5	2
NC	Iredell	1.32	668	28.2	8.1	24.7	73.9	80.2	895	273
NC	Jackson	2.62	355	33.4	11.1	24.1	74.6	79.6	3365	1026
NC	Johnston	-1.16	2221	33.9	10.5	27.7	73.2	79.4	204	62
NC	Jones	-1.59	2419	34.8	12.1	31.4	71.3	78.3	45	14
NC	Lee	-0.68	1930	30.2	10.3	23.5	73.3	80	324	99
NC	Lenoir	-1.71	2475	32.4	11.4	33.2	70.6	77.8	77	24
NC	Lincoln	1.49	600	27.2	10	22.9	73.3	78.9	879	268
NC	Macon	3.33	266	26.3	8.1	23	74.5	80.8	3085	940
NC	Madison	1.92	490	28.8	8.7	21.4	73.9	79	2649	807
NC	Martin	-2.93	2892	35.8	12	27.8	69.5	76.4	45	14
NC	McDowell	2.21	430	33.6	10.6	29.4	73.2	79.2	1811	552
NC	Mecklenburg	0.82	903	25.6	8.5	20.4	75.6	80.7	687	209
NC	Mitchell	1.55	585	28.7	9	24.4	72.8	79.1	3130	954
NC	Montgomery	1.37	646	32.6	10.7	27.5	71.8	78	522	159
NC	Moore	0.12	1356	27.2	7.8	22.5	75.3	80.9	426	130
NC	Nash	-1.39	2318	33.6	10.7	28.3	71.9	78.5	187	57
NC	New Hanover	1.25	710	25.5	10.2	20.6	75.5	80.8	22	7
NC	Northampton	-0.65	1913	34.3	12.1	31.9	68.9	77	97	30
NC	Onslow	0.74	935	30.2	9.9	24	74.5	79.6	42	13
NC	Orange	-1.39	2319	22.6	6.5	16.5	77.4	81.5	604	184
NC	Pamlico	1.00	814	28	9.8	25.2	73	78.5	13	4
NC	Pasquotank	0.43	1122	33.4	10.9	25.9	73.7	78.3	8	3
NC	Pender	0.52	1054	32.2	10.7	23.7	74.3	79.5	37	11
NC	Perquimans	0.50	1073	34	9.7	26.6	73	78.8	12	4
NC	Person	1.33	662	33.1	11	27	72.2	78.3	565	172
NC	Pitt	-1.74	2485	35.6	9.3	25.3	72.9	78	46	14
NC	Polk	1.84	512	22.8	7	23	74.9	80.8	1220	372
NC	Randolph	-0.01	1447	29.6	9.6	29.5	73.6	79.7	649	198
NC	Richmond	0.89	865	31.7	10.7	29.8	70.7	77.1	335	102
NC	Robeson	-1.52	2389	40.9	13.3	38.5	68.7	76.8	150	46
NC	Rockingham	0.10	1369	33.3	10	29.6	71.7	77.9	703	214
NC	Rowan	-0.10	1528	31.6	10.8	29.2	73.4	79.3	746	227
NC	Rutherford	0.45	1106	31.2	9.9	29.8	71.4	78	1114	340
NC	Sampson	-1.63	2440	35.8	10.9	28.4	70.9	77.6	124	38
NC	Scotland	-0.69	1935	36	13.4	28.4	70.5	76.9	252	77
NC	Stanly	0.68	964	26.6	9.6	30.8	73.2	79.4	515	157
NC	Stokes	0.02	1422	27.9	8.3	25	73.1	79.5	976	297
NC	Surry	1.24	716	31.9	11.2	26.7	72.8	79	1231	375
NC	Swain	2.97	311	32.5	12.1	28.5	72	78.6	3171	966
NC	Transylvania	2.40	388	24.5	7.4	22.8	75.5	82.1	2824	861
NC	Tyrrell	0.67	970	32	11.1	28	71.6	77.6	5	1
NC	Union	-0.34	1702	27.9	8.3	22.4	75.2	79.8	566	173
NC	Vance	0.05	1404	32.8	12.1	32	69.5	76.5	384	117
NC	Wake	0.23	1278	25.7	7.8	18.5	77.6	82	324	99
NC	Warren	-0.25	1634	36.8	12.6	29.8	70.4	76.9	301	92

HEALTHIEST PLACES TO LIVE

ST	COUNTY	USDA	AMEN	OBES	DIAB	INACT	M AGE	W AGE	ALT ft	ALT m
NC	Washington	0.31	1210	34.9	12	28.4	71.6	77.6	15	4
NC	Watauga	1.82	519	24.9	8.8	20.8	76.7	80.8	3298	1005
NC	Wayne	-1.41	2326	32.8	10.9	31.4	71.6	77.6	126	38
NC	Wilkes	1.88	502	30.2	10	30.7	72.9	79	1490	454
NC	Wilson	-1.23	2253	32.2	11.2	30.9	71.1	77.6	128	39
NC	Yadkin	0.20	1308	30.1	9.4	27.6	73.5	79.3	934	285
NC	Yancey	1.37	647	27.9	7.8	26.5	74.5	79.8	3365	1026
ND	Adams	-1.82	2515	30.6	7.5	26.2	75.7	81.6	2654	809
ND	Barnes	-2.83	2869	26.7	5.6	25.6	75.9	81.3	1394	425
ND	Benson	-3.08	2921	33.3	9.7	33	74.3	81.1	1549	472
ND	Billings	-0.76	1982	29.2	6.9	26.3	75.7	82.2	2591	790
ND	Bottineau	-3.44	2994	31.8	8.1	26.1	74.4	80.2	1584	483
ND	Bowman	-1.01	2139	30	7.5	29.5	75.7	81.6	2974	906
ND	Burke	-2.07	2608	28.8	7.8	30.1	76.5	81.9	2108	643
ND	Burleigh	-2.01	2584	25	6.9	21.1	77.4	83	1900	579
ND	Cass	-4.84	3096	28.2	7	22.3	77.2	82.9	1008	307
ND	Cavalier	-3.52	3007	31.3	7	27	75	81.2	1549	472
ND	Dickey	-2.96	2900	29.5	7.5	28.4	75.8	82	1534	468
ND	Divide	-2.06	2602	29.8	6.5	30.5	76.5	81.9	2146	654
ND	Dunn	0.20	1309	30.6	8.8	31.3	75.7	82.2	2259	689
ND	Eddy	-2.47	2771	26.9	7.4	29.9	75.2	81.1	1517	462
ND	Emmons	-1.81	2510	32.1	7.5	28.6	74.6	80.6	1893	577
ND	Foster	-2.53	2793	28.4	7	27.5	75.2	81.1	1531	467
ND	Golden Valley	-1.55	2401	30.2	6.6	30.2	75.7	82.2	2696	822
ND	Grand Forks	-5.01	3100	30.9	7.4	23	76.5	81.4	1015	309
ND	Grant	-1.79	2503	37.9	7	29.8	75.7	81.6	2239	682
ND	Griggs	-3.18	2942	28.1	6.5	24.3	75.2	81.1	1449	442
ND	Hettinger	-1.81	2511	27.2	7	29.1	75.7	81.6	2571	784
ND	Kidder	-1.40	2323	30.7	7.3	29.6	75.2	81.3	1852	564
ND	LaMoure	-3.35	2978	26.8	6.5	25.8	75.8	82	1543	470
ND	Logan	-2.59	2808	33	7.7	32	75.2	81.3	2002	610
ND	McHenry	-3.30	2965	32.7	7.8	36.1	74.4	80.2	1541	470
ND	McIntosh	-2.21	2655	32.9	6.7	31.4	75.2	81.3	2052	626
ND	McKenzie	-0.05	1483	33.5	8.3	28.6	75.7	82.2	2249	685
ND	McLean	-1.41	2327	30.9	7.3	29.4	75.8	80.8	1966	599
ND	Mercer	-1.60	2425	31.5	8.1	27.1	75.8	80.8	2015	614
ND	Morton	-1.30	2283	30.9	7.1	26	74.6	80.6	2049	624
ND	Mountrail	-1.35	2301	35	8.3	33.3	75.7	81.4	2190	668
ND	Nelson	-3.72	3040	30.2	7.2	28.1	75.2	81.1	1487	453
ND	Oliver	-2.18	2646	29.1	7.4	24.7	77.4	83	2030	619
ND	Pembina	-5.18	3104	32.7	8	29.7	75.8	81.4	888	271
ND	Pierce	-2.72	2844	31.9	7.4	31.6	74.3	81.1	1576	480
ND	Ramsey	-3.10	2930	31.9	6.8	24.9	75	81.2	1493	455
ND	Ransom	-4.21	3085	31.6	7.5	28.2	75.9	81.3	1199	365
ND	Renville	-2.70	2841	26.6	6.8	25.1	74.4	80.2	1713	522
ND	Richland	-3.81	3049	32.3	6.4	27.8	76.8	82.2	1022	311
ND	Rolette	-2.21	2656	39.5	13.3	35.4	74.4	80.2	1799	548

ST	COUNTY	USDA	AMEN	OBES	DIAB	INACT	M AGE	W AGE	ALT ft	ALT m
ND	Sargent	-3.61	3024	30.2	8	29.1	75.8	82	1239	378
ND	Sheridan	-1.89	2543	30.7	7.3	29.5	74.3	81.1	1865	568
ND	Sioux	-0.96	2109	41.8	13.5	32.3	74.6	80.6	2029	618
ND	Slope	-0.78	1997	28.8	6.8	30.3	75.7	81.6	2845	867
ND	Stark	-1.74	2486	29.2	7.8	27.1	75.7	81.6	2498	761
ND	Steele	-3.56	3012	32.9	6.9	26.3	75.2	81.1	1266	386
ND	Stutsman	-1.79	2504	30	7.7	26.9	75.2	81.3	1674	510
ND	Towner	-3.99	3067	29.7	7.1	24.6	75	81.2	1562	476
ND	Traill	-5.12	3102	32.6	6.3	29.8	76.5	81.4	943	287
ND	Walsh	-3.95	3061	32.5	6.6	27.3	75.8	81.4	1124	343
ND	Ward	-2.01	2585	30.2	8.1	27.4	75.7	81.4	1934	589
ND	Wells	-2.27	2682	28.6	6.4	27.4	74.3	81.1	1681	512
ND	Williams	-2.01	2586	30.1	7.3	30.8	76.5	81.9	2205	672
NE	Adams	-2.36	2720	29.7	7.3	23.5	76.8	81.8	1949	594
NE	Antelope	-2.49	2781	28.9	8	27.3	75.3	81.4	1872	570
NE	Arthur	-0.25	1635	27.4	7.3	26.8	76.1	80.2	3671	1119
NE	Banner	-0.75	1972	30.4	7.9	26.9	75.8	80.7	4655	1419
NE	Blaine	-0.81	2017	29.7	7	28.4	75.6	81.2	2651	808
NE	Boone	-1.21	2243	28.6	6.9	28.1	75.6	80.5	1904	580
NE	Box Butte	-0.02	1456	31.7	8.2	25.4	75.4	80.3	4169	1271
NE	Boyd	-2.64	2825	28.2	6.2	28.7	75.6	80.9	1726	526
NE	Brown	-1.10	2190	28.6	8	27.1	75.6	81.2	2601	793
NE	Buffalo	0.04	1412	29.6	7	23.1	76.7	81.7	2185	666
NE	Burt	-1.73	2480	30.9	8.1	31.5	74.2	79.8	1226	374
NE	Butler	-3.37	2981	27.9	6.3	27.7	75.5	81.1	1543	470
NE	Cass	-2.12	2626	28.2	8.1	26	76.1	81.2	1165	355
NE	Cedar	-2.01	2587	27.9	6.9	28.6	76.5	82	1486	453
NE	Chase	-1.47	2364	26.1	6.8	26.4	76.1	81.4	3335	1017
NE	Cherry	-0.74	1969	27.3	6.5	28.6	75.6	81.2	3201	976
NE	Cheyenne	-1.68	2462	29.1	6.8	24	75.8	80.7	4268	1301
NE	Clay	-3.36	2980	34.7	8.4	30.3	75.9	80.7	1772	540
NE	Colfax	-0.72	1962	32.6	7.9	28.2	75.5	81.1	1498	457
NE	Cuming	-0.77	1990	29.3	6.6	28.4	75.7	81.6	1438	438
NE	Custer	-1.40	2324	29.5	6.8	29.3	75.6	81.2	2616	797
NE	Dakota	-1.76	2494	34.5	9.3	30.9	74.8	79.6	1227	374
NE	Dawes	-0.39	1747	28.4	7.1	24.3	75.4	80.3	3827	1166
NE	Dawson	0.56	1036	32.1	8.4	26.4	75.6	80.9	2519	768
NE	Deuel	-0.61	1886	27.9	6.5	28.2	76.1	81.4	3731	1137
NE	Dixon	-1.71	2476	33.9	6.7	30.3	74.8	79.6	1406	429
NE	Dodge	-0.55	1843	29.8	7.9	29	75.2	81.5	1301	397
NE	Douglas	-1.92	2553	27.1	8.1	23.6	75.6	80.7	1159	353
NE	Dundy	-1.93	2559	30.2	8.2	30.4	76.1	81.4	3287	1002
NE	Fillmore	-4.00	3069	29.1	6.9	26.7	75.9	80.7	1636	499
NE	Franklin	-1.56	2408	28.5	7.8	31.8	75.6	80.3	2038	621
NE	Frontier	0.29	1226	33.3	7	30.7	76	81	2645	806
NE	Furnas	-1.63	2441	33.2	8.2	25.7	75.6	80.3	2287	697
NE	Gage	-2.26	2679	32.9	8.2	27	76.3	80.9	1366	416

HEALTHIEST PLACES TO LIVE

ST	COUNTY	USDA	AMEN	OBES	DIAB	INACT	M AGE	W AGE	ALT ft	ALT m
NE	Garden	2.14	444	27.9	7.8	29.8	76.1	80.2	3804	1159
NE	Garfield	-1.42	2334	27.2	6.8	23.8	76.2	80.7	2281	695
NE	Gosper	-1.08	2182	28.6	7.6	25.8	75.6	80.9	2452	747
NE	Grant	-0.08	1512	25.4	6.9	29.8	76.1	80.2	3773	1150
NE	Greeley	-0.60	1880	33.1	7.6	28.3	76.2	80.7	2052	625
NE	Hall	-1.83	2519	31.6	8	26.1	75.1	80.8	1931	589
NE	Hamilton	-2.83	2870	31.1	6.9	27.8	77.1	81.3	1798	548
NE	Harlan	-0.41	1765	26.9	6.7	27.9	75.6	80.3	2133	650
NE	Hayes	-2.55	2798	28.3	6.5	28.2	76.1	81.4	3023	922
NE	Hitchcock	-0.97	2111	32.9	7.5	31	76	81	2858	871
NE	Holt	-1.67	2454	28.7	7.4	30.8	75.6	80.9	2041	622
NE	Hooker	-1.64	2443	33.4	7.3	26.7	76.1	80.2	3386	1032
NE	Howard	0.30	1215	29.4	6.4	28.9	76.2	80.7	1917	584
NE	Jefferson	-2.42	2748	30.7	8.1	30.6	75.9	80.7	1434	437
NE	Johnson	-2.60	2811	33.2	7.8	28.9	75.4	80.8	1243	379
NE	Kearney	-3.34	2973	26.9	6	24.7	75.6	80.3	2141	653
NE	Keith	1.50	599	28.4	6.9	21.7	76.1	80.2	3353	1022
NE	Keya Paha	-3.69	3033	28.7	7.1	32.7	75.6	80.9	2271	692
NE	Kimball	-0.08	1513	28.7	7.6	24.3	75.8	80.7	4933	1504
NE	Knox	-1.32	2289	27.8	7.2	29.5	75.3	81.4	1595	486
NE	Lancaster	-2.55	2799	27.4	7.4	20.3	77.8	82.3	1296	395
NE	Lincoln	0.25	1254	31.8	8	27.4	76.1	81.4	2983	909
NE	Logan	-1.41	2328	27.6	6.9	26.6	76.1	80.2	2988	911
NE	Loup	-1.42	2335	29.2	7.5	27.1	75.6	81.2	2424	739
NE	Madison	-0.53	1834	28.5	7.5	23.4	75.6	80.8	1703	519
NE	McPherson	-0.90	2070	29.8	7.9	28.1	76.1	80.2	3326	1014
NE	Merrick	-2.29	2688	34.9	7.8	26.8	75.6	80.5	1712	522
NE	Morrill	1.63	565	28.3	9.8	26.6	74.4	80.9	4004	1220
NE	Nance	-0.42	1771	28	8	29.5	75.6	80.5	1736	529
NE	Nemaha	-1.88	2535	33.2	7.3	29	75.4	80.8	1049	320
NE	Nuckolls	-1.85	2526	30.3	6.8	27.6	76.8	81.8	1719	524
NE	Otoe	-2.36	2721	32.2	7.7	27.2	76.6	80.9	1149	350
NE	Pawnee	-2.50	2785	31.2	8	31.5	75.4	80.8	1276	389
NE	Perkins	-2.24	2667	26.8	6.9	29	76.1	81.4	3393	1034
NE	Phelps	-2.21	2657	30.9	6.8	25.2	75.6	80.9	2324	708
NE	Pierce	-2.58	2806	31.7	7.2	32.6	75.3	81.4	1718	524
NE	Platte	-0.60	1881	27.9	6.9	23.6	77.2	82.1	1620	494
NE	Polk	-3.13	2933	33.7	8.3	28.4	77.1	81.3	1633	498
NE	Red Willow	-1.76	2495	30.8	7.6	24.2	76	81	2551	777
NE	Richardson	-1.91	2550	33.1	8.3	31.5	75.4	80.8	1022	312
NE	Rock	-1.06	2173	30.9	7.8	29.5	75.6	80.9	2391	729
NE	Saline	-3.04	2912	32.9	7.4	27.2	76.9	81.8	1466	447
NE	Sarpy	-2.03	2590	28.9	7.7	20.8	77.6	80.9	1121	342
NE	Saunders	-2.60	2812	29.3	7.1	24.8	76.6	81.5	1290	393
NE	Scotts Bluff	1.11	770	32.5	8.7	27	74.4	80.9	4149	1265
NE	Seward	-3.21	2951	29.1	8	23	76.7	81.5	1499	457
NE	Sheridan	2.00	472	27	7.8	29.7	74.4	80.9	3829	1167

ST	COUNTY	USDA	AMEN	OBES	DIAB	INACT	M AGE	W AGE	ALT ft	ALT m
NE	Sherman	0.26	1247	31.4	6.7	29.3	76.2	80.7	2157	657
NE	Sioux	-0.67	1924	28.4	6.5	27.5	75.4	80.3	4450	1356
NE	Stanton	-0.61	1887	32.5	6.5	30.8	75.7	81.6	1609	490
NE	Thayer	-3.12	2931	29.5	7.6	27.5	75.9	80.7	1563	476
NE	Thomas	-1.61	2431	33.3	7.2	27.7	75.6	81.2	2979	908
NE	Thurston	-1.96	2569	37.1	12.9	34.2	74.2	79.8	1345	410
NE	Valley	-0.06	1495	29.5	8	28.6	76.2	80.7	2202	671
NE	Washington	-2.35	2711	29.4	7.3	21.7	77	81.2	1200	366
NE	Wayne	-4.02	3071	29	6.8	25.8	76.5	82	1611	491
NE	Webster	-1.88	2536	30.5	8.5	31.1	76.8	81.8	1880	573
NE	Wheeler	-2.04	2597	26.8	6.9	28.6	76.2	80.7	2104	641
NE	York	-4.05	3075	35	7.4	28.1	76.9	81.8	1642	500
NH	Belknap	0.80	912	26.4	8	21.7	76	82	755	230
NH	Carroll	0.93	849	24.7	7.3	20	77.1	82.4	1033	315
NH	Cheshire	0.26	1248	28.2	7.8	21.3	77.4	81.4	1041	317
NH	Coos	-0.09	1520	30.8	8	27.8	74.3	80.4	1857	566
NH	Grafton	0.32	1206	23.7	7.1	19	78.8	82	1492	455
NH	Hillsborough	0.07	1391	26.7	7.9	21.8	77.3	81.4	652	199
NH	Merrimack	0.02	1423	25.3	6.9	20	77.1	81.4	729	222
NH	Rockingham	0.34	1193	25.3	6.8	20.1	77.8	81.7	266	81
NH	Strafford	-0.10	1529	29.3	8.3	22.9	76.5	81	423	129
NH	Sullivan	-0.17	1574	28.8	7.8	25	75.6	81.2	1179	359
NJ	Atlantic	-0.04	1476	28	8.8	24.6	73.6	79.8	48	15
NJ	Bergen	1.20	733	21.6	6.8	23.3	79.3	83.5	192	59
NJ	Burlington	-1.30	2284	27.2	8.4	23.4	76.5	81.3	70	21
NJ	Camden	-1.15	2216	27.8	9.2	27.9	74	79.7	86	26
NJ	Cape May	0.07	1392	24.9	8.4	22.3	74.2	80.2	13	4
NJ	Cumberland	0.38	1157	33.2	10.2	30.7	72.7	78.6	47	14
NJ	Essex	-0.02	1457	25.8	9.2	27.5	73.8	79.8	234	71
NJ	Gloucester	-0.61	1888	26.7	9.4	25.1	74.6	80	78	24
NJ	Hudson	0.49	1081	23.9	8.3	28.6	75.8	81.3	37	11
NJ	Hunterdon	0.83	898	20.5	6.2	18.4	79.4	82.7	400	122
NJ	Mercer	-0.80	2009	24.8	8.7	25.2	76.2	81.4	130	40
NJ	Middlesex	-0.57	1862	23.5	8.1	27.1	78	82.4	85	26
NJ	Monmouth	0.64	990	21.3	7.5	21.2	77.3	81.6	111	34
NJ	Morris	1.30	677	21.4	6.6	20.5	79.5	82.2	636	194
NJ	Ocean	0.66	979	26.7	8.6	24	76	81.8	85	26
NJ	Passaic	1.30	678	24.2	8.2	27.4	76.3	81.1	587	179
NJ	Salem	-0.20	1600	33.8	9.3	30.6	73.4	78.7	44	13
NJ	Somerset	-1.44	2346	21.3	6.2	21.2	78.7	82.5	196	60
NJ	Sussex	1.30	679	26.4	7.4	21.8	77.2	80.6	806	246
NJ	Union	0.14	1341	22	8.2	25.2	77.2	81.1	127	39
NJ	Warren	0.95	838	27.1	7.5	25.4	76.7	80.7	604	184
NM	Bernalillo	3.77	216	19.9	6	15.9	74.8	81.1	5967	1819
NM	Catron	6.24	53	24.6	6.3	19.3	73.3	79.8	7377	2248
NM	Chaves	3.87	207	29.6	7.5	25.9	73	79.7	4233	1290
NM	Cibola	3.04	302	32.3	11.2	26	73.4	80.4	7096	2163

ST	COUNTY	USDA	AMEN	OBES	DIAB	INACT	M AGE	W AGE	ALT ft	ALT m
NM	Colfax	3.70	226	21.1	6.2	23.7	75.4	80.3	7214	2199
NM	Curry	0.94	842	27.1	8.6	27.4	74.2	79.1	4437	1352
NM	De Baca	3.43	254	23	6.7	26.4	72.9	79.6	4435	1352
NM	Dona Ana	4.77	146	25.6	6.9	17.5	76.3	80.9	4463	1360
NM	Eddy	4.97	127	31.2	9.9	26.9	73.8	80.1	3739	1140
NM	Grant	6.45	50	23.8	6	19.2	74.7	80.6	5823	1775
NM	Guadalupe	2.66	346	25	6.3	22.9	72.9	79.6	5179	1578
NM	Harding	1.28	690	28.3	6.2	20.5	75.4	80.3	5044	1537
NM	Hidalgo	3.37	262	24.1	6.1	23.5	73.2	79.8	4735	1443
NM	Lea	1.79	525	31.7	7.8	29.8	73.2	78.9	3784	1153
NM	Lincoln	4.26	178	20.8	5.5	20	76.3	81.8	5852	1784
NM	Los Alamos	3.04	303	18.8	5.3	14.4	80.1	83	7655	2333
NM	Luna	2.87	324	27.6	7.1	21.4	73.2	79.8	4514	1376
NM	McKinley	3.39	259	35.9	12.4	25.9	71.5	79.5	6942	2116
NM	Mora	5.22	96	21.5	6.7	21.8	75.4	81.8	7166	2184
NM	Otero	4.00	198	25.9	7.8	22	75.6	79.7	5301	1616
NM	Quay	1.66	554	24.7	6.1	27.3	72.9	79.6	4323	1318
NM	Rio Arriba	5.23	95	24.5	6.3	22.4	71	79.5	7657	2334
NM	Roosevelt	1.44	620	27.2	5.9	28	73.6	79.3	4240	1292
NM	San Juan	2.83	329	29.6	8.5	24.1	73.9	80.1	6047	1843
NM	San Miguel	3.73	218	22.7	6.4	19	72.7	79.8	5930	1807
NM	Sandoval	3.66	228	24.3	6.4	19.1	76.4	81.1	6720	2048
NM	Santa Fe	3.02	306	14.1	3.9	12	78.1	82.9	6924	2110
NM	Sierra	6.72	41	26.5	6.1	24.3	73.3	79.8	5445	1660
NM	Socorro	3.13	292	26.9	7.3	21.8	74.3	79.4	5989	1825
NM	Taos	4.16	189	18.8	5.9	15.7	75.4	81.8	8533	2601
NM	Torrance	4.02	197	25.2	6.5	23.8	74.3	79.4	6455	1967
NM	Union	0.99	820	24.3	5.9	24.6	75.4	80.3	5423	1653
NM	Valencia	3.04	304	27.5	7	24.1	73.4	79.6	5424	1653
NV	Carson City	7.29	27	23.1	7.1	19.8	74	79.6	5780	1762
NV	Churchill	5.42	85	28.9	7.3	26	75.1	80.1	4754	1449
NV	Clark	4.86	140	26	8.8	25.6	74.1	79.7	3305	1008
NV	Douglas	7.61	22	21.7	6.3	16.4	79.1	82.7	6047	1843
NV	Elko	2.05	460	30.6	7.2	24.7	75	79.7	6144	1873
NV	Esmeralda	4.12	192	28.6	7.4	23.2	72.2	78.8	5670	1728
NV	Eureka	1.92	491	26.8	7.2	25.6	74.9	80.3	6211	1893
NV	Humboldt	3.87	208	29.4	7	24.4	74.7	80.1	5085	1550
NV	Lander	3.67	227	26.9	7.6	24.3	74.9	80.3	6000	1829
NV	Lincoln	3.86	211	26.3	8.7	22.9	74.1	79.7	5266	1605
NV	Lyon	5.70	74	30	7.4	25.3	74.5	79.9	5207	1587
NV	Mineral	5.71	73	32	9.9	28.2	72.2	78.8	5872	1790
NV	Nye	4.97	128	31	7.9	28.7	72.2	78.8	5823	1775
NV	Pershing	4.23	184	29	7.7	26	74.7	80.1	4891	1491
NV	Storey	5.11	113	22.7	7.4	22.4	74.5	79.9	5565	1696
NV	Washoe	6.77	40	22.6	6.4	17.2	75.2	80.3	5359	1633
NV	White Pine	3.04	305	30	7.5	24	74.9	80.3	6825	2080
NY	Albany	0.30	1216	24.2	7.1	22.4	76.1	80.8	770	235

ST	COUNTY	USDA	AMEN	OBES	DIAB	INACT	M AGE	W AGE	ALT ft	ALT m
NY	Allegany	-0.90	2071	28.8	8.5	25.7	75.6	79.9	1826	557
NY	Bronx	1.04	799	27.3	9.6	30.1	73.9	80.5	77	24
NY	Broome	-0.84	2029	29.5	8.4	23.6	75.5	81.2	1317	401
NY	Cattaraugus	-0.32	1689	28.8	9.1	26	74.5	80	1700	518
NY	Cayuga	-1.44	2347	24.3	7.9	24.9	76	80.8	781	238
NY	Chautauqua	-0.26	1644	28.1	7.6	24.6	75.7	80.4	1376	419
NY	Chemung	-1.13	2209	26.3	8.8	26.2	75.4	80	1303	397
NY	Chenango	-1.41	2329	27	7.1	23.9	74.9	79.8	1448	441
NY	Clinton	-0.34	1703	28.9	7.6	24	75.8	80.5	918	280
NY	Columbia	-0.33	1691	25.3	6.7	21.1	75.9	80.6	620	189
NY	Cortland	-1.55	2402	26.7	7.8	26.7	75.2	80.2	1479	451
NY	Delaware	0.35	1188	27.4	7.6	26.3	75	80	1824	556
NY	Dutchess	-0.07	1502	27.3	9	22.5	77.4	81.6	537	164
NY	Erie	-0.70	1944	28.4	9	25.6	75.3	80.2	936	285
NY	Essex	-0.26	1645	27.4	7.9	22.4	75.6	80.7	1541	470
NY	Franklin	-0.63	1898	28.2	8.2	25.4	75	80.1	1397	426
NY	Fulton	-0.24	1632	28.5	7.9	25.9	75.2	81.1	1222	372
NY	Genesee	-2.94	2893	27.8	8.7	23.7	76.3	81.2	834	254
NY	Greene	0.31	1211	28.2	8.2	25.1	73.8	80	1420	433
NY	Hamilton	0.24	1266	24.7	8.6	21.4	75.6	80.7	1985	605
NY	Herkimer	-1.59	2420	31.9	8	26.1	75.4	79.8	1534	468
NY	Jefferson	-1.27	2270	31.3	8.7	26.8	75.8	80.7	544	166
NY	Kings	-0.17	1575	24.5	9.5	27.6	76.8	82.3	40	12
NY	Lewis	-2.79	2859	28.3	8.4	26.1	75.4	81	1300	396
NY	Livingston	-0.91	2076	27.4	8.3	24.3	76.5	81.2	1046	319
NY	Madison	-0.94	2096	26.3	7.1	22.4	76	80.5	1224	373
NY	Monroe	-0.75	1973	30.1	8.5	20.4	76.9	81.4	492	150
NY	Montgomery	-2.63	2820	30	7.4	27.9	74.3	80.7	712	217
NY	Nassau	0.76	930	20.8	7.3	22.3	79.4	83.3	94	29
NY	New York	-0.31	1682	15.2	7.2	16.4	78.7	83.7	48	15
NY	Niagara	-0.52	1828	28.4	8.1	28.1	74.9	80.1	459	140
NY	Oneida	-1.65	2445	28.7	8.1	25.7	75.5	80.7	899	274
NY	Onondaga	-2.26	2680	28.2	8.4	21.6	76.3	81.3	780	238
NY	Ontario	-0.67	1925	26.2	7.7	19.2	76.9	81.7	918	280
NY	Orange	0.09	1371	25.9	8.1	25.9	76.3	80.9	634	193
NY	Orleans	-0.58	1872	29.4	8	27.5	75.5	80.6	476	145
NY	Oswego	-0.23	1621	33.7	9.2	26.1	74.9	79.3	575	175
NY	Otsego	-0.77	1991	28.1	7.6	23.9	75.7	81.3	1559	475
NY	Putnam	0.37	1170	27.9	7	22.5	78.6	82.6	649	198
NY	Queens	0.01	1430	22.2	9	28	79	83.7	54	17
NY	Rensselaer	-0.49	1810	28.7	8	23.3	75.8	80.3	823	251
NY	Richmond	0.23	1279	27.3	8.7	28.8	76.6	81.4	87	27
NY	Rockland	0.77	925	25.2	8.7	24.3	78.7	82.8	422	129
NY	Saratoga	0.11	1360	25.8	7.1	23.4	78	82.3	730	222
NY	Schenectady	-2.06	2603	27.9	8.7	24.3	76	81.2	713	217
NY	Schoharie	-0.30	1669	27.5	7.9	26.8	75.7	81.2	1503	458
NY	Schuyler	-0.03	1466	27.3	7.1	28.8	76.2	80.5	1312	400

ST	COUNTY	USDA	AMEN	OBES	DIAB	INACT	M AGE	W AGE	ALT ft	ALT m
NY	Seneca	-1.08	2183	30.9	8	31.1	75.4	80.4	608	185
NY	St. Lawrence	-2.11	2619	31.8	9.3	30.5	74.5	79.1	804	245
NY	Steuben	-0.76	1983	30.9	9.7	25	75.4	80.8	1602	488
NY	Suffolk	1.52	593	25.3	7.1	22.2	77.6	81.7	76	23
NY	Sullivan	0.14	1342	26.2	8.6	23.8	74.6	79.9	1428	435
NY	Tioga	-1.05	2164	28.3	7.5	25	76	80.6	1248	380
NY	Tompkins	-0.28	1655	23.1	7	21.7	77.7	81.4	1200	366
NY	Ulster	0.70	961	26.5	7.5	22.9	76.6	80.9	1134	346
NY	Warren	0.00	1441	29.3	8.2	19.8	76.7	81.4	1285	392
NY	Washington	-0.64	1907	28.2	8.9	30	76.1	80.2	590	180
NY	Wayne	-0.51	1817	29.4	8.7	23.3	75.6	80.7	434	132
NY	Westchester	0.80	913	17	6.7	18.6	79.2	83.3	340	104
NY	Wyoming	-2.69	2838	28.7	7.8	22.7	74.9	80.5	1479	451
NY	Yates	-0.03	1467	24.4	7.5	26.1	76	81.5	1035	315
OH	Adams	-1.84	2521	30.7	9.1	33.6	72.2	77.8	850	259
OH	Allen	-2.37	2726	36.6	9.7	26.2	74.9	79.7	842	257
OH	Ashland	-2.84	2873	30.1	10.1	28.6	75.7	80.5	1122	342
OH	Ashtabula	-0.92	2084	30.6	9.1	30.7	73.7	79.1	891	272
OH	Athens	-0.01	1448	32.2	11.4	28.7	73.7	79.3	806	246
OH	Auglaize	-3.25	2957	34.4	9.1	25.4	75.8	80.9	918	280
OH	Belmont	0.13	1349	30.6	9.9	28.5	73.5	79.4	1107	337
OH	Brown	-0.08	1514	33.8	10.2	32.4	73.5	78.7	879	268
OH	Butler	-1.65	2446	31.2	11.3	26	74.9	79	788	240
OH	Carroll	0.01	1431	30	9.1	23.6	75	80.2	1128	344
OH	Champaign	-2.35	2712	33.4	9.2	25.7	74.2	79.1	1117	341
OH	Clark	-2.03	2591	31.8	10.4	29.1	73.5	78.5	1050	320
OH	Clermont	-0.06	1496	29.5	9	24.4	75.6	79.5	819	249
OH	Clinton	-2.07	2609	28.7	9.8	31.7	74.7	80	1017	310
OH	Columbiana	-0.25	1636	35.6	11.4	28.1	74.2	79.4	1136	346
OH	Coshocton	-0.64	1908	31.1	9.5	29.5	74.5	79.6	946	288
OH	Crawford	-3.71	3037	33.9	9.6	27.1	73.8	79.6	1001	305
OH	Cuyahoga	-0.63	1899	27.8	9.5	25	74	79.7	852	260
OH	Darke	-3.31	2968	31.6	9.4	30.6	75	81.2	1037	316
OH	Defiance	-2.60	2813	28.8	9.9	27.5	75.6	80.7	727	222
OH	Delaware	-1.60	2426	25.5	8.8	21.6	77.5	81.2	942	287
OH	Erie	-0.91	2077	28.6	9.8	27.6	75.3	80.1	665	203
OH	Fairfield	-0.17	1576	30.7	9.7	27.3	75.6	79.8	938	286
OH	Fayette	-3.20	2948	29.8	9.9	30.4	73.2	78.6	970	296
OH	Franklin	-2.43	2754	30.7	10.5	25.5	73.7	79	833	254
OH	Fulton	-3.29	2962	30.1	11.1	26.1	75.8	81.1	734	224
OH	Gallia	-1.02	2146	32.2	10.4	38	72.1	79.3	732	223
OH	Geauga	-2.45	2764	23.6	8	19.9	78.1	82.5	1166	355
OH	Greene	-1.97	2574	29.6	9.3	22.7	76.5	80.5	966	294
OH	Guernsey	0.55	1042	30.1	9.7	30.8	73.4	79.4	962	293
OH	Hamilton	-1.39	2320	26.9	9.2	24.4	73.9	79.4	708	216
OH	Hancock	-2.63	2821	29.7	8.4	24.5	76.5	81.3	805	245
OH	Hardin	-3.57	3016	31	10.5	26.4	73.7	79.8	968	295

81

ST	COUNTY	USDA	AMEN	OBES	DIAB	INACT	M AGE	W AGE	ALT ft	ALT m
OH	Harrison	-0.01	1449	31.6	11.6	28.8	73.7	79	1102	336
OH	Henry	-2.68	2834	33	9.5	28.6	75.6	81	689	210
OH	Highland	-1.49	2371	31.9	9.3	33.6	73.1	78.9	983	299
OH	Hocking	-0.68	1931	33.9	10.9	27.3	73.4	79	907	277
OH	Holmes	-0.95	2105	30.6	8.9	26.7	73.5	78.5	1079	329
OH	Huron	-3.09	2927	31.8	10.1	31.7	74.6	79.4	883	269
OH	Jackson	-1.28	2275	33.8	11.2	37.5	71.4	78.2	782	238
OH	Jefferson	-0.77	1992	36.2	12	31.5	72.6	78.3	1073	327
OH	Knox	-2.89	2885	27.9	10.1	25.9	74.8	79.8	1114	340
OH	Lake	-0.42	1772	28.5	10.6	24.6	76.1	81	765	233
OH	Lawrence	-1.08	2184	39.5	11.3	35.4	71.7	77.4	756	230
OH	Licking	-0.55	1844	31.9	11.2	24.9	75.1	79.6	1030	314
OH	Logan	-1.38	2314	32.6	10.8	29.7	74.5	79.4	1114	340
OH	Lorain	-0.33	1692	31.6	10.4	27.5	75.6	80.3	774	236
OH	Lucas	-0.87	2051	31.3	10.3	27.5	73.4	78.8	629	192
OH	Madison	-3.07	2920	31.1	11.3	32.6	74.9	79.5	985	300
OH	Mahoning	-1.72	2478	28.9	9.3	26.8	73.3	79.6	1087	331
OH	Marion	-3.93	3057	31.6	10.4	30.4	74	78.8	928	283
OH	Medina	-3.16	2938	27.2	8.5	23	77.4	81.3	1019	311
OH	Meigs	-3.23	2953	31.2	9.6	31.2	71.9	78.5	759	231
OH	Mercer	-1.88	2537	27.4	9.4	26.1	75.7	80.7	872	266
OH	Miami	-2.33	2702	30	10.2	28.4	75.5	80.3	953	290
OH	Monroe	-0.21	1609	33.7	9.8	30.9	74.4	79.8	1033	315
OH	Montgomery	-2.23	2664	30.9	10.9	24.6	73.9	79.6	902	275
OH	Morgan	0.28	1233	35.2	10.4	29.7	73.2	79.8	885	270
OH	Morrow	-2.67	2831	29.8	9	31.6	74.5	79.1	1167	356
OH	Muskingum	0.42	1129	28.5	11	30.3	73.9	79.3	891	272
OH	Noble	0.63	1001	33.1	9.4	27.5	74.4	79.8	964	294
OH	Ottawa	-1.41	2330	33.3	9.5	24	75.1	79.9	589	180
OH	Paulding	-2.67	2832	29.9	8.9	29.3	74.4	80.2	714	218
OH	Perry	0.20	1310	33.2	9.9	31.9	72.8	79.6	944	288
OH	Pickaway	-2.21	2658	33.3	10.6	29.9	74.1	79.2	768	234
OH	Pike	-0.79	2005	32.2	10.5	35.2	71.4	78.4	833	254
OH	Portage	-2.17	2642	29.4	8.6	28.3	75.8	80.1	1098	335
OH	Preble	-1.97	2575	30	9.9	28.5	74.7	79.8	1035	315
OH	Putnam	-3.70	3036	30.8	8.8	26.8	76.3	81.6	732	223
OH	Richland	-2.88	2883	29.4	9.3	27	74.8	79.4	1195	364
OH	Ross	-1.10	2191	34.2	10.1	28.8	73.3	78.6	840	256
OH	Sandusky	-2.54	2795	31.8	10.6	26.3	74.6	79.7	650	198
OH	Scioto	-0.97	2112	33.7	10.2	30.3	71.3	78.3	784	239
OH	Seneca	-3.37	2982	29.8	9	28.5	74.8	79.9	811	247
OH	Shelby	-2.44	2758	29.8	9.6	29.2	75.4	80.3	994	303
OH	Stark	-2.50	2786	31.7	9.8	25.8	75.6	80.4	1108	338
OH	Summit	-2.40	2740	28.5	9.4	23.6	74.8	80	1023	312
OH	Trumbull	-2.12	2627	29.6	9.4	29.2	73.7	79.5	973	297
OH	Tuscarawas	-0.33	1693	33.4	9.8	28.4	75.3	80.3	1019	311
OH	Union	-3.50	3005	33.9	8.9	26.4	75.3	79.8	982	299

HEALTHIEST PLACES TO LIVE

ST	COUNTY	USDA	AMEN	OBES	DIAB	INACT	M AGE	W AGE	ALT ft	ALT m
OH	Van Wert	-3.60	3021	34.5	9.9	23.5	75.2	80.5	766	233
OH	Vinton	-0.64	1909	30.9	9.9	29.3	71.9	78.5	834	254
OH	Warren	-1.09	2187	26.1	9.2	22.1	76.7	80.5	848	259
OH	Washington	0.21	1299	33.1	9.9	22.5	74.7	79.5	822	251
OH	Wayne	-3.22	2952	31.7	8.9	23.5	75.4	80.4	1071	326
OH	Williams	-2.97	2904	30.3	9.2	23.7	75.8	80.7	832	254
OH	Wood	-2.80	2861	29.7	8.4	25	76.4	81.3	677	206
OH	Wyandot	-3.19	2946	32.5	10.6	30.5	75.3	80.2	847	258
OK	Adair	1.00	815	36.5	13.1	32.5	71.3	77.7	1068	325
OK	Alfalfa	-0.17	1577	31.8	9.7	32.1	74.4	79.7	1267	386
OK	Atoka	3.20	281	32.1	11.3	28.9	71.3	77.3	660	201
OK	Beaver	0.70	962	32.6	8.8	31.2	74.4	79.8	2568	783
OK	Beckham	-0.40	1757	34.8	9.9	33.3	72	77.9	1953	595
OK	Blaine	-0.20	1601	33.4	9.8	30.8	73.6	79.4	1486	453
OK	Bryan	2.03	465	33	10.2	31	72.7	78	615	188
OK	Caddo	0.95	839	33.6	10.4	32.6	72	78.5	1416	432
OK	Canadian	-0.10	1530	32.1	10.6	29.2	75.7	79.9	1350	412
OK	Carter	1.18	737	34.7	9.1	34.8	71.7	77.7	914	279
OK	Cherokee	2.39	390	36.4	10.6	31.2	73.2	78.6	855	261
OK	Choctaw	0.29	1227	34.2	11.1	33.4	71.3	77.3	492	150
OK	Cimarron	1.56	580	31.8	9.1	34.7	74.4	79.8	4139	1262
OK	Cleveland	1.06	787	29.5	9.4	26.1	75	79.8	1144	349
OK	Coal	0.88	869	32.8	10.3	31.9	71.1	78.1	684	208
OK	Comanche	2.29	416	32.8	9.8	31.3	73.2	78.4	1309	399
OK	Cotton	0.88	870	34	9.7	35.7	71.7	78.1	1005	306
OK	Craig	-1.49	2372	34.7	10.9	32.7	73.2	79	803	245
OK	Creek	0.58	1031	33.9	10.1	32.4	72.1	78.2	832	254
OK	Custer	0.46	1100	31.3	9.6	34.6	73.3	79.7	1729	527
OK	Delaware	0.72	945	31.9	11.1	34.9	73.3	79	945	288
OK	Dewey	0.16	1332	32.6	10	32.7	73.3	79.7	1873	571
OK	Ellis	1.11	771	30.8	9.4	32.8	74.4	79.8	2298	700
OK	Garfield	-1.25	2265	32.5	8.4	28.9	73.9	79.3	1167	356
OK	Garvin	0.38	1158	29.4	9.9	33.7	71.6	78.1	1004	306
OK	Grady	-0.25	1637	37.4	8.4	28	73.1	78.9	1220	372
OK	Grant	-1.01	2140	33.6	9.1	29	74.7	80.3	1122	342
OK	Greer	0.74	936	32.8	10.2	33.9	72.4	78.7	1653	504
OK	Harmon	-0.46	1795	32.5	9.8	34.4	72	77.9	1687	514
OK	Harper	0.51	1063	30.9	10	34.6	74.4	79.8	1982	604
OK	Haskell	2.00	473	33	10	33.9	72.3	78.8	617	188
OK	Hughes	-0.05	1484	32.9	11.7	31.2	71.6	77.3	825	251
OK	Jackson	-0.05	1485	34.5	11.4	32.7	73.7	78.1	1393	425
OK	Jefferson	1.29	683	34.1	10.2	34.4	71.7	78.1	900	274
OK	Johnston	1.67	550	30.3	10.7	33	71.1	78.1	847	258
OK	Kay	0.05	1405	36.9	10.9	31.3	73	78.7	1069	326
OK	Kingfisher	-0.77	1993	35.7	10.3	30.5	73.6	79.4	1121	342
OK	Kiowa	1.99	476	32.6	10.5	34.5	72.4	78.7	1502	458
OK	Latimer	0.89	866	34.5	10.7	34.3	72.3	78.8	876	267

ST	COUNTY	USDA	AMEN	OBES	DIAB	INACT	M AGE	W AGE	ALT ft	ALT m
OK	Le Flore	1.31	671	31.9	10.4	36.9	71.3	78.1	830	253
OK	Lincoln	0.13	1350	30.9	10.4	39.8	72.4	78.5	935	285
OK	Logan	-0.27	1648	32.5	10.2	29.8	74.5	79.8	1036	316
OK	Love	1.34	658	29.3	11.2	31.7	73	78.8	804	245
OK	Major	-1.49	2373	30.9	8.9	32.4	74.4	79.7	1421	433
OK	Marshall	2.54	368	34.9	9.7	31	73	78.8	741	226
OK	Mayes	0.21	1300	34.9	10.8	37	73.1	79.7	712	217
OK	McClain	0.64	991	33.7	9.8	27.8	74.6	79.8	1114	340
OK	McCurtain	2.08	454	33.7	10.1	37.5	70.2	77.5	632	193
OK	McIntosh	1.21	729	36.9	9.7	34.8	72.2	79.4	660	201
OK	Murray	1.34	659	34.2	10.1	31.2	71.6	78.1	1046	319
OK	Muskogee	0.45	1107	32.3	11	35.4	71.9	78.3	597	182
OK	Noble	-0.04	1477	34.2	9.9	31.3	74.7	80.3	1015	309
OK	Nowata	-0.36	1725	33	10.3	29	73.2	79	760	232
OK	Okfuskee	0.34	1194	33.3	11.1	36.3	71.6	77.3	837	255
OK	Oklahoma	0.24	1267	29.7	9.9	30.1	73.2	78.8	1143	348
OK	Okmulgee	-0.87	2052	35.3	9.9	33.2	70.8	78.1	722	220
OK	Osage	1.17	743	31.7	10.1	34.1	74.4	80	932	284
OK	Ottawa	0.03	1414	34.7	11.2	34.8	72.2	78.4	839	256
OK	Pawnee	0.01	1432	35.1	12.4	37.2	74	79	888	271
OK	Payne	0.42	1130	31.1	9.6	28.1	76.2	79.9	938	286
OK	Pittsburg	1.64	558	32.6	11	33.8	72.2	78.4	739	225
OK	Pontotoc	1.04	800	37	10.4	34.7	72.9	78.2	971	296
OK	Pottawatomie	0.26	1249	34.5	9.8	34.5	72.7	77.9	1024	312
OK	Pushmataha	1.75	538	31	10.9	33.8	70.2	77.5	808	246
OK	Roger Mills	-0.28	1656	33.8	9.5	34.2	73.3	79.7	2149	655
OK	Rogers	0.23	1280	32.2	10.3	30.8	75	79.2	674	205
OK	Seminole	0.58	1032	37	10.3	34.6	71.3	78.2	927	283
OK	Sequoyah	2.55	367	36.4	12.6	38.1	71.7	78.8	695	212
OK	Stephens	1.13	761	31	8.6	28.7	73.4	78.8	1101	336
OK	Texas	2.01	468	29.8	8.6	30.6	74.4	79.8	3171	966
OK	Tillman	0.41	1135	33.1	10.9	32.5	71.7	78.1	1189	362
OK	Tulsa	-0.30	1670	28.9	9.3	28.3	73.3	78.2	682	208
OK	Wagoner	0.05	1406	30.6	11.2	33.8	74.8	80	599	183
OK	Washington	0.96	834	31.3	9	29	75.1	80.3	729	222
OK	Washita	-0.30	1671	28.3	9	28.5	72	78.5	1632	497
OK	Woods	-1.14	2211	29.4	8.4	30.4	74.4	79.7	1573	479
OK	Woodward	-0.65	1914	31.3	9.6	31.5	74.5	80.4	1941	591
OR	Baker	2.42	386	26.3	7.9	18.8	75.7	80.2	4359	1329
OR	Benton	3.10	296	22.4	6.8	14.8	78.7	81.9	787	240
OR	Clackamas	3.64	234	26.1	7.9	16.9	77.8	81.4	2160	658
OR	Clatsop	4.97	129	25.7	7.6	18.7	76.6	80.5	862	263
OR	Columbia	4.98	125	27.9	7.7	18.9	75.5	80.8	761	232
OR	Coos	5.53	83	30	8	20.5	74	79.3	932	284
OR	Crook	5.06	116	27.6	7.9	18.9	75.6	80.1	4355	1328
OR	Curry	6.47	46	30.2	7.6	21.6	74.8	80.2	1633	498
OR	Deschutes	6.10	56	20	6.6	15.3	78.4	81.7	4577	1395

HEALTHIEST PLACES TO LIVE

ST	COUNTY	USDA	AMEN	OBES	DIAB	INACT	M AGE	W AGE	ALT ft	ALT m
OR	Douglas	6.78	39	31.3	9.2	20.6	74.1	80.7	2109	643
OR	Gilliam	0.45	1108	27.2	7.5	17.8	75.9	80.8	1934	590
OR	Grant	0.44	1116	24.2	7.6	18.4	75.9	80.4	4696	1431
OR	Harney	3.45	252	26.2	7.7	19.5	75.9	80.4	4848	1478
OR	Hood River	4.54	158	22.3	7.4	16.8	76.3	81.5	3018	920
OR	Jackson	4.50	164	22.8	6.6	13.9	76.2	81.5	3182	970
OR	Jefferson	4.99	122	28.4	7.7	21	74.6	79.2	3261	994
OR	Josephine	4.26	179	25	8.1	20.7	73.9	80.3	2418	737
OR	Klamath	5.15	107	26.5	7.3	20.4	74.4	78.7	4982	1518
OR	Lake	4.19	188	25.5	7.7	19.8	74.4	78.7	5132	1564
OR	Lane	4.29	177	27	7.1	16.6	76.1	81.1	2146	654
OR	Lincoln	6.06	58	27	7.4	19	75.5	80.3	704	215
OR	Linn	3.65	231	29.1	7.7	20.1	75.2	80.1	2071	631
OR	Malheur	1.68	548	26.4	7.7	21	74.2	80	4291	1308
OR	Marion	3.51	244	30.3	8.1	19	75.8	80.6	1553	473
OR	Morrow	3.34	265	26	8.3	24.1	75.6	80.5	2355	718
OR	Multnomah	4.33	174	24.1	7.5	16.4	75.3	80.2	1025	313
OR	Polk	3.28	274	29.7	7.6	18.9	77.7	82.2	862	263
OR	Sherman	1.61	566	25.3	7.6	17.8	75.9	80.8	1846	563
OR	Tillamook	5.54	81	26.5	7.4	18.9	75.8	80.8	1113	339
OR	Umatilla	1.64	559	34.1	8.7	24.2	75.6	80.5	2632	802
OR	Union	1.38	641	27.5	7.4	18.1	76.3	80.5	4331	1320
OR	Wallowa	2.68	343	25.4	6.9	19.3	75.7	80.2	4447	1355
OR	Wasco	3.38	260	32.9	7.6	19.4	75.9	80.8	2497	761
OR	Washington	2.65	347	23.9	6.1	16.5	78.9	82.5	743	227
OR	Wheeler	2.79	333	25.8	7.7	18.8	75.6	80.5	3742	1141
OR	Yamhill	3.25	275	27.2	6.9	18.7	76.6	80.6	678	207
PA	Adams	-0.13	1549	26.1	8.9	27.1	76.1	80.5	758	231
PA	Allegheny	0.47	1095	28.4	8.4	24.6	74.7	80.2	1043	318
PA	Armstrong	0.36	1176	33.9	8.6	26	74.8	79.7	1208	368
PA	Beaver	0.64	992	31.1	9.2	26.6	74.6	80.4	1053	321
PA	Bedford	-0.67	1926	29.5	9.4	25.9	75.2	80.6	1458	444
PA	Berks	-0.73	1964	29	7.9	23.6	76	81.5	566	172
PA	Blair	-0.86	2045	31.9	9.1	29.3	73.4	80	1538	469
PA	Bradford	0.29	1228	34	8.1	27.7	75.2	80.6	1368	417
PA	Bucks	0.01	1433	23.9	8	22.1	77.1	81.4	337	103
PA	Butler	-0.25	1638	26.5	8.6	22.5	75.9	80.8	1241	378
PA	Cambria	-0.23	1622	36.3	11.5	29.7	74.3	80.1	1931	588
PA	Cameron	0.73	942	28.8	8.8	25.9	75.2	80	1671	509
PA	Carbon	0.67	971	29.7	9.3	26.3	73.6	79.5	1244	379
PA	Centre	-0.40	1758	26.8	8.4	20.4	77.8	81.3	1472	449
PA	Chester	-1.53	2395	20.8	7.5	18.5	77.9	82.2	442	135
PA	Clarion	-0.30	1672	32.4	9.9	28.5	74.9	80.3	1396	426
PA	Clearfield	0.81	910	29.1	9	23.7	74.8	80.8	1636	499
PA	Clinton	0.47	1096	31.9	8	28.4	74.3	79.8	1438	438
PA	Columbia	-0.05	1486	35.7	8.6	27.4	74.9	80.8	972	296
PA	Crawford	-1.99	2579	28.6	10.1	24.9	74.8	80.1	1299	396

ST	COUNTY	USDA	AMEN	OBES	DIAB	INACT	M AGE	W AGE	ALT ft	ALT m
PA	Cumberland	-0.57	1863	27.2	9.1	22.7	77	81.3	713	217
PA	Dauphin	1.07	783	31.9	9.3	27.2	74.8	80.1	681	208
PA	Delaware	-0.69	1936	26.5	8.9	23.6	74.8	80	235	72
PA	Elk	0.07	1393	31.5	9.4	28.4	74.9	80.7	1769	539
PA	Erie	-0.57	1864	29.4	8.6	28.8	75.3	80.3	1158	353
PA	Fayette	0.27	1238	35.2	11.4	32.9	73.4	80	1488	453
PA	Forest	-1.09	2188	31.7	10	24.4	74.9	80.7	1570	479
PA	Franklin	-0.57	1865	31.1	8.6	24.9	76.1	81.4	893	272
PA	Fulton	-1.20	2237	29.7	8.9	26	74.6	80.4	1118	341
PA	Greene	0.22	1287	28	9.1	33.6	74.7	79.8	1196	365
PA	Huntingdon	0.15	1337	30.6	9.3	30.6	74.6	79.8	1136	346
PA	Indiana	0.40	1140	29.3	8.5	29.3	76.2	81	1426	435
PA	Jefferson	-0.93	2087	29.5	10.7	28.8	74.9	80.3	1569	478
PA	Juniata	-0.34	1704	30.4	9.4	26.6	74.6	80.8	865	264
PA	Lackawanna	0.16	1333	25.6	8.1	28.3	74	80.3	1456	444
PA	Lancaster	0.45	1109	29.3	8.1	21.3	76.8	81.4	462	141
PA	Lawrence	0.24	1268	29.6	9.5	27.7	74.5	80.6	1093	333
PA	Lebanon	-0.66	1920	30.7	9	22.7	75.7	80.9	612	187
PA	Lehigh	-0.40	1759	28.9	9.3	24.1	76.2	81.8	589	179
PA	Luzerne	0.30	1217	29.7	8.8	29.7	73.3	79.8	1268	386
PA	Lycoming	0.33	1199	30.1	8.5	27.5	74.9	80	1290	393
PA	McKean	-1.11	2196	32.2	9.1	27.7	74.3	80	1917	584
PA	Mercer	-2.78	2855	29.8	10.1	23.9	74.7	80.2	1211	369
PA	Mifflin	-0.19	1589	30.6	9.3	28.3	74.7	80.3	1072	327
PA	Monroe	0.94	843	29.2	9	25.6	75.6	80.4	1241	378
PA	Montgomery	-0.53	1835	25	7.3	20.7	77.7	82	287	87
PA	Montour	0.11	1361	29.2	9.4	28.1	75.4	80.5	688	210
PA	Northampton	-0.04	1478	29.7	7.1	23.7	76.5	81.8	578	176
PA	Northumberland	0.72	946	31.7	8.1	29.6	74.3	80.2	774	236
PA	Perry	-0.45	1788	31.3	10	26.2	74.9	79.8	841	256
PA	Philadelphia	-0.46	1796	31.4	11.1	29.6	69.2	77.6	114	35
PA	Pike	1.26	706	30.8	9	23.9	77.3	82.3	1234	376
PA	Potter	-2.42	2749	30.5	9.1	26.9	75.2	80	1996	608
PA	Schuylkill	0.49	1082	31.8	8.8	31.7	73.2	79.5	1052	321
PA	Snyder	-0.63	1900	31.3	9.9	24	75.1	81.2	855	261
PA	Somerset	0.01	1434	31.4	9	26.8	74.6	80.8	2193	668
PA	Sullivan	0.01	1435	33.6	9.2	27.4	74.8	80.7	1774	541
PA	Susquehanna	0.25	1255	26.8	9.9	25.5	74.7	80.1	1424	434
PA	Tioga	-0.25	1639	31.5	8.6	25.9	75.8	80.4	1709	521
PA	Union	-1.08	2185	30.2	9	24.4	76	80.5	956	291
PA	Venango	-0.86	2046	31.4	7.9	27.2	74.5	80.1	1376	419
PA	Warren	-0.71	1952	28.3	9.5	28.3	75.4	79.9	1623	495
PA	Washington	0.40	1141	29	9.3	24.5	75.1	80.6	1139	347
PA	Wayne	0.44	1117	27.4	8.9	23.9	74.3	80	1463	446
PA	Westmoreland	0.88	871	28	8.6	26.9	75.8	80.9	1312	400
PA	Wyoming	0.68	965	30.4	8.5	24.3	74.8	80.7	1256	383
PA	York	-0.58	1873	31.6	8.9	22.6	76.1	81.6	595	182

HEALTHIEST PLACES TO LIVE

ST	COUNTY	USDA	AMEN	OBES	DIAB	INACT	M AGE	W AGE	ALT ft	ALT m
RI	Bristol	1.36	649	20.5	5.2	19	77	82.6	32	10
RI	Kent	1.30	680	26.7	7.8	24.5	75.9	81	286	87
RI	Newport	2.14	445	21.4	6.1	18.6	77.9	81.7	102	31
RI	Providence	0.97	827	27	8.3	27.1	75.7	81.4	362	110
RI	Washington	2.64	349	20.9	5.8	18.7	78.1	82	156	48
SC	Abbeville	-0.61	1889	32.6	11.5	31.6	72	78.1	575	175
SC	Aiken	-0.04	1479	32.8	10	25.1	73.6	79.2	363	111
SC	Allendale	-0.27	1649	34.7	14	34.7	68.7	76.2	148	45
SC	Anderson	0.71	953	30.1	10.7	28.8	71.8	79	756	231
SC	Bamberg	-0.75	1974	41.5	12.6	33.1	68.7	76.2	159	48
SC	Barnwell	-0.21	1610	37.2	11.8	31	70.4	76.5	232	71
SC	Beaufort	1.66	555	21.4	7	17.2	78	83.3	10	3
SC	Berkeley	0.71	954	37.7	12.3	30.1	73.9	79.2	45	14
SC	Calhoun	0.20	1311	39.6	12.9	32.8	71.9	78.1	214	65
SC	Charleston	1.45	613	27.5	9.7	23.6	73.8	80	13	4
SC	Cherokee	-0.31	1683	30.6	11	30.7	70.1	76.7	690	210
SC	Chester	-0.04	1480	31.8	11.3	33	70.2	77.9	490	149
SC	Chesterfield	-0.38	1736	34.9	11.4	32.5	69.7	76.8	326	99
SC	Clarendon	1.15	751	37	12.3	32	70.8	77.4	103	31
SC	Colleton	0.67	972	34.1	12	32.6	69.7	77.4	50	15
SC	Darlington	0.28	1234	35.7	12.6	33.4	69.9	76.8	176	54
SC	Dillon	-0.68	1932	38.7	11.9	37.3	67.9	75.4	101	31
SC	Dorchester	-1.11	2197	29.6	10.1	26.5	74.1	79.4	62	19
SC	Edgefield	-0.25	1640	35.6	10.1	25.6	72	77.6	432	132
SC	Fairfield	0.67	973	39.1	14	35.1	69	76.8	406	124
SC	Florence	-0.56	1853	34.5	11.8	32.9	70.7	77.1	85	26
SC	Georgetown	1.49	601	35.9	11	29.6	73.7	79	21	6
SC	Greenville	1.83	515	28	9.4	24.3	74.1	79.9	1081	329
SC	Greenwood	-0.11	1536	34.7	10.1	30.4	72.5	78.5	535	163
SC	Hampton	-0.69	1937	41.1	14.3	30	69.9	76.7	82	25
SC	Horry	0.88	872	29.1	10.2	24.4	73.7	79.8	50	15
SC	Jasper	0.59	1024	39.7	12.9	30.2	71.1	77	31	9
SC	Kershaw	0.27	1239	31.6	9.7	27.1	73	78.9	297	90
SC	Lancaster	0.09	1372	32.5	11	31.4	72.9	79.1	519	158
SC	Laurens	-0.35	1715	37.2	10.9	31.8	71.2	77.7	605	184
SC	Lee	-1.00	2133	38.2	13.1	34.9	68.3	75.4	217	66
SC	Lexington	0.99	821	31.2	9.1	25.4	74.5	80	389	119
SC	Marion	-0.15	1561	38.4	13.3	33.6	68.8	76	55	17
SC	Marlboro	0.27	1240	42.7	12.7	33.1	68.1	75.3	147	45
SC	McCormick	0.81	911	35.2	11.9	25.3	72	78.1	411	125
SC	Newberry	0.18	1321	36.8	10.7	30.4	71.7	78.5	433	132
SC	Oconee	3.55	242	31.1	10	24.5	74	79.9	1094	333
SC	Orangeburg	0.25	1256	41	13.5	32.2	69.4	76.9	183	56
SC	Pickens	3.02	307	28.3	9.5	26.6	74.2	79.7	1122	342
SC	Richland	0.56	1037	30.6	11.2	26.4	73.1	78.8	256	78
SC	Saluda	0.02	1424	33.2	11	31.7	72.6	78.2	484	147
SC	Spartanburg	0.52	1055	30	9.9	27.5	72	78.4	769	234

ST	COUNTY	USDA	AMEN	OBES	DIAB	INACT	M AGE	W AGE	ALT ft	ALT m
SC	Sumter	0.45	1110	36.7	12.8	31.7	71.6	78.5	162	49
SC	Union	-0.80	2010	35.8	11.9	33.6	69.3	77.1	499	152
SC	Williamsburg	-0.88	2060	41.9	13.4	31.4	67.8	75.6	53	16
SC	York	0.45	1111	29.4	9	25.5	74	79.2	618	188
SD	Aurora	-2.83	2871	29.6	6.5	34.1	74.9	81.2	1573	479
SD	Beadle	-3.25	2958	32.9	6	29.3	75.8	81.4	1331	406
SD	Bennett	0.50	1074	36.9	11.7	28.7	71	78.3	3168	966
SD	Bon Homme	-1.59	2421	30.4	7.5	30.1	75	80.9	1432	437
SD	Brookings	-2.06	2604	27	6	22.6	77	81.8	1710	521
SD	Brown	-2.72	2845	31.9	6.8	29.5	76.3	82.4	1337	408
SD	Brule	-1.54	2399	34.6	6.5	32.3	75	80.8	1663	507
SD	Buffalo	-1.59	2422	41.2	17.2	36.8	75.8	81.4	1650	503
SD	Butte	0.43	1123	31	7	30.5	74.8	80.5	3019	920
SD	Campbell	-1.45	2354	29.4	6.7	33	74.1	80.3	1807	551
SD	Charles Mix	-1.23	2254	35.6	9.6	29	75	80.9	1567	478
SD	Clark	-2.27	2683	32.7	6.9	28.7	74.9	80.6	1705	520
SD	Clay	-1.87	2533	32.5	6.4	23.6	77.4	82.7	1230	375
SD	Codington	-1.73	2481	30	6.3	26.6	76.2	82.2	1813	553
SD	Corson	-0.71	1953	41.7	13	31.6	72.9	79.9	2088	636
SD	Custer	0.97	828	25.9	6.6	24	71.1	78.5	4234	1290
SD	Davison	-3.29	2963	28	6.7	27.2	76.2	81.6	1382	421
SD	Day	-1.21	2244	31.9	6.9	28.5	74.9	81.2	1739	530
SD	Deuel	-1.68	2463	33.1	6.5	26.7	76.2	82.2	1771	540
SD	Dewey	0.62	1011	42.3	15.5	33.9	72.9	79.9	2004	611
SD	Douglas	-3.59	3020	31.8	6.7	31.6	74.9	81.2	1564	477
SD	Edmunds	-2.68	2835	39.2	6.5	27.1	74.1	80.3	1696	517
SD	Fall River	1.89	500	32.3	8.3	21.5	71.1	78.5	3596	1096
SD	Faulk	-2.32	2696	28.8	6.9	29.2	76.3	82.4	1627	496
SD	Grant	-2.49	2782	32.2	8.7	28.9	76.2	82.2	1441	439
SD	Gregory	-0.64	1910	30.6	7.8	29.5	75	80.8	1919	585
SD	Haakon	-0.30	1673	30	7.1	27.5	76.6	81.5	2287	697
SD	Hamlin	-1.37	2308	30.1	7.5	28.3	74.9	80.6	1738	530
SD	Hand	-3.20	2949	31.3	6.8	31.9	75.8	81.4	1652	504
SD	Hanson	-3.42	2990	29.1	6.2	25.8	76.2	81.6	1338	408
SD	Harding	-0.65	1915	30.6	6.7	30.2	74.8	80.5	3077	938
SD	Hughes	0.07	1394	29.6	8.4	21.3	76.2	81.5	1718	524
SD	Hutchinson	-3.33	2971	31.8	6.4	27.5	74.9	81.2	1391	424
SD	Hyde	-2.39	2735	37.2	8	30	76.3	82.4	1849	564
SD	Jackson	-0.75	1975	34.1	10.9	30.8	71	78.3	2525	770
SD	Jerauld	-2.91	2888	28.9	5.5	29.8	75.8	81.4	1641	500
SD	Jones	-1.48	2366	31.9	6.9	30.6	76.6	81.5	2070	631
SD	Kingsbury	-1.92	2554	27.1	5.7	29	74.9	80.6	1667	508
SD	Lake	-1.86	2529	32.3	6.9	26.6	76.8	82.3	1704	519
SD	Lawrence	1.76	531	22.8	5.7	23.6	77	81.3	4968	1514
SD	Lincoln	-3.91	3055	26.3	5.8	22.8	77.3	81.4	1380	421
SD	Lyman	-1.28	2276	36.7	9.3	32.1	76.2	81.5	1765	538
SD	Marshall	-1.65	2447	28.6	8.1	29.2	74.9	81.2	1559	475

ST	COUNTY	USDA	AMEN	OBES	DIAB	INACT	M AGE	W AGE	ALT ft	ALT m
SD	McCook	-3.05	2916	26.6	7	27.7	76.2	81.6	1513	461
SD	McPherson	-1.98	2577	29.2	6.4	25.8	74.1	80.3	1827	557
SD	Meade	-1.66	2448	25.9	7.5	27	74.8	80.5	2760	841
SD	Mellette	-0.76	1984	36.7	12.8	33.1	71	78.3	2219	676
SD	Miner	-3.45	2997	30.8	6.3	33.9	76.2	81.6	1489	454
SD	Minnehaha	-2.58	2807	29.1	6.9	23.6	77.1	82.3	1544	471
SD	Moody	-2.96	2901	32.5	7.3	27	76.8	82.3	1629	497
SD	Pennington	1.27	693	26.2	7.3	22.1	76.6	81.5	3562	1086
SD	Perkins	-0.73	1965	29.3	7.3	30.6	74.8	80.5	2611	796
SD	Potter	-1.38	2315	28.1	6.7	26.8	72.9	79.9	1928	588
SD	Roberts	-1.68	2464	36.8	9.5	29.2	74.9	81.2	1320	402
SD	Sanborn	-3.47	2999	35.4	6.9	33.2	75.8	81.4	1295	395
SD	Shannon	-0.10	1531	40.9	16.8	32.4	71.1	78.5	3101	945
SD	Spink	-3.62	3026	35.9	7	30.7	74.9	81.2	1314	400
SD	Stanley	-0.15	1562	33.1	7.5	30.6	76.6	81.5	1868	570
SD	Sully	0.20	1312	35.3	6.4	27	76.6	81.5	1799	548
SD	Todd	-0.98	2119	41	14.4	31.5	71	78.3	2697	822
SD	Tripp	-2.25	2672	36.7	9.1	30.9	75	80.8	2096	639
SD	Turner	-3.48	3002	31.3	6.5	30.7	76.9	81.5	1384	422
SD	Union	-1.78	2500	29.9	5.9	23.7	77.4	82.7	1253	382
SD	Walworth	-1.45	2355	33.2	8.8	30.5	74.1	80.3	1916	584
SD	Yankton	-1.76	2496	33.2	7.2	23.4	76.9	81.5	1333	406
SD	Ziebach	-0.55	1845	43.3	14.1	34.5	72.9	79.9	2278	694
TN	Anderson	1.36	650	31.2	10.5	31.5	73.7	79.2	1299	396
TN	Bedford	-0.55	1846	34.1	11.8	30.5	71.9	79	842	257
TN	Benton	1.13	762	34.1	11.2	30.3	70.6	77.8	470	143
TN	Bledsoe	-0.56	1854	32.8	11.1	34.6	72.7	79.1	1601	488
TN	Blount	1.25	711	33.3	9.5	26.4	74.1	79.6	1420	433
TN	Bradley	-0.17	1578	29.5	11.6	30.2	73.3	79.2	848	258
TN	Campbell	1.87	506	34.9	11.4	34.5	70.9	77.4	1561	476
TN	Cannon	-2.75	2851	31.7	9.6	31.8	71.5	78.4	980	299
TN	Carroll	-1.91	2551	37.5	11.1	33	70.1	77.2	469	143
TN	Carter	2.93	319	34.7	10.8	31.7	72.4	78.6	2655	809
TN	Cheatham	-0.23	1623	31.5	9.3	32.1	73.5	78.8	588	179
TN	Chester	-2.01	2588	36.4	11.1	28.3	72.9	78.2	492	150
TN	Claiborne	1.57	577	30.6	10.3	34.4	71.1	77.7	1478	451
TN	Clay	1.29	684	32.7	10.5	28.6	71.2	77.1	783	239
TN	Cocke	1.31	672	36.9	11.4	33.4	69.9	76.7	1725	526
TN	Coffee	-0.89	2064	33.4	11.1	25.6	72.3	78.5	1093	333
TN	Crockett	-2.21	2659	34.4	11.9	32.2	70.7	77.4	339	103
TN	Cumberland	0.54	1047	28.2	9.5	25.6	74.7	80.6	1784	544
TN	Davidson	0.33	1200	29.8	9.5	26.9	73.3	79.2	579	177
TN	Decatur	0.34	1195	31	10.5	34.4	70.6	78.2	474	144
TN	DeKalb	1.23	718	32.1	10	29	71.5	78.4	872	266
TN	Dickson	-0.83	2024	30.1	10.4	31.5	72.4	78.8	706	215
TN	Dyer	-0.39	1748	36	10.8	34.2	71.2	77.7	292	89
TN	Fayette	-1.18	2228	35.3	11.9	30.4	72.3	78.3	397	121

ST	COUNTY	USDA	AMEN	OBES	DIAB	INACT	M AGE	W AGE	ALT ft	ALT m
TN	Fentress	-0.05	1487	35.6	11.7	32.7	69.5	77.1	1484	452
TN	Franklin	1.68	549	34.2	9.4	33	73.5	78.9	1158	353
TN	Gibson	-1.86	2530	37.3	11	37.3	70.3	77.5	371	113
TN	Giles	-1.46	2359	36.5	9.9	30	72.2	78.9	831	253
TN	Grainger	1.45	614	32	10.4	32.9	71.2	77.2	1289	393
TN	Greene	0.14	1343	32.5	10.1	33	72.6	77.8	1548	472
TN	Grundy	0.02	1425	30.7	9.9	31.8	68.8	77.9	1706	520
TN	Hamblen	1.52	594	32.9	11.7	32.7	72.4	78.3	1247	380
TN	Hamilton	1.16	746	30.5	9.5	26.7	73.4	79.5	978	298
TN	Hancock	0.38	1159	31.3	10.9	34.9	71.2	77.2	1515	462
TN	Hardeman	-1.05	2165	38.6	11.4	33.8	70.7	77.2	459	140
TN	Hardin	0.44	1118	30.3	9.4	33.9	71.5	78.1	507	154
TN	Hawkins	1.21	730	34.6	11.3	31.5	72.6	78.6	1416	432
TN	Haywood	-1.70	2473	36.3	12.1	32.6	68.8	77	333	101
TN	Henderson	0.82	904	32.3	9.1	31.5	71.3	77.3	500	152
TN	Henry	0.06	1400	34.7	10.6	32.3	71.6	77.9	469	143
TN	Hickman	-2.18	2647	32.4	10.5	31.8	71.7	79	679	207
TN	Houston	0.56	1038	34	10.4	29.3	72.4	78.3	564	172
TN	Humphreys	0.61	1018	31.6	11.4	30.7	72.1	78.5	565	172
TN	Jackson	0.86	884	35	11.6	32.5	71.3	77.6	756	231
TN	Jefferson	1.39	636	32.3	10.5	31.4	73	78.7	1151	351
TN	Johnson	0.74	937	32	10.8	31.2	70.8	77.4	2915	888
TN	Knox	0.62	1012	30.5	10.3	27.3	74.3	79.5	1009	307
TN	Lake	-0.36	1726	35.2	11.9	37.3	71.8	77.9	277	84
TN	Lauderdale	0.05	1407	36	10.9	34.8	69.8	76.4	304	93
TN	Lawrence	-0.89	2065	30.1	10.7	32.2	71.5	78.6	876	267
TN	Lewis	-0.80	2011	31.7	10.3	36	71.1	77.6	842	257
TN	Lincoln	-1.20	2238	34.1	9.2	33.6	72.8	79	848	258
TN	Loudon	1.14	755	31.3	10.7	28.7	74.2	80	911	278
TN	Macon	-2.11	2620	35.2	11.5	28.8	71	77.4	858	262
TN	Madison	-1.44	2348	34.3	10.9	28.8	72.7	78.9	434	132
TN	Marion	0.83	899	31.7	9.4	35.6	71.2	77.8	1321	403
TN	Marshall	-0.89	2066	30.7	9.6	32.9	72.4	79.1	818	249
TN	Maury	-0.19	1590	33	10.6	30	72.8	78.5	730	222
TN	McMinn	-0.35	1716	33.8	10.7	32.6	71.9	78.3	913	278
TN	McNairy	-1.69	2469	37.3	11	32.1	71.4	78.4	490	149
TN	Meigs	1.30	681	34.3	11.5	33.6	71.1	78	812	248
TN	Monroe	1.51	598	34	10.4	31	72.5	78.7	1439	438
TN	Montgomery	-0.51	1818	32.8	12.4	30.5	74.3	79.1	538	164
TN	Moore	0.37	1171	30.9	9.8	28.6	72.8	79	988	301
TN	Morgan	-0.52	1829	32.3	9.9	29	71.5	77.7	1496	456
TN	Obion	-0.71	1954	32.5	11.4	35.2	71.8	77.9	354	108
TN	Overton	0.20	1313	33.2	9.6	33.8	71.2	77.1	1187	362
TN	Perry	0.43	1124	31.3	9.7	30.2	70.6	78.2	602	183
TN	Pickett	1.67	551	32.1	10.3	31.6	71.2	77.1	1055	321
TN	Polk	1.67	552	33.4	11.2	33.2	70.9	77.7	1365	416
TN	Putnam	0.24	1269	32.7	9.5	28.1	73.4	79	1182	360

HEALTHIEST PLACES TO LIVE

ST	COUNTY	USDA	AMEN	OBES	DIAB	INACT	M AGE	W AGE	ALT ft	ALT m
TN	Rhea	1.33	663	34.2	10.2	30.6	71.1	78	1146	349
TN	Roane	1.22	726	35.4	11.3	33.9	73.2	79.4	909	277
TN	Robertson	-1.92	2555	32.2	11.5	33.1	72.8	78.5	664	202
TN	Rutherford	-0.85	2039	29.1	10.6	27.4	75.2	79.5	678	207
TN	Scott	0.28	1235	31.8	10.2	36.4	70.7	77.1	1514	461
TN	Sequatchie	-0.44	1779	35.8	9.6	30.7	72.7	79.1	1649	503
TN	Sevier	1.76	532	30.3	10.5	28.2	73.6	79.6	1978	603
TN	Shelby	-0.44	1780	33.8	11.7	28.6	71.4	77.7	284	87
TN	Smith	0.87	877	32.4	10.8	31.5	71.3	77.6	692	211
TN	Stewart	0.98	823	33	10.2	32.6	72.4	78.3	509	155
TN	Sullivan	1.27	694	35.3	12	29.4	72.6	79	1688	515
TN	Sumner	0.25	1257	30	10	28.1	74.9	79.4	691	211
TN	Tipton	-0.38	1737	35.6	11	32.4	72.2	78	320	98
TN	Trousdale	-0.30	1674	32.8	10.4	34.7	71	77.4	640	195
TN	Unicoi	0.36	1177	33.2	10.4	30.3	71.4	78.6	2735	834
TN	Union	1.35	652	31.9	9.9	31.6	71.1	77.9	1227	374
TN	Van Buren	-1.32	2290	33	10.2	32.9	71.6	78.2	1547	471
TN	Warren	-1.45	2356	34.9	10.1	30.8	71.4	78	1111	339
TN	Washington	0.67	974	29.5	10.2	28.6	72.5	79.6	1700	518
TN	Wayne	-0.71	1955	32.2	9.6	29.4	71.1	77.6	785	239
TN	Weakley	-1.62	2436	31.9	10.1	34.9	72.9	78.4	399	121
TN	White	-0.76	1985	33.2	10.1	34.6	71.6	78.2	1207	368
TN	Williamson	-0.87	2053	23.8	8.2	18.8	77.9	82	778	237
TN	Wilson	-0.82	2020	29.8	9.3	28.6	74.7	78.9	664	203
TX	Anderson	1.07	784	32.7	10.7	32	69.8	77.8	378	115
TX	Andrews	0.68	966	29.6	8.9	27.1	73.9	78.9	3177	968
TX	Angelina	1.92	492	32.1	9.5	28.8	73.1	78.7	230	70
TX	Aransas	3.71	223	27.8	8.6	26.5	73.9	81.3	8	2
TX	Archer	-0.33	1694	28.1	10	27.4	74.9	81.1	1071	327
TX	Armstrong	0.36	1178	29	8.6	26.9	74.6	79.8	3125	952
TX	Atascosa	0.90	860	29.6	8.5	28	74.6	80.4	434	132
TX	Austin	1.38	642	29.5	9	25.9	74.5	80.2	240	73
TX	Bailey	0.91	855	28.8	8.9	28.2	73.1	78.8	3874	1181
TX	Bandera	5.83	70	29.8	9.1	28.9	76.4	81.2	1684	513
TX	Bastrop	0.94	844	30.8	9.5	26.3	74	79.3	465	142
TX	Baylor	1.70	545	27.7	8.8	26.6	72.6	79	1254	382
TX	Bee	-0.36	1727	28.4	9.7	25.9	74.2	79.4	240	73
TX	Bell	1.26	707	28.7	10.4	28.3	74.5	79.7	668	203
TX	Bexar	2.63	352	28.2	8.7	22.5	74.9	80.7	818	249
TX	Blanco	4.05	195	28.3	8.6	25.1	76.6	81.3	1334	407
TX	Borden	2.39	391	28.1	8.7	27	72.4	77.8	2542	775
TX	Bosque	0.84	893	27.4	8.2	24.8	73.8	79.5	830	253
TX	Bowie	0.79	916	32.8	9.7	29.4	72.4	78.4	316	96
TX	Brazoria	1.31	673	26.9	9.9	25.9	75.3	78.8	26	8
TX	Brazos	0.59	1025	30.2	9.1	22.9	77.1	80.4	284	87
TX	Brewster	4.58	155	27.2	8	25.1	75	80.8	3614	1102
TX	Briscoe	1.76	533	28.5	8.7	25.3	74.6	79.8	2791	851

ST	COUNTY	USDA	AMEN	OBES	DIAB	INACT	M AGE	W AGE	ALT ft	ALT m
TX	Brooks	-0.34	1705	28.7	8.7	28.3	73.4	78.6	187	57
TX	Brown	0.35	1189	31	8.9	27.2	72.4	78.9	1522	464
TX	Burleson	1.40	632	32.5	9.8	30.8	74.7	79.4	319	97
TX	Burnet	4.36	171	28.5	8.4	25.7	76.9	82.3	1159	353
TX	Caldwell	0.51	1064	32.3	8.8	24.8	73.5	79.4	497	151
TX	Calhoun	1.86	510	29.5	8.8	24.9	73.8	78.9	12	4
TX	Callahan	0.33	1201	30.7	8.4	24	73.1	79.5	1801	549
TX	Cameron	2.46	377	27.2	8.5	22.8	76.9	83	26	8
TX	Camp	0.71	955	31.2	10.4	26.6	71.3	78.3	353	107
TX	Carson	1.21	731	31.1	9.2	25.5	74.6	79.8	3349	1021
TX	Cass	0.63	1002	30.6	9.9	32.3	71.7	78.4	319	97
TX	Castro	1.23	719	29.6	8.8	29.1	73.7	79.3	3770	1149
TX	Chambers	1.57	578	28.2	8.7	29.8	74.1	79.8	15	5
TX	Cherokee	1.25	712	33	10.3	29.6	71.9	79	391	119
TX	Childress	1.02	805	29.6	9.4	25.9	72.2	77.9	1765	538
TX	Clay	-0.36	1728	29.4	8.7	31.5	73.2	79.6	954	291
TX	Cochran	-0.12	1540	30.1	9.1	27.9	73.1	78.8	3784	1153
TX	Coke	3.73	219	31.7	8.4	29.9	73.2	78.8	2127	648
TX	Coleman	2.14	446	27.7	8.3	31.8	73.1	79.5	1705	520
TX	Collin	1.01	811	24.3	7.6	22.1	79.7	82.5	613	187
TX	Collingsworth	0.01	1436	30	9	27.6	73.2	78.9	2137	651
TX	Colorado	1.72	542	29.1	9.3	29	73.5	79.3	237	72
TX	Comal	3.25	276	25.7	8.3	25	76.8	81.8	1026	313
TX	Comanche	0.36	1179	28.2	8.6	27.1	72.9	79.5	1360	415
TX	Concho	2.30	413	30.4	8.7	25.6	73.6	78.3	1859	566
TX	Cooke	0.63	1003	33	9.8	27.2	74.8	80.6	839	256
TX	Coryell	1.01	812	29.8	10.8	28.2	74.9	79.8	953	291
TX	Cottle	-0.19	1591	29.8	9	28.5	73.2	78.7	1808	551
TX	Crane	1.34	660	29.8	9.4	28	73.4	78.5	2566	782
TX	Crockett	1.64	560	29.9	8.7	26.2	73.4	78.5	2438	743
TX	Crosby	2.45	381	27.9	8.9	29.6	72.9	78.7	2925	892
TX	Culberson	3.62	236	28.1	8.8	26.2	76.3	82	4130	1259
TX	Dallam	0.22	1288	27.4	8.9	28.8	73.7	78.9	4150	1265
TX	Dallas	0.64	993	30.5	10.2	25.3	75.1	80.3	511	156
TX	Dawson	-0.24	1633	31.1	9.8	28.8	73.1	78.8	2954	900
TX	Deaf Smith	0.94	845	30.4	8.6	28	72.4	79.1	4046	1233
TX	Delta	-0.59	1877	29	9.2	28.2	73.8	80	453	138
TX	Denton	1.40	633	29.4	9.4	24.6	77.3	80.9	643	196
TX	DeWitt	0.50	1075	28.4	9.1	25.2	73.3	79.2	283	86
TX	Dickens	0.38	1160	30.5	9.1	27	73.2	78.7	2395	730
TX	Dimmit	0.48	1088	28.9	9	26.3	72.2	78.1	609	186
TX	Donley	0.86	885	30.4	9.3	27.5	74.6	79.8	2672	814
TX	Duval	0.96	835	30.3	8.8	26.3	73.4	78.6	487	148
TX	Eastland	0.24	1270	29.4	9.1	27.2	72.9	79.5	1514	462
TX	Ector	2.50	370	32	9.5	27.8	72.2	78	3018	920
TX	Edwards	3.15	287	29.3	8.9	27.4	73.7	79.9	2129	649
TX	El Paso	4.46	165	23.7	8.3	21.7	76.3	82	4069	1240

ST	COUNTY	USDA	AMEN	OBES	DIAB	INACT	M AGE	W AGE	ALT ft	ALT m
TX	Ellis	0.24	1271	29.7	8.9	25.2	75	78.9	533	162
TX	Erath	0.03	1415	28	9.2	25.5	73.9	79.6	1251	381
TX	Falls	0.34	1196	30.6	10.6	29.6	70.9	76.7	430	131
TX	Fannin	0.22	1289	29.8	9.2	30.9	72.9	78.4	595	181
TX	Fayette	1.04	801	29	8.6	26	74.1	79.9	362	110
TX	Fisher	0.30	1218	30.5	8.5	28.3	72.9	78.9	1997	609
TX	Floyd	0.86	886	28.6	9.6	28.7	73.8	79	3140	957
TX	Foard	0.03	1416	29.5	9.6	28.3	73.2	78.7	1497	456
TX	Fort Bend	-0.52	1830	25.5	8.6	21.4	77.8	81.8	83	25
TX	Franklin	0.76	931	27.2	8.8	30.1	73.8	80	404	123
TX	Freestone	0.40	1142	31.7	9.5	28.1	73.4	79.1	385	117
TX	Frio	0.40	1143	28.6	8.5	29.7	72.9	78.7	581	177
TX	Gaines	0.84	894	30.7	9.2	29.2	73.9	78.9	3320	1012
TX	Galveston	1.87	507	29.2	9.5	24.6	73.4	78.7	12	4
TX	Garza	1.11	772	32.1	9.1	28.6	73.2	79.3	2518	768
TX	Gillespie	2.59	362	28	8.2	25.7	76.4	81.6	1832	558
TX	Glasscock	0.23	1281	28.6	8.8	27.5	75.9	81.1	2654	809
TX	Goliad	1.61	567	29.2	9	25.6	73.3	79.8	199	61
TX	Gonzales	0.68	967	31.6	9.5	28.2	72.1	79.1	342	104
TX	Gray	0.79	917	31.1	10.3	37.6	73.2	78.9	3006	916
TX	Grayson	0.78	922	26.5	8.6	25.6	73.6	79.1	707	216
TX	Gregg	0.21	1301	32.3	10.2	29.6	71.8	78.7	332	101
TX	Grimes	0.74	938	33.4	9.4	25.7	73.1	78.5	299	91
TX	Guadalupe	0.58	1033	29.8	8.2	23.9	76.5	81.1	564	172
TX	Hale	-0.07	1503	29.4	8.6	28.5	73.8	79	3407	1038
TX	Hall	0.27	1241	28.5	9	26.2	72.2	77.9	2059	628
TX	Hamilton	-0.65	1916	29.3	8.5	29	73.8	79.5	1200	366
TX	Hansford	0.05	1408	28.2	8.8	28.5	74.2	79.8	3137	956
TX	Hardeman	0.14	1344	29.8	8.8	26.9	72.2	77.9	1518	463
TX	Hardin	1.04	802	30.2	10.6	29.2	73.5	78.3	71	22
TX	Harris	-0.04	1481	28.5	9	23.3	75.8	80.5	85	26
TX	Harrison	0.52	1056	33.9	10.2	32.9	72.3	78.3	312	95
TX	Hartley	0.51	1065	30.7	9.8	27.8	73.7	78.9	3947	1203
TX	Haskell	2.04	463	29	8.7	26.6	72.6	79	1535	468
TX	Hays	2.18	438	29.4	8.6	26.3	77	80.8	978	298
TX	Hemphill	1.27	695	27.5	8.5	28.4	73.8	79.3	2523	769
TX	Henderson	2.72	338	25.6	9.2	28.4	73	79.2	410	125
TX	Hidalgo	0.46	1101	30	10.2	23.8	77.8	83.4	129	39
TX	Hill	0.83	900	32.8	9.3	31.2	72.7	79.1	631	192
TX	Hockley	0.37	1172	29.6	8.6	30.6	72.9	78.7	3485	1062
TX	Hood	1.35	653	30.4	8.6	23.9	75.7	80	872	266
TX	Hopkins	0.17	1325	32.7	10.2	28.8	73.6	78.9	477	145
TX	Houston	0.11	1362	31	10.1	26.3	72.3	77.8	302	92
TX	Howard	2.23	428	31.5	9.1	28.9	72.4	77.8	2525	769
TX	Hudspeth	4.00	199	28.2	8.8	29.2	76.3	82	4437	1352
TX	Hunt	1.05	795	31.1	10.3	30.4	73.1	78.7	541	165
TX	Hutchinson	1.90	498	31.3	8.9	26.2	73.8	79.3	3060	933

PEGGY FORNEY

ST	COUNTY	USDA	AMEN	OBES	DIAB	INACT	M AGE	W AGE	ALT ft	ALT m
TX	Irion	0.11	1363	28.6	8.8	27.8	74.3	79.9	2406	733
TX	Jack	0.35	1190	30.4	9.5	27.3	74.9	81.1	1091	332
TX	Jackson	-0.02	1458	30.4	8.9	26.1	73.7	79.7	57	17
TX	Jasper	2.25	424	30.1	10.1	33.7	72.9	78.2	155	47
TX	Jeff Davis	5.93	65	26.5	8.8	22.6	76.3	82	4906	1495
TX	Jefferson	1.04	803	31.5	10.7	30.2	72.4	78.4	12	4
TX	Jim Hogg	-1.01	2141	29.1	8.7	27	73.4	78.6	542	165
TX	Jim Wells	1.45	615	31.5	8.7	26	72.8	79.8	215	66
TX	Johnson	0.12	1357	31.1	10.1	29.1	74.2	78.8	791	241
TX	Jones	1.55	586	31	9.6	29.3	72.9	78.9	1690	515
TX	Karnes	1.38	643	30.4	9.3	28.4	72.1	79.1	353	108
TX	Kaufman	0.63	1004	35.8	9.3	31.8	72.7	77.6	430	131
TX	Kendall	4.72	148	23.8	7.8	23.9	76.5	81.2	1558	475
TX	Kenedy	3.14	291	29.2	8.8	26.8	73.8	78.4	28	8
TX	Kent	0.45	1112	28.9	8.5	26.6	72.9	78.9	2113	644
TX	Kerr	4.52	161	29.5	9.2	22.1	75.5	81.5	2005	611
TX	Kimble	1.02	806	27.1	8.3	25.4	75.5	81	2031	619
TX	King	0.40	1144	28.5	8.7	26.3	73.2	78.7	1805	550
TX	Kinney	3.80	215	29.5	8.6	27	74.2	80.1	1240	378
TX	Kleberg	3.15	288	30	8.7	26.8	73.6	79.6	48	15
TX	Knox	0.62	1013	28.2	9.4	26.3	72.6	79	1453	443
TX	La Salle	0.71	956	29.6	8.6	26.8	72.9	78.7	429	131
TX	Lamar	0.36	1180	25.8	9.4	31	72.5	78.2	492	150
TX	Lamb	1.31	674	31.7	8.5	26.5	72.1	78.6	3636	1108
TX	Lampasas	2.81	331	30.5	8.4	25.5	75.4	79.8	1231	375
TX	Lavaca	-0.08	1515	27.8	8.7	26.5	74.2	80.6	252	77
TX	Lee	0.88	873	31	9.4	28.7	74.6	80.2	409	125
TX	Leon	0.36	1181	31.1	9.7	30.3	73.8	79.3	346	105
TX	Liberty	0.08	1381	30.5	9.1	31.3	71	77.3	71	22
TX	Limestone	1.12	766	28.6	9.7	26.6	71	77.7	495	151
TX	Lipscomb	-0.43	1775	29	8.7	30.1	73.8	79.3	2604	794
TX	Live Oak	2.67	344	28.6	8.7	28.1	74.6	80.4	246	75
TX	Llano	3.75	217	27.4	9.1	26.9	76.6	81.3	1230	375
TX	Loving	3.31	272	28.1	8.5	25.4	72.2	78	2954	900
TX	Lubbock	1.14	756	27.4	8.3	26.2	74	79.2	3232	985
TX	Lynn	1.32	669	29.4	9.2	27.7	72.9	78.7	3083	940
TX	Madison	0.22	1290	31.5	10	27	72.8	78.4	278	85
TX	Marion	1.40	634	30.9	10.3	28.9	71.7	78.4	266	81
TX	Martin	0.91	856	29.1	8.6	26.4	72.4	77.8	2779	847
TX	Mason	1.54	588	27.6	8.4	27	76.4	81.6	1631	497
TX	Matagorda	1.54	589	28.3	9.8	27	73.4	77.9	26	8
TX	Maverick	0.52	1057	29.8	9	29	74.2	80.1	794	242
TX	McCulloch	2.36	395	28.4	8.9	29.3	73.6	78.3	1681	512
TX	McLennan	0.76	932	30	9.3	24.9	73.4	79.2	572	174
TX	McMullen	1.76	534	29.9	8.9	27	72.9	78.7	330	101
TX	Medina	0.68	968	29.6	9.2	24.9	75.3	79.8	960	292
TX	Menard	0.51	1066	30.5	8.6	26.3	76.4	81.6	2101	640

ST	COUNTY	USDA	AMEN	OBES	DIAB	INACT	M AGE	W AGE	ALT ft	ALT m
TX	Midland	1.42	628	26.5	7.7	29.5	75.9	81.1	2765	843
TX	Milam	0.72	947	32.2	9.8	30.1	73.3	78.2	406	124
TX	Mills	-0.43	1776	29.2	8.5	25.2	73.8	79.5	1462	446
TX	Mitchell	2.47	376	31.4	9.7	28.5	72.1	78	2180	665
TX	Montague	-0.57	1866	29.2	8.7	28.7	73.2	79.6	971	296
TX	Montgomery	1.58	574	26.3	8.6	22.3	75.6	80.2	208	63
TX	Moore	2.46	378	31.4	8.9	30.3	73.7	78.9	3503	1068
TX	Morris	0.41	1136	31.8	10.7	29.4	71.3	78.3	350	107
TX	Motley	-0.22	1616	29.1	8.9	27.3	73.2	78.7	2330	710
TX	Nacogdoches	2.12	448	29.7	9.3	26.5	72.6	78.8	330	101
TX	Navarro	0.57	1035	32.5	9.1	30.3	72.3	78.9	402	122
TX	Newton	1.44	621	31.3	10	30.4	71.1	77.4	167	51
TX	Nolan	2.11	451	30.4	9.3	28.3	72.1	78	2353	717
TX	Nueces	3.33	267	30.2	9.8	23.7	74.3	80.5	55	17
TX	Ochiltree	0.39	1153	28.5	8.3	26.4	74.2	79.8	2920	890
TX	Oldham	1.19	735	30.3	9	28.4	72.4	79.1	3697	1127
TX	Orange	0.44	1119	29.7	10	33.9	71.5	78	12	4
TX	Palo Pinto	1.45	616	29.6	9.2	26.2	72.6	79.1	1042	318
TX	Panola	1.35	654	30.2	9.7	26.3	72.1	78.9	287	88
TX	Parker	0.14	1345	31.2	9.8	29.7	74.4	79.3	974	297
TX	Parmer	1.93	489	30.7	8.6	28.2	73.7	79.3	4052	1235
TX	Pecos	4.40	168	29.4	8.9	28.1	73.2	78.7	3133	955
TX	Polk	1.84	513	32.8	9.4	29.2	69.8	78.6	237	72
TX	Potter	2.60	360	33.9	9.4	30.8	71.7	77.4	3389	1033
TX	Presidio	3.06	299	24.8	8.2	25.5	75	80.8	4287	1307
TX	Rains	0.78	923	30.1	9	27.1	73.6	78.9	454	138
TX	Randall	2.36	396	25.8	8.9	21.4	75.6	80.2	3623	1104
TX	Reagan	0.60	1022	28.6	8.9	28.7	75.9	81.1	2650	808
TX	Real	3.48	248	29.4	9	26.9	73.7	79.9	2043	623
TX	Red River	-0.11	1537	31.3	10	31.3	72.5	78.1	400	122
TX	Reeves	2.84	327	30.4	9.5	27.3	73.2	78.7	2981	909
TX	Refugio	2.56	366	29.3	9.1	28.2	73.3	79.8	42	13
TX	Roberts	-0.41	1766	28.5	8.6	27.7	73.8	79.3	2830	863
TX	Robertson	0.63	1005	31.6	10.1	28.2	72.8	78.4	379	116
TX	Rockwall	1.39	637	26.5	8.4	27.3	76.9	80.8	523	159
TX	Runnels	1.18	738	34	8.8	26.5	73.2	78.8	1828	557
TX	Rusk	1.88	503	31.4	9.8	27.6	73	78.9	403	123
TX	Sabine	2.13	447	31.3	8.8	28.1	71.8	78.2	243	74
TX	San Augustine	1.96	482	30.4	10.3	29.7	71.8	78.2	272	83
TX	San Jacinto	2.18	439	29.7	9.4	29.6	71.7	78.4	214	65
TX	San Patricio	1.97	479	29.6	9.9	27.8	73.7	79.9	60	18
TX	San Saba	2.92	320	29.3	8.9	29.8	76.4	81.6	1445	440
TX	Schleicher	0.08	1382	29.4	8.6	26.5	73.6	78.3	2370	722
TX	Scurry	1.44	622	29.2	8.3	29.1	73.2	79.3	2357	718
TX	Shackelford	-0.09	1521	28.4	8.5	26.7	72.6	79.1	1545	471
TX	Shelby	2.45	382	32.6	10	31.6	71.3	77.6	296	90
TX	Sherman	-0.65	1917	29.2	8.6	27.7	73.7	78.9	3524	1074

ST	COUNTY	USDA	AMEN	OBES	DIAB	INACT	M AGE	W AGE	ALT ft	ALT m
TX	Smith	0.72	948	28.5	8.7	25.7	75	81	445	136
TX	Somervell	1.17	744	28.7	8.7	27.2	73.9	79.6	817	249
TX	Starr	1.99	477	29.2	8.5	28.9	74.1	80	359	109
TX	Stephens	1.38	644	28.3	8.4	27.7	72.6	79.1	1282	391
TX	Sterling	0.27	1242	28.8	8.5	27.5	73.2	78.8	2482	756
TX	Stonewall	0.61	1019	29.2	9	28	72.9	78.9	1750	533
TX	Sutton	1.47	607	28.1	8.5	26	75.5	81	2252	686
TX	Swisher	0.42	1131	29.4	9.1	29	74.6	79.8	3452	1052
TX	Tarrant	1.02	807	27.6	8.7	22.8	75.3	79.9	656	200
TX	Taylor	2.04	464	28.6	8.9	32.9	73.6	79	2008	612
TX	Terrell	3.17	285	26.7	8.6	29.5	75	80.8	2398	731
TX	Terry	1.11	773	30.5	9.4	30.9	73.1	78.8	3337	1017
TX	Throckmorton	-0.79	2006	29.4	8.6	27.4	72.6	79	1363	416
TX	Titus	0.84	895	33	9	27.1	72.5	78.1	358	109
TX	Tom Green	2.62	356	29.5	9.1	25.5	74.3	79.9	2080	634
TX	Travis	3.24	279	24.7	8	19.2	77.6	81.4	726	221
TX	Trinity	1.45	617	32.3	9.8	31.4	71.7	78.4	248	76
TX	Tyler	1.18	739	28.7	9.8	28.8	72.4	78.4	203	62
TX	Upshur	0.28	1236	30.4	10.3	34.9	72.3	78.4	383	117
TX	Upton	1.02	808	28.9	8.7	27.6	73.4	78.5	2743	836
TX	Uvalde	4.26	180	30	9.1	27	73.7	79.9	1190	363
TX	Val Verde	5.20	101	29.2	9	25.4	75.5	81	1686	514
TX	Van Zandt	0.42	1132	29.4	9.5	29.5	73.6	79.2	466	142
TX	Victoria	-0.82	2021	30.4	9.2	24.9	74.5	80.1	87	27
TX	Walker	1.07	785	32.5	9.6	27.9	73.9	78.8	277	84
TX	Waller	1.28	691	31.4	9.8	30.1	73.8	78.8	203	62
TX	Ward	1.46	610	28.6	8.9	29.6	73.4	78.5	2612	796
TX	Washington	1.43	626	29.2	8.8	27.1	73.7	80.2	304	93
TX	Webb	1.12	767	29.2	9.1	27.7	75.3	81.8	588	179
TX	Wharton	-0.99	2124	30.5	9.8	27.6	73.2	79.2	101	31
TX	Wheeler	0.31	1212	29.4	9.1	28	73.2	78.9	2454	748
TX	Wichita	0.80	914	31.1	10.6	30.3	72.5	78.7	1046	319
TX	Wilbarger	0.88	874	30.4	9.2	25.9	73.2	78.7	1231	375
TX	Willacy	1.85	511	29.5	8.8	28.1	73.8	78.4	23	7
TX	Williamson	0.91	857	26.8	7.3	19.7	79.3	82.7	751	229
TX	Wilson	0.44	1120	29.3	9.6	26.4	74.3	79.6	458	140
TX	Winkler	1.31	675	30.8	9.4	27.4	72.2	78	2914	888
TX	Wise	0.87	878	31.3	8.6	29.1	73.8	79	879	268
TX	Wood	1.37	648	30.1	9	28.8	73.3	80.3	442	135
TX	Yoakum	0.21	1302	29.9	8.5	28	73.9	78.9	3661	1116
TX	Young	0.51	1067	29.9	9.6	26.6	73.3	78.8	1179	359
TX	Zapata	2.36	397	30.2	8	27.9	74.1	80	436	133
TX	Zavala	0.49	1083	29.6	8.7	27.4	72.2	78.1	691	211
UT	Beaver	2.39	392	26.5	7.5	22.3	75.2	79.9	6359	1938
UT	Box Elder	3.29	273	26.8	7.6	22	76.8	81	4839	1475
UT	Cache	2.63	353	23.8	6.5	17.9	78.8	81.8	6306	1922
UT	Carbon	3.13	293	24.1	7.8	25.1	74.6	80.2	7129	2173

HEALTHIEST PLACES TO LIVE

ST	COUNTY	USDA	AMEN	OBES	DIAB	INACT	M AGE	W AGE	ALT ft	ALT m
UT	Daggett	4.30	176	27.7	7	19.4	75	79.8	7536	2297
UT	Davis	5.54	82	24.7	6.8	16.5	78.2	81.1	4589	1399
UT	Duchesne	3.73	220	27.6	8.6	24.5	75	79.8	7792	2375
UT	Emery	0.83	901	28.5	7.3	20.8	75.7	80	5846	1782
UT	Garfield	4.00	200	24.8	7	23.2	75.2	79.9	6778	2066
UT	Grand	2.08	455	19.9	5.8	18.2	75.7	80	5752	1753
UT	Iron	2.37	394	25.2	7.1	19.5	76.2	80.3	6376	1943
UT	Juab	1.91	496	29.1	7.2	21.2	75.4	80.2	5528	1685
UT	Kane	2.97	312	24.1	7.5	21.6	74.9	80.2	5736	1748
UT	Millard	2.69	342	28.5	6.6	21	75.2	79.9	5412	1650
UT	Morgan	3.72	221	22.3	6.8	18.2	78.8	81.8	6736	2053
UT	Piute	3.87	209	24.3	6.9	24.4	75.2	79.9	7786	2373
UT	Rich	5.03	119	26.6	7.2	19.9	78.8	81.8	6822	2079
UT	Salt Lake	4.21	187	24.4	7.5	18.4	77.1	81.3	5577	1700
UT	San Juan	3.60	239	28.3	8.7	29	74.9	80.2	5658	1725
UT	Sanpete	4.44	166	26.7	7.3	23.3	75.4	80.2	7311	2228
UT	Sevier	3.66	229	26	8	21.9	75.5	79.8	7550	2301
UT	Summit	4.96	131	15.7	4.5	13	78.7	82.8	8472	2582
UT	Tooele	2.83	330	29.5	9.6	22.1	76.1	79.5	4788	1459
UT	Uintah	3.53	243	28.6	8.6	27.2	75	80.6	6258	1908
UT	Utah	4.93	135	25.5	7.3	16.4	78.5	81.7	6264	1909
UT	Wasatch	4.92	136	23.5	6.3	15.5	77.5	80.5	8034	2449
UT	Washington	2.57	364	24	6.5	17.1	78.8	83.5	5072	1546
UT	Wayne	0.92	853	24.6	6.8	20.3	75.5	79.8	6110	1862
UT	Weber	3.71	224	27.1	8	19.3	76.3	80.5	5649	1722
VA	Accomack	1.16	747	33.6	10.5	29.2	71.5	77.6	19	6
VA	Albemarle	-0.02	1459	27.1	8.7	19.1	77.8	81.7	741	226
VA	Alexandria	-2.25	2673	20.2	7.8	18.7	78.3	83.6	112	34
VA	Alleghany	1.77	527	26	8.4	23.8	72.8	79	2000	610
VA	Amelia	-1.52	2390	32.5	9.4	25	72.4	78.7	303	92
VA	Amherst	0.83	902	29.9	10.4	24.9	73.2	79.4	1129	344
VA	Appomattox	-0.69	1938	31.8	10.8	26.4	73.1	79.7	658	201
VA	Arlington	-2.25	2674	19.4	7.5	17.6	79.7	83.3	207	63
VA	Augusta	-0.12	1541	26.5	8.7	25.1	75.1	80.6	1870	570
VA	Bath	2.19	434	27.7	9	25.3	75.1	80.6	2213	674
VA	Bedford	1.39	638	25.3	7.7	28.3	75.8	80.9	1050	320
VA	Bedford City	1.39	639	30.5	10	23.8	75.8	80.9	973	297
VA	Bland	-0.85	2040	30.6	9.4	24.9	72.5	78.8	2705	825
VA	Botetourt	1.15	752	28.8	9	20.7	75.7	80.4	1483	452
VA	Bristol	-0.23	1624	28.1	9	24.7	72.8	79.4	1771	540
VA	Brunswick	-1.44	2349	36.2	12.2	28.9	69.9	76.6	279	85
VA	Buchanan	-1.61	2432	33.6	12.3	30.8	69	76.7	1876	572
VA	Buckingham	-0.31	1684	32.6	10.9	28.1	71.3	76.9	500	152
VA	Buena Vista	0.64	994	29.1	8.8	23.7	74.3	80.4	999	304
VA	Campbell	-0.38	1738	31.8	9.5	23.5	74.7	80.1	692	211
VA	Caroline	-1.22	2249	30.8	10.5	23.5	71.7	78.9	162	49
VA	Carroll	0.67	975	31	10	28.5	73	79	2470	753

ST	COUNTY	USDA	AMEN	OBES	DIAB	INACT	M AGE	W AGE	ALT ft	ALT m
VA	Charles City	0.59	1026	33.6	11.3	30.2	72	77.8	63	19
VA	Charlotte	-1.49	2374	30.7	9.8	25.6	71.1	78.1	491	150
VA	Charlottesville	-0.02	1460	26.9	9.2	26.8	75.6	81.5	453	138
VA	Chesapeake	0.48	1089	27.2	9.1	22	74.6	79.6	13	4
VA	Chesterfield	-0.84	2030	26.5	9.1	21.8	75.3	79.7	200	61
VA	Clarke	-1.75	2490	28.4	8.8	23.4	75.2	79.8	631	192
VA	Colonial Hghts	-0.84	2031	28.2	9	22.3	75	80.5	75	23
VA	Covington	1.77	528	28.8	9.5	24.9	72.8	79	1397	426
VA	Craig	-0.60	1882	27	8.1	24.7	72.8	79	2175	663
VA	Culpeper	-1.15	2217	32.2	9.8	23.9	74.7	79.6	380	116
VA	Cumberland	-1.50	2379	33.8	11	27.8	72.4	78.7	335	102
VA	Danville	-0.30	1675	31.1	10.1	28.7	70.2	76.9	516	157
VA	Dickenson	0.61	1020	31.4	9.6	29	70.2	77.4	1896	578
VA	Dinwiddie	-1.34	2296	33.3	10.4	24.1	71.3	78.6	220	67
VA	Emporia	-0.78	1998	33.5	11.5	28.7	70.5	75.4	103	31
VA	Essex	0.48	1090	32.7	10.8	27.4	72.4	79.2	87	26
VA	Fairfax	-1.31	2285	23.2	8.1	18.7	81.1	83.8	266	81
VA	Fairfax City	-1.31	2286	28.1	9	26.6	76.6	82.1	390	119
VA	Falls Church	-1.31	2287	26.1	8.9	21.7	79.7	83.3	324	99
VA	Fauquier	-1.53	2396	26.4	8.7	20.5	76.7	80.8	528	161
VA	Floyd	-1.05	2166	27.6	9.2	23.3	73.4	78.9	2581	787
VA	Fluvanna	-0.51	1819	29.6	9.6	21.3	76	80.3	387	118
VA	Franklin	1.92	493	29.6	9.4	24.4	74.6	80.2	1198	365
VA	Franklin City	-0.94	2097	32.8	10.3	30.5	72.8	78.9	31	10
VA	Frederick	-0.38	1739	28.2	8.5	26	75.3	80.5	916	279
VA	Fredericksburg	-0.97	2113	29.7	9.7	25	73.5	80.6	103	31
VA	Galax	0.67	976	29.8	8.8	24.4	72.3	77.9	2487	758
VA	Giles	0.09	1373	28.8	9.7	27.4	72.5	78.8	2479	756
VA	Gloucester	1.27	696	28.6	8.5	24.3	75	80.7	44	13
VA	Goochland	-1.06	2174	26.5	9.2	21.4	75.6	81.2	276	84
VA	Grayson	1.20	734	28.9	9.6	26.3	72.3	77.9	3015	919
VA	Greene	-0.44	1781	30.5	8.7	23.2	74.7	80.1	1167	356
VA	Greensville	-0.78	1999	34.1	12	29.9	70.5	75.4	147	45
VA	Halifax	0.53	1052	33.9	11.8	31.3	70.6	78	461	140
VA	Hampton	1.27	697	36.7	11.8	27.6	74.4	79.1	4	1
VA	Hanover	-2.08	2613	26.4	8.4	19.9	76.5	80.8	181	55
VA	Harrisonburg	1.25	713	29.1	9.2	25.5	75.6	80.5	1357	414
VA	Henrico	-0.93	2088	28.5	8.7	25.6	75.6	80.3	142	43
VA	Henry	-0.28	1657	28.7	10.4	31.3	71.2	78.3	913	278
VA	Highland	0.30	1219	27.2	8.4	21.8	75.1	80.6	2850	869
VA	Hopewell	0.26	1250	33.5	11	29.1	71.7	77.5	98	30
VA	Isle of Wight	0.51	1068	31	11.4	26.9	72.8	78.9	53	16
VA	James City	1.15	753	27	8	20.1	78.1	82.5	65	20
VA	King & Queen	-0.13	1550	34.1	10.6	27.7	73.3	79	87	26
VA	King George	-0.17	1579	28	9.5	21.5	74.7	79.7	88	27
VA	King William	-0.06	1497	29.7	9.4	28.1	73.3	79	89	27
VA	Lancaster	1.33	664	31.6	9.9	28.6	72.5	78.7	44	13

HEALTHIEST PLACES TO LIVE

ST	COUNTY	USDA	AMEN	OBES	DIAB	INACT	M AGE	W AGE	ALT ft	ALT m
VA	Lee	-1.36	2303	34.2	10.6	33.2	70.4	77	1776	541
VA	Lexington	0.64	995	29.2	9.5	23.7	74.3	80.4	1055	322
VA	Loudoun	-0.63	1901	22.8	7.9	21	79	82.2	461	140
VA	Louisa	-0.68	1933	31.7	9.9	29.1	73.4	80.2	362	110
VA	Lunenburg	-2.17	2643	34.3	11.3	31.4	71.1	78.1	431	131
VA	Lynchburg	-0.38	1740	31.8	10.7	29.3	74.3	79.2	743	226
VA	Madison	-0.76	1986	31.9	8.3	24.2	74.7	80.1	1015	309
VA	Manassas	-0.94	2098	28.4	9.9	24.9	76.5	80.4	249	76
VA	Manassas Park	-0.94	2099	29.7	9.5	25.9	76.5	80.4	235	72
VA	Martinsville	-0.28	1658	33.5	10.8	27.6	71.2	78.3	897	274
VA	Mathews	1.11	774	29.1	9	24.4	75	80.7	4	1
VA	Mecklenburg	-0.03	1468	32.4	10.8	27.8	70.9	78	360	110
VA	Middlesex	1.27	698	28.6	9.2	28.1	72.4	79.2	54	16
VA	Montgomery	0.27	1243	28.5	7.7	22.3	75.8	79.6	2022	616
VA	Nelson	0.36	1182	26.4	9.1	22.7	73.1	79.7	1150	350
VA	New Kent	0.24	1272	28.6	9.8	21.2	78.1	82.5	89	27
VA	Newport News	1.27	699	33.5	11.2	29.2	73.1	79.1	10	3
VA	Norfolk	0.48	1091	32.9	10.9	26.6	70.9	77.5	9	3
VA	Northampton	1.29	685	30.2	11.3	28.7	71.5	77.6	18	6
VA	Northumberland	1.19	736	34.6	9.7	26.7	73	79.5	54	16
VA	Norton	0.25	1258	28	9	24	71.1	77.1	2246	684
VA	Nottoway	-1.57	2410	32.7	10.3	27.2	71.6	77.6	372	114
VA	Orange	-0.89	2067	31.8	9.7	24.5	75.1	80.1	420	128
VA	Page	0.94	846	32.2	8.9	26.4	73.9	80	1402	427
VA	Patrick	1.27	700	30.4	9.7	24.9	73.4	78.9	1577	481
VA	Petersburg	-1.34	2297	37.8	13.5	32.5	66.9	76.2	95	29
VA	Pittsylvania	-0.30	1676	29.4	10.2	26.8	72.5	79.3	703	214
VA	Poquoson	1.27	701	28.3	8.5	21.9	78.3	81.3	3	1
VA	Portsmouth	0.48	1092	39.1	12	29	70.7	76.9	8	2
VA	Powhatan	-1.85	2527	27.1	8.8	26.9	75.9	80.1	275	84
VA	Prince Edward	-1.67	2455	32	9.9	29	71.5	77	462	141
VA	Prince George	0.26	1251	33.9	11.8	28.4	74.9	79.3	88	27
VA	Prince William	-0.94	2100	26.8	9.4	21.3	77.5	80.6	270	82
VA	Pulaski	1.29	686	26.9	9.8	23.5	72.9	78.8	2178	664
VA	Radford	0.27	1244	27.8	9.3	22.8	74.5	79.7	1861	567
VA	Rappahannock	-0.84	2032	26.3	8.5	24.5	73.9	80	1031	314
VA	Richmond	0.64	996	32.5	9.9	29.2	72.5	78.7	82	25
VA	Richmond City	-0.93	2089	31.4	11.4	28	69.2	78.6	160	49
VA	Roanoke	0.01	1437	27	9.2	22.8	76	80.5	1680	512
VA	Roanoke City	0.01	1438	34.4	10.5	26.5	71.2	78.8	1038	316
VA	Rockbridge	0.64	997	29	8.7	27.4	74.3	80.4	1606	489
VA	Rockingham	1.25	714	26.6	8	20.1	75.8	81	1706	520
VA	Russell	-0.38	1741	30.2	10.4	33.4	71.3	77.5	2239	682
VA	Salem	0.01	1439	27.9	9	22.4	75	80.6	1087	331
VA	Scott	-0.47	1802	28.2	8.2	30	71.9	78.2	1822	555
VA	Shenandoah	-0.77	1994	30.3	8.8	27.1	74.8	80.4	1240	378
VA	Smyth	-1.55	2403	32.7	8.2	23.3	71.7	78.1	2679	816

ST	COUNTY	USDA	AMEN	OBES	DIAB	INACT	M AGE	W AGE	ALT ft	ALT m
VA	Southampton	-0.94	2101	28.5	11.6	27.2	72	77.8	65	20
VA	Spotsylvania	-0.97	2114	28	9.5	20	75.4	80.8	282	86
VA	Stafford	-0.12	1542	29.2	8.4	20.4	76.2	79.5	212	65
VA	Staunton	-0.12	1543	29	9.1	24.2	73.7	79.7	1527	465
VA	Suffolk	0.17	1326	31.9	11.2	26.4	72.6	78	42	13
VA	Surry	0.79	918	34.5	11.7	26.2	72	77.8	77	24
VA	Sussex	-1.11	2198	32.8	11.5	29.9	70.5	75.4	95	29
VA	Tazewell	-0.56	1855	32.7	10.2	36.1	70.8	78.4	2697	822
VA	Virginia Beach	1.18	740	26.5	8.7	24.6	76.8	81	9	3
VA	Warren	1.07	786	28.4	9.7	23.9	75.2	79.8	860	262
VA	Washington	-0.23	1625	27.6	9.8	28.4	73.3	78.9	2170	662
VA	Waynesboro	-0.12	1544	28.9	9.1	25.3	74	80.9	1356	413
VA	Westmoreland	0.25	1259	29.3	10.4	28.9	73	79.5	68	21
VA	Williamsburg	1.15	754	29.4	9.8	23.7	78.1	82.5	55	17
VA	Winchester	-0.38	1742	29.5	9.3	24.5	73.9	80.6	748	228
VA	Wise	0.25	1260	35.4	10.2	37.5	71.1	77.1	2296	700
VA	Wythe	0.11	1364	29.3	9.2	24.5	73.2	78.6	2474	754
VA	York	1.27	702	27.8	9.1	22.1	78.3	81.3	33	10
VT	Addison	-0.28	1659	22.8	5.6	18.5	77.1	82.3	849	259
VT	Bennington	-0.81	2018	22.9	5.9	19.5	76.8	81.5	1710	521
VT	Caledonia	-1.16	2222	25.5	7.1	20.7	76.1	81.4	1350	411
VT	Chittenden	0.09	1374	20.1	5.2	15	77.5	82.1	685	209
VT	Essex	-1.01	2142	26.1	6.6	23	75.4	80.3	1595	486
VT	Franklin	-0.30	1677	27.9	7.2	24.4	76.4	81.1	671	205
VT	Grand Isle	-0.16	1568	26.2	5.5	18.1	76.4	81.1	106	32
VT	Lamoille	-0.82	2022	25.4	6.6	17.4	77.8	81.4	1284	391
VT	Orange	-0.57	1867	27.3	6.7	20	76.3	81.1	1269	387
VT	Orleans	0.09	1375	28.5	6.9	24.5	75.4	80.3	1319	402
VT	Rutland	-0.35	1717	28	6.9	22.2	76.1	81.5	1256	383
VT	Washington	-0.63	1902	22.3	6.2	17	77.7	81.2	1338	408
VT	Windham	0.04	1413	23.1	5.6	15.8	76.7	81.9	1353	412
VT	Windsor	0.14	1346	24.2	6.4	19.1	77.2	81.7	1273	388
WA	Adams	-1.34	2298	36.8	10.4	26.7	74.2	79.4	1590	485
WA	Asotin	1.22	727	29.2	9	22.8	75.4	81.6	2773	845
WA	Benton	1.58	575	31.1	8.7	19.8	77.4	80.6	958	292
WA	Chelan	1.56	581	24.2	7.3	19.1	77.8	81.9	3944	1202
WA	Clallam	6.52	45	28.4	8.2	17.6	76.2	81.6	1501	458
WA	Clark	4.25	181	28.8	8.2	18.8	77.3	81.4	727	221
WA	Columbia	1.84	514	29.1	9	17.4	77.1	80.8	2805	855
WA	Cowlitz	4.54	159	37	8.8	22.3	74.6	79.3	1345	410
WA	Douglas	0.42	1133	27.7	7.8	20	76.3	81.1	2237	682
WA	Ferry	2.31	411	25.4	6.4	23.5	75.7	80.4	3275	998
WA	Franklin	-0.39	1749	30.7	9.5	20.5	75.4	79.2	931	284
WA	Garfield	2.31	412	34.6	10.7	24.5	77.1	80.8	2721	829
WA	Grant	0.62	1014	32.4	8.7	22.9	75.5	79.7	1400	427
WA	Grays Harbor	3.94	203	32.7	10.3	23.7	73.7	79	515	157
WA	Island	3.41	255	26.3	7.8	15.5	79.8	83.1	157	48

HEALTHIEST PLACES TO LIVE

ST	COUNTY	USDA	AMEN	OBES	DIAB	INACT	M AGE	W AGE	ALT ft	ALT m
WA	Jefferson	5.31	89	24.8	6.4	15.7	77.8	83.2	2186	666
WA	King	4.53	160	22.3	6.6	16.7	78.6	82.8	1842	561
WA	Kitsap	2.61	358	29.3	7.3	18	77.7	80.9	295	90
WA	Kittitas	3.33	268	26.4	7.1	18.5	77.2	81.3	3169	966
WA	Klickitat	1.97	480	27.4	7.3	21.4	76.3	81	2020	616
WA	Lewis	3.40	258	34.7	9	21.2	75.1	79.8	1900	579
WA	Lincoln	0.56	1039	32.3	7.2	21.5	75.7	80.4	2148	655
WA	Mason	5.20	102	30.8	7.9	20.6	75.3	79.8	1052	321
WA	Okanogan	1.36	651	27.5	7.9	22	75.4	81.1	3741	1140
WA	Pacific	4.85	141	32.6	10.2	22.1	74.8	80.3	581	177
WA	Pend Oreille	3.33	269	30.7	7.7	19.7	74.5	80	3454	1053
WA	Pierce	4.62	153	30.7	9.2	20.2	75.5	80.4	2244	684
WA	San Juan	4.35	172	19.2	4.9	13.1	77.3	81.1	180	55
WA	Skagit	4.94	133	27.4	6.8	17.3	76.9	81.1	2403	732
WA	Skamania	-0.04	1482	32	7.4	20.4	76.3	81	2892	881
WA	Snohomish	4.68	151	28.1	7.8	19.1	77.3	81.1	2135	651
WA	Spokane	1.33	665	27.8	7.9	20.2	76.2	80.5	2388	728
WA	Stevens	2.58	363	27.1	7.7	22.3	74.5	80	2738	835
WA	Thurston	3.32	270	28.4	8.2	18.5	77	81.3	492	150
WA	Wahkiakum	3.25	277	29.3	9.1	20.1	74.8	80.3	676	206
WA	Walla Walla	1.06	788	28.7	8.5	16.3	76.4	80.9	1198	365
WA	Whatcom	5.26	93	24.2	6.8	15.5	77.7	82.2	3024	922
WA	Whitman	2.23	429	28	8.2	21	77.1	80.8	2076	633
WA	Yakima	1.48	604	32.3	8.9	24	75	80.1	2834	864
WI	Adams	-2.43	2755	32.7	7.9	24.9	74.7	80	984	300
WI	Ashland	-0.63	1903	29.5	7.8	20.4	74.4	80.9	1281	390
WI	Barron	-2.86	2879	31.1	6.9	23.7	75.8	81.2	1199	365
WI	Bayfield	-0.56	1856	29.1	7.1	21.2	76.2	80.9	1117	340
WI	Brown	-1.36	2304	29.5	7.9	20.1	77.4	82	746	227
WI	Buffalo	-1.17	2226	32.4	7.9	23.3	76.8	81.8	947	289
WI	Burnett	-2.24	2668	31.6	7.7	22.8	75.5	81.1	994	303
WI	Calumet	-1.49	2375	30.2	6.9	18.6	78.3	82.3	853	260
WI	Chippewa	-2.36	2722	31.5	8.3	17.4	76.7	81	1064	324
WI	Clark	-4.34	3089	31.1	6.8	24.1	75.7	81.2	1166	355
WI	Columbia	-0.52	1831	30.6	7.3	26.3	76.7	81.6	914	278
WI	Crawford	-0.55	1847	28.2	7.7	22	75.1	80.2	937	286
WI	Dane	-0.17	1580	23.9	6.1	17.7	78.7	82.5	957	292
WI	Dodge	-1.83	2520	35.8	7.4	23.7	76.1	80.8	920	280
WI	Door	-0.15	1563	31.7	6.7	19.8	78.2	82.7	676	206
WI	Douglas	-0.66	1921	29.4	7.4	20.9	74.6	80.6	1061	323
WI	Dunn	-1.54	2400	29.1	6.5	23.9	76.3	81.6	983	300
WI	Eau Claire	-3.16	2939	28.2	6.5	23.2	77.3	81.9	987	301
WI	Florence	-2.61	2817	28.2	6.9	22.4	75.8	80.6	1391	424
WI	Fond du Lac	-1.92	2556	30.7	7.3	25	76.5	81.4	940	287
WI	Forest	-2.56	2803	31	8.7	24.2	75.8	80.6	1594	486
WI	Grant	-0.46	1797	29.1	7.6	19.5	76.2	80.8	931	284
WI	Green	-2.32	2697	25.5	6.7	18.1	76.5	81.2	924	282

ST	COUNTY	USDA	AMEN	OBES	DIAB	INACT	M AGE	W AGE	ALT ft	ALT m
WI	Green Lake	-1.58	2413	30.1	8	23.9	76.3	81	857	261
WI	Iowa	-0.98	2120	29.9	8.2	23.6	76.6	81.5	1006	307
WI	Iron	-0.70	1945	27.8	7.5	21.4	75.3	80.7	1531	467
WI	Jackson	-0.87	2054	30.4	8.4	24.1	74.8	79.6	983	300
WI	Jefferson	-1.63	2442	32.1	7.9	21.8	76.8	82.5	848	259
WI	Juneau	-0.43	1777	29.9	7.9	22.8	74.1	80.1	949	289
WI	Kenosha	-0.45	1789	28.3	7.9	23.3	75.3	80	739	225
WI	Kewaunee	0.17	1327	33.8	7.9	24	76.3	81.6	732	223
WI	La Crosse	-0.69	1939	24.1	7.2	18.4	76.9	81.9	891	272
WI	Lafayette	-1.53	2397	31	7.2	21.5	75.8	81.2	954	291
WI	Langlade	-3.13	2934	30.1	7.6	22.3	75.1	80.9	1535	468
WI	Lincoln	-2.98	2905	28.7	8	23	76	81	1476	450
WI	Manitowoc	-0.37	1731	31.1	7	22.2	77	81.6	775	236
WI	Marathon	-3.30	2966	30.7	7.9	26	77.8	82.6	1307	398
WI	Marinette	-2.16	2640	30.3	7.1	25.3	75.1	81.2	906	276
WI	Marquette	-2.25	2675	33.3	7.1	25.5	74.9	80.2	840	256
WI	Menominee	-3.38	2984	35.5	12.4	30.8	75.1	80.9	1051	320
WI	Milwaukee	-0.40	1760	32.1	9.9	26.6	73.9	79.7	700	213
WI	Monroe	-1.36	2305	28.7	8.2	24.6	74.4	80.1	1050	320
WI	Oconto	-1.95	2566	27.6	6.9	23.9	75.9	81.3	872	266
WI	Oneida	-2.19	2650	26.8	6.9	20.4	76	81.3	1603	489
WI	Outagamie	-3.35	2979	28.7	8.8	21.6	77.8	82.4	774	236
WI	Ozaukee	-0.39	1750	25.7	6.9	17.5	78.6	82.7	777	237
WI	Pepin	-0.71	1956	28.7	7.8	25.1	76.8	81.8	910	277
WI	Pierce	-1.21	2245	25.8	7.2	21	77.3	82.1	1025	312
WI	Polk	-2.73	2849	28.4	6.9	19	76.1	81.7	1121	342
WI	Portage	-2.54	2796	27.7	6.9	23	77.3	81.8	1111	339
WI	Price	-2.66	2830	31.9	7.8	24.3	75.3	80.7	1534	468
WI	Racine	-0.51	1820	31.2	7.8	24.6	75.7	80.6	759	231
WI	Richland	-1.29	2279	31.3	7.8	24	76.2	81.1	953	290
WI	Rock	-2.62	2819	31	8	23.7	75.8	80.5	887	270
WI	Rusk	-2.32	2698	28.7	7.4	25.4	74.8	80.2	1250	381
WI	Sauk	-1.01	2143	29.7	8	23.5	76.2	81.9	981	299
WI	Sawyer	-1.42	2336	26.6	7.7	21.9	75.5	80.4	1377	420
WI	Shawano	-3.40	2986	30.2	8.1	25.4	76.3	81	979	298
WI	Sheboygan	-0.37	1732	28.6	7.7	22.4	76.7	81.2	845	257
WI	St. Croix	-1.37	2309	27.9	7	17	77.8	82.2	1065	324
WI	Taylor	-3.39	2985	27.2	7.7	24.2	76	81.1	1398	426
WI	Trempealeau	-1.42	2337	32.9	7.6	24.9	75.4	81.2	930	283
WI	Vernon	-0.66	1922	27.9	7.2	22.9	75.2	80.4	1061	324
WI	Vilas	-1.58	2414	26.2	6.4	23.2	77	81.8	1672	510
WI	Walworth	-2.46	2766	25.3	6.8	21.3	77.2	80.8	927	283
WI	Washburn	-2.26	2681	30.6	8.5	21	75.6	81.2	1178	359
WI	Washington	-2.63	2822	28.1	6.6	21.8	77.6	82.5	982	299
WI	Waukesha	-2.11	2621	25.6	5.9	18.5	78.7	82.2	894	272
WI	Waupaca	-2.48	2779	32.4	7.4	21.6	74.3	80.2	873	266
WI	Waushara	-2.61	2818	32.9	8.1	23.2	75.2	80.6	945	288

HEALTHIEST PLACES TO LIVE

ST	COUNTY	USDA	AMEN	OBES	DIAB	INACT	M AGE	W AGE	ALT ft	ALT m
WI	Winnebago	-1.37	2310	29.4	7.7	19.4	76.6	81.5	788	240
WI	Wood	-2.44	2759	26.3	7.5	18.5	77	82.7	1081	330
WV	Barbour	0.22	1291	34.1	10.8	28.1	72.8	79.2	1668	508
WV	Berkeley	-0.55	1848	31.2	10.5	29.2	73.4	78.7	642	196
WV	Boone	-1.90	2548	34.3	13.8	40.2	69.9	76.7	1340	408
WV	Braxton	-0.55	1849	34.4	12.5	33.6	71.9	78.3	1186	361
WV	Brooke	0.38	1161	36.3	13	34.1	73.8	78.8	1003	306
WV	Cabell	0.11	1365	33	12.9	30.4	71.3	78.2	751	229
WV	Calhoun	-2.37	2727	34.9	10.5	30.8	72.1	78.7	966	295
WV	Clay	-0.51	1821	37.3	13.4	33.2	71.9	78.3	1167	356
WV	Doddridge	-2.52	2791	32.3	11.1	36.3	73	78.9	1051	320
WV	Fayette	-0.13	1551	33.9	12.1	33.4	71.1	77.8	1957	596
WV	Gilmer	-2.64	2826	36.6	11.5	34.2	72.1	78.7	1004	306
WV	Grant	1.46	611	34.9	12.1	28.9	73.9	79.3	2076	633
WV	Greenbrier	-0.20	1602	29	10.2	29.7	73.3	78.7	2627	801
WV	Hampshire	0.69	963	35.1	9.9	30.3	73.3	79.2	1201	366
WV	Hancock	0.39	1154	32.6	11.7	27.3	73.9	79	998	304
WV	Hardy	0.82	905	32.8	11.2	26.8	73.9	79.3	1742	531
WV	Harrison	-1.36	2306	32.4	11.7	31.2	72.7	79.3	1190	363
WV	Jackson	-0.08	1516	35.8	11.7	28.7	74.2	79	806	246
WV	Jefferson	-1.12	2204	34.5	10.6	27.5	74.6	79.1	512	156
WV	Kanawha	-0.12	1545	31.8	11.3	30.4	72	78.3	1015	309
WV	Lewis	-0.98	2121	30.4	11.1	31.9	72	78.5	1216	371
WV	Lincoln	-1.05	2167	38.4	10.7	37.7	70.6	76.6	911	278
WV	Logan	-1.03	2152	37.8	13.6	42.7	68.9	76.4	1355	413
WV	Marion	-0.52	1832	35	10.9	32.1	73.9	79	1218	371
WV	Marshall	-0.34	1706	33.1	10.2	34.7	73.8	80.2	1108	338
WV	Mason	-0.05	1488	36.8	10.7	32.3	71.9	78.6	721	220
WV	McDowell	-1.88	2538	32.6	14.2	42.1	66.3	74.7	1869	570
WV	Mercer	-1.67	2456	34.3	11	33.6	71	77.5	2462	750
WV	Mineral	0.68	969	34	10.8	30.8	73.8	79.3	1281	390
WV	Mingo	-1.12	2205	31.4	11.7	40	68.7	75.9	1249	381
WV	Monongalia	-0.07	1504	27.8	9.6	24.9	75.4	80.1	1280	390
WV	Monroe	-1.38	2316	29.6	11.7	30.1	72.6	79.2	2308	704
WV	Morgan	0.41	1137	31.4	11	29.2	74.1	80	888	271
WV	Nicholas	0.02	1426	36.2	11.2	32.9	73	78.5	2051	625
WV	Ohio	-0.13	1552	30.3	10.8	28.9	74.2	79.8	1084	331
WV	Pendleton	0.82	906	34.8	10.8	30.8	73.3	78.6	2567	783
WV	Pleasants	-0.12	1546	31.2	11	29.7	73.3	79	860	262
WV	Pocahontas	-0.42	1773	30.9	10.8	27.4	73.3	78.6	3215	980
WV	Preston	-0.84	2033	33.9	9.6	32.1	73.4	79.8	2020	616
WV	Putnam	-0.43	1778	29.4	10.4	27.7	75.5	79.3	792	241
WV	Raleigh	-0.13	1553	34	11.9	34.4	72.4	78.6	2241	683
WV	Randolph	-1.61	2433	33.6	11.3	32.7	73.3	79.2	2938	896
WV	Ritchie	-2.42	2750	33.8	11.3	33.8	73.3	79	939	286
WV	Roane	-1.66	2449	34.2	12.9	32.2	72	78	939	286
WV	Summers	0.67	977	34.7	11	33.1	72.6	79.2	2147	654

ST	COUNTY	USDA	AMEN	OBES	DIAB	INACT	M AGE	W AGE	ALT ft	ALT m
WV	Taylor	-0.01	1450	32.4	11	35.2	73.8	78.8	1341	409
WV	Tucker	-0.29	1663	32.8	10.5	35.5	72.8	79.2	2776	846
WV	Tyler	-0.22	1617	33.2	10.9	28.1	73	78.9	938	286
WV	Upshur	-1.52	2391	30.4	12.5	30.1	73.3	78.7	1807	551
WV	Wayne	-0.19	1592	35.5	11.8	31	72.3	77.9	856	261
WV	Webster	-2.35	2713	34.8	11.5	35.6	72	78.5	2404	733
WV	Wetzel	-0.91	2078	33.9	10.6	30.5	73.7	79.7	1125	343
WV	Wirt	-0.34	1707	37.3	12.7	28.1	72	78	866	264
WV	Wood	-0.19	1593	32	11.7	31	74.9	79.5	794	242
WV	Wyoming	-1.37	2311	35.8	14.3	40.9	69.5	76.6	1898	579
WY	Albany	4.91	138	22	5.7	19.4	77.2	81.1	7464	2275
WY	Big Horn	2.49	371	27.6	7	25.7	75	80.6	5422	1653
WY	Campbell	0.79	919	31.3	7.9	27.5	75.9	81.5	4501	1372
WY	Carbon	5.41	86	29.9	7.5	31.2	75.2	80	7294	2223
WY	Converse	2.86	325	28.4	6.7	23.7	75.9	81.2	5426	1654
WY	Crook	2.57	365	22.7	6.1	22.2	75.9	81.5	4270	1301
WY	Fremont	3.71	225	24.6	7.3	24.6	73.3	79.7	7037	2145
WY	Goshen	2.00	474	26.8	6.7	29.2	76.3	80.9	4650	1417
WY	Hot Springs	1.08	782	24.2	7.3	22.9	76.1	81.5	6124	1867
WY	Johnson	2.78	335	23.3	7.2	21.9	76.6	81.5	5557	1694
WY	Laramie	3.05	301	25.1	7.9	23.4	74.9	79.8	5987	1825
WY	Lincoln	5.12	111	21.4	7.8	20.7	76.8	81.4	7381	2250
WY	Natrona	2.49	372	27.2	7.1	23.6	74.9	81.1	6069	1850
WY	Niobrara	-0.01	1451	23.7	6.3	28.5	76.3	80.9	4532	1381
WY	Park	3.96	202	21.7	6	21.2	76.1	81.5	7529	2295
WY	Platte	4.10	193	24.6	8.6	26.8	75.9	81.2	5155	1571
WY	Sheridan	2.17	441	24.5	7.5	19.1	76.6	81.5	5151	1570
WY	Sublette	5.29	91	25.7	5.8	23.2	76.8	81.4	8045	2452
WY	Sweetwater	2.63	354	29.1	7.1	24.4	74.8	80.5	6869	2094
WY	Teton	5.39	87	13.8	4.4	10.6	79.9	84.7	8044	2452
WY	Uinta	3.32	271	30.3	7	23.1	75.7	80.9	7249	2210
WY	Washakie	1.10	777	24	7.2	23.8	75	80.6	5211	1588
WY	Weston	-0.91	2079	28.4	6.3	26.9	75.9	81.5	4452	1357

CHAPTER 6

Natural Amenities Ratings for 3,108
Lower Forty-Eight Counties

There's no way to remove the observer – us – from our perceptions of the world. - Stephen Hawking

This blue book section ranks the 3,108 lower forty-eight counties by USDA-defined natural amenities. Here is what the USDA has to say about its Natural Amenities Scale.

> The natural amenities scale is a measure of the physical characteristics of a county area that enhance the location as a place to live. The scale was constructed by combining six measures of climate, topography, and water area that reflect environmental qualities most people prefer. These measures are warm winter, winter sun, temperate summer, low summer humidity, topographic variation, and water area. The data are available for counties in the lower forty-eight States.[1]

> The six measures used in the natural amenities composite score were selected on the basis of a conception of the environmental qualities most people prefer, availability of measures, simplicity, nonredundancy, and the correlation to population change. Hawaii and Alaska were not included, as data were not always available. Because it is difficult to handle a number of separate indicators in a given analysis, a simple additive

scale was developed, with some adjustment for the interrelationships among the measures.

Warm winter (average January temperature)

People are attracted to areas with warm winters. Southern areas of the country generally have the warmest winters, while the upper Midwest and the Rocky Mountains experience the coldest. Coastal areas are generally warmer than inland. This measure, and the others relating to climate, was drawn from the Area Resources tape issued at the time by the Center for National Health Statistics, U.S. Department of Health and Human Services.

Winter sun (average January days of sun)

Brochures almost inevitably show sunny skies. The Southwest has the sunniest Januaries while the Pacific Northwest has the cloudiest. Some areas around the Great Lakes also have frequent January overcast.

Temperate summer (low winter-summer temperature gap)

While less so with the widespread use of air conditioning, summer heat is still a drawback. Places warm in the winter tend to be hot in the summer: the correlation coefficient between average January and average July temperatures is 0.74 for counties. What seems most desirable is a temperate climate, with relatively little temperature gain between January and July.

One possible measure of temperate climate would be the gain in temperature between January and July, with a low gain indicating a more favorable climate. However, places cold in the winter tend to have greater gains in temperature between winter and summer. The size of the variance in average July temperature across counties is only 20 percent of the size of variance in average January temperature. This means that the temperature difference between January and July is largely redundant with the January temperature measure.

To solve this problem, the residual of a simple regression of July temperature on January temperature was used to reflect low gain in temperature, i.e., a temperate climate. In effect, we asked how much higher or lower the July temperature is, given what one would predict on the basis of the January temperature. Since residuals are not correlated with independent variables, this produced a measure of temperate climate not at all redundant with the January temperature measure.

Mountainous areas and areas along the west coast tend to have the most temperate summers according to this measure. The Central and Southern Plains, southern Arizona, and the Imperial Valley in California have the least temperate summers.

Summer humidity (low average July humidity)

Humidity, which adds to summer discomfort, is relatively low in the West, except along the coast. July humidity is high in much of the Southeast (although humidity tends to be lower in southern Florida than in northern Florida and southern Georgia).

Topographic variation (topography scale)

In general, the more varied the topography, the more appealing the setting. To measure topography, we drew on a topographic map in The National Atlas of the United States of America (1970). This map delineated five basic land formations: plains, tablelands, plains with hills or mountains, open hills or mountains, and hills and mountains. Within each of these broad categories, land was distinguished by its degree of variation. For example, the "plains" category ranged from "flat plains" to "irregular plains," and the "hills and mountains" category ranged from "hills" to "high mountains." A total of 21 categories were delineated. We created a county map overlay and mapped the topography onto the county map. Where a county had more than one type of land formation, we assigned the highest of the categories that applied, provided this higher category appeared to apply to at least 25 percent of the county area. At the high end of the scale, the resulting county map reproduces the principal mountain ranges in the country and, at the low end, the coastal plains.

Water area (water area as proportion of total county area)

Coastal areas and areas with lakes are more pleasant than areas lacking surface water. Coding water area proved a problem, however. In this data tape, from the Bureau of the Census, coastal waters, because the boundaries extend out 3 miles, are inevitably large and dwarf inland lakes in their surface area. The problem is particularly distorting in the Great Lakes, as the entire water area within U.S. boundaries is assigned to counties along the shores.

Two adjustments were made to reduce what seemed to be the undue influence of coastal waters. First, we limited the amount of water area measured to a maximum of 250 square miles. This reduced the outlier problem in the Great Lakes, but still left the measure as one that discriminated coastal from inland counties but gave inland lakes and ponds little weight. The second adjustment was to take the logarithm of the percentage of county area in water, a transformation that accentuates differences at the low end and reduces them at the high end. Implicit in the transformation is the assumption that a difference between 5 percent and 10 percent in water surface area improves the attractiveness of an area as much as a difference between 10 and 20 percent.[2]

You may notice the USDA study was done back in 1999. However, mountain ranges don't move very much and hot and humid places in summer are generally hot and humid from year to year. So the variables the USDA study measured stay relatively constant over the decades. Other than shrinking water areas in some parts of the West, things are pretty much the same as they were in 1999.

While the overall USDA rating provides valuable information, it is important to note that this is an average of the six measures. Be aware that the average can mask certain characteristics of a county. For example, at #11 out of 3,108, Lake County, Colorado is rated very highly for natural amenities. And Lake County does indeed have everything, except a Bermuda shorts winter. Based on the overall rating, it might be assumed the county has a "warm winter" but that's definitely not the case. While there are 370 counties that have a colder mean January temperature than Lake County, there are 2,737 counties that have a warmer mean January temperature. And, although Lake County has many comfortable sunny dry winter days, a Canadian arctic cold air mass can occasionally drop the winter temperatures to below -20 degrees. As a result, you don't often see Bermuda shorts in Lake County during the winter months.

So, it's a good idea to drill down a little deeper on those counties that bubble to the top of your list. Based upon your specific interests and activities, you may find certain counties to be more desirable than others. The complete USDA natural amenities dataset can be downloaded in Excel format from this web page.

http://www.ers.usda.gov/data-products/natural-amenities-scale.aspx

The blue book dataset headers are as follows:

ABBREVIATION	DESCRIPTION
ST	State
COUNTY	County
USDA	USDA numerical rating with +11.17 denoting the highest number of natural amenities and -6.40 denoting the lowest number of natural amenities
AMEN	Numerical amenity ranking of the USDA natural amenities data with +11.17 being #1 and -6.40 being #3,108. #1 denotes highest ranking and #3,108 denotes lowest ranking
OBES	% obesity among adults ≥ 20
DIAB	% diabetes among adults ≥ 20
INACT	% leisure-time physical inactivity among adults ≥ 20
M AGE	Longevity for men in years
W AGE	Longevity for women in years
ALT ft.	Mean county altitude in feet
ALT m.	Mean county altitude in meters

Lower Forty-Eight Counties Ranked by USDA-defined Natural Amenities

ST	COUNTY	USDA	AMEN	OBES	DIAB	INACT	M AGE	W AGE	ALT ft	ALT m
CA	Ventura	11.17	1	22.9	6.8	16.8	78.1	82.6	2690	820
CA	Humboldt	11.15	2	25.9	8.1	18.9	73.9	79.1	1754	535
CA	Santa Barbara	10.97	3	19.9	6.6	15.8	78.3	83.1	1823	556
CA	Mendocino	10.93	4	22.6	6.3	17	75.6	80.8	1827	557
CA	Del Norte	10.75	5	27.2	7.6	18.1	72.8	79.8	2189	667
CA	San Francisco	10.52	6	17.2	7.3	17	77.6	83.8	236	72
CA	Los Angeles	10.33	7	21.4	7.7	18.9	77.4	82.5	2265	691
CA	San Diego	9.78	8	22.8	7.3	17.4	77.6	82.4	1975	602
CA	Monterey	9.24	9	22.3	7.3	16	78	82.6	1464	446
CA	Orange	8.74	10	20.5	7.1	16.4	79.3	83.6	725	221

ST	COUNTY	USDA	AMEN	OBES	DIAB	INACT	M AGE	W AGE	ALT ft	ALT m
CO	Lake	8.52	11	17.7	5.1	18.9	77.1	81.6	10931	3332
CA	Santa Cruz	8.49	12	19.5	6.1	12.4	78.1	82.6	939	286
CA	Contra Costa	8.36	13	24.2	6.9	17.3	78.3	82.4	486	148
CA	Calaveras	8.27	14	25.6	6.7	19.3	76.6	81.6	2430	741
CA	Mariposa	8.25	15	24.1	7.2	19.4	76.3	81.1	3637	1108
CA	Mono	8.21	16	20.3	6.5	13.6	77	80.7	7760	2365
CA	San Mateo	8.19	17	19.8	6.5	16.1	79.8	84.5	669	204
CA	Marin	8.14	18	15	5.4	12.1	80.8	84.5	426	130
CO	Summit	8.08	19	15.1	4.7	12.3	79.3	83	10481	3195
CA	Sonoma	7.93	20	22.7	6.1	14.2	77.8	82.1	729	222
CA	San Luis Obispo	7.87	21	21.5	5.9	14.2	77.9	82.2	1552	473
NV	Douglas	7.61	22	21.7	6.3	16.4	79.1	82.7	6047	1843
CA	Napa	7.53	23	22.1	6.2	15.1	77.2	81.9	935	285
AZ	Gila	7.50	24	26.5	8.7	23.1	72.9	79.6	4662	1421
CO	Grand	7.47	25	18.3	5.2	16.9	78.2	82	9259	2822
CA	Alpine	7.41	26	24.9	7.9	19.4	77	80.7	7732	2357
NV	Carson City	7.29	27	23.1	7.1	19.8	74	79.6	5780	1762
CA	Nevada	7.26	28	20.1	5.5	12.9	78	81.8	4139	1262
CA	Amador	7.23	29	24.8	8	16.6	76.3	81.1	2655	809
CA	Stanislaus	7.21	30	30.2	8.2	23.9	74.8	79.4	491	150
CO	San Juan	7.16	31	18.8	5.3	18.4	75.6	80.9	11344	3458
AZ	Cochise	7.13	32	23.8	7.2	22.3	75.8	81.1	4635	1413
CO	Park	7.11	33	17.7	5	19.2	77.1	81.6	9672	2948
CA	Tuolumne	7.10	34	23.1	6	18.1	77	80.7	5653	1723
CA	Inyo	7.08	35	23.1	6.9	16.7	75.5	81.1	4163	1269
CO	Gilpin	6.97	36	19.2	5.4	18.7	77.1	81.8	9303	2836
CO	Clear Creek	6.96	37	17.7	5.1	17.3	78.2	82	10296	3138
CO	Hinsdale	6.90	38	18.9	5.3	18.3	75.7	81.2	10935	3333
OR	Douglas	6.78	39	31.3	9.2	20.6	74.1	80.7	2109	643
NV	Washoe	6.77	40	22.6	6.4	17.2	75.2	80.3	5359	1633
NM	Sierra	6.72	41	26.5	6.1	24.3	73.3	79.8	5445	1660
CA	Riverside	6.64	42	27.5	8.9	21.5	75.8	81.3	1857	566
CA	Lake	6.55	43	26.5	7.8	16.6	73.2	78.4	2327	709
CA	Plumas	6.55	44	23.9	6.6	18.4	76.3	81.5	5309	1618
WA	Clallam	6.52	45	28.4	8.2	17.6	76.2	81.6	1501	458
OR	Curry	6.47	46	30.2	7.6	21.6	74.8	80.2	1633	498
CO	Chaffee	6.46	47	15.9	4.6	15.6	77.1	81.1	9959	3035
CA	Imperial	6.45	48	24.6	7.3	22.6	75.1	81.7	415	126
CO	Jackson	6.45	49	20.5	5.4	17.9	78.6	83.3	8919	2719
NM	Grant	6.45	50	23.8	6	19.2	74.7	80.6	5823	1775
CA	Lassen	6.35	51	26.4	7.6	18.9	75.5	79.8	5361	1634
CO	Teller	6.29	52	17.8	6	18.7	77.9	81.8	9181	2798
NM	Catron	6.24	53	24.6	6.3	19.3	73.3	79.8	7377	2248
CO	Pitkin	6.14	54	14.2	4.7	12.7	80	84.2	10010	3051
CA	El Dorado	6.10	55	20.4	6.5	14.1	77.2	81.5	4256	1297
OR	Deschutes	6.10	56	20	6.6	15.3	78.4	81.7	4577	1395

ST	COUNTY	USDA	AMEN	OBES	DIAB	INACT	M AGE	W AGE	ALT ft	ALT m
CO	Ouray	6.08	57	17	5.4	15	75.7	81.2	8980	2737
OR	Lincoln	6.06	58	27	7.4	19	75.5	80.3	704	215
FL	Monroe	6.05	59	19.4	6.1	18.1	76	81.8	3	1
CA	Fresno	6.03	60	29.2	9.3	21	75.2	80.2	3364	1025
CA	Madera	6.00	61	29.9	8.5	20.4	74.6	80.2	3089	942
CA	Placer	6.00	62	20.3	6.5	13.8	79	82.8	3812	1162
AZ	Santa Cruz	5.95	63	21.8	6.1	16.7	74.3	81	4548	1386
CA	Santa Clara	5.95	64	21.1	7.4	16.6	80.6	83.9	1226	374
TX	Jeff Davis	5.93	65	26.5	8.8	22.6	76.3	82	4906	1495
CA	Sierra	5.90	66	23.4	6.9	17.7	76.3	81.5	5746	1751
CA	Solano	5.88	67	26.7	9.7	21.2	76.1	81	167	51
AZ	Mohave	5.84	68	27.9	9.5	28	72	78.5	3769	1149
CO	La Plata	5.83	69	15.9	4.6	15.5	77.9	82.2	7988	2435
TX	Bandera	5.83	70	29.8	9.1	28.9	76.4	81.2	1684	513
CO	Boulder	5.82	71	14.5	4.6	11.3	77.6	81.4	7381	2250
CO	Mineral	5.79	72	18.7	5.2	17.2	75.7	81.2	10492	3198
NV	Mineral	5.71	73	32	9.9	28.2	72.2	78.8	5872	1790
NV	Lyon	5.70	74	30	7.4	25.3	74.5	79.9	5207	1587
CA	Shasta	5.69	75	28	7.1	18.9	73.9	79.1	2997	913
CA	Tulare	5.65	76	31.1	7.9	24.5	74.1	79.4	4352	1326
CO	Larimer	5.62	77	18.5	5	14.2	79.2	82.7	7725	2355
CO	Custer	5.61	78	20.2	5.4	20.5	74.9	79.9	9062	2762
CO	Jefferson	5.61	79	18.7	5.2	15.7	77.6	81.4	7056	2151
CO	Archuleta	5.58	80	16.5	5	16.7	76.8	81.4	8265	2519
OR	Tillamook	5.54	81	26.5	7.4	18.9	75.8	80.8	1113	339
UT	Davis	5.54	82	24.7	6.8	16.5	78.2	81.1	4589	1399
OR	Coos	5.53	83	30	8	20.5	74	79.3	932	284
FL	Miami-Dade	5.48	84	23.9	8.6	23.6	76.6	82.8	5	1
NV	Churchill	5.42	85	28.9	7.3	26	75.1	80.1	4754	1449
WY	Carbon	5.41	86	29.9	7.5	31.2	75.2	80	7294	2223
WY	Teton	5.39	87	13.8	4.4	10.6	79.9	84.7	8044	2452
FL	Martin	5.34	88	21.7	6.2	18.9	77.7	83.4	21	6
WA	Jefferson	5.31	89	24.8	6.4	15.7	77.8	83.2	2186	666
CO	Routt	5.29	90	13.5	3.8	11.1	78.6	83.3	8197	2499
WY	Sublette	5.29	91	25.7	5.8	23.2	76.8	81.4	8045	2452
CO	Rio Grande	5.26	92	21.1	6	22.5	75.7	81.2	9029	2752
WA	Whatcom	5.26	93	24.2	6.8	15.5	77.7	82.2	3024	922
FL	Lee	5.23	94	26.4	8.6	22.3	76.4	83.1	15	5
NM	Rio Arriba	5.23	95	24.5	6.3	22.4	71	79.5	7657	2334
NM	Mora	5.22	96	21.5	6.7	21.8	75.4	81.8	7166	2184
AZ	Yavapai	5.21	97	22	6.6	19.1	75.8	81.6	4508	1374
AZ	Graham	5.20	98	32.5	9.6	27.3	74.6	79.5	4541	1384
CA	San Benito	5.20	99	23.9	7	16.1	77.7	82	1939	591
CO	Huerfano	5.20	100	20.1	5.5	23.1	74.5	80.1	7507	2288
TX	Val Verde	5.20	101	29.2	9	25.4	75.5	81	1686	514
WA	Mason	5.20	102	30.8	7.9	20.6	75.3	79.8	1052	321

ST	COUNTY	USDA	AMEN	OBES	DIAB	INACT	M AGE	W AGE	ALT ft	ALT m
AZ	Greenlee	5.18	103	35.4	8.7	25	74.6	79.5	5710	1740
CO	Douglas	5.15	104	15.7	4.6	11.1	80.3	83.5	6876	2096
CO	El Paso	5.15	105	21	6	18.2	76.6	81.1	6423	1958
FL	Glades	5.15	106	35.9	10.2	33	74.2	80.1	29	9
OR	Klamath	5.15	107	26.5	7.3	20.4	74.4	78.7	4982	1518
CO	San Miguel	5.14	108	16.4	5.4	13.7	75.6	80.9	7943	2421
FL	Palm Beach	5.14	109	22.2	8	21.6	77.1	83.5	15	5
CA	Alameda	5.13	110	20.1	7.3	16.6	77.7	82.3	864	263
WY	Lincoln	5.12	111	21.4	7.8	20.7	76.8	81.4	7381	2250
CA	Butte	5.11	112	24.8	8	16.3	74	80	1558	475
NV	Storey	5.11	113	22.7	7.4	22.4	74.5	79.9	5565	1696
CA	Yolo	5.10	114	26.1	7.8	16.5	76.9	81.5	340	104
FL	Charlotte	5.10	115	27.2	8.7	19.4	76.2	83.1	27	8
OR	Crook	5.06	116	27.6	7.9	18.9	75.6	80.1	4355	1328
FL	Pinellas	5.05	117	24	8.2	19.5	74.7	81.4	21	6
FL	St. Lucie	5.03	118	26.9	10.9	24.3	75.1	81.5	23	7
UT	Rich	5.03	119	26.6	7.2	19.9	78.8	81.8	6822	2079
FL	Collier	5.00	120	22.1	7.2	16.2	80.2	86	11	3
CA	Modoc	4.99	121	24.7	6.7	18.9	75.5	79.8	4979	1517
OR	Jefferson	4.99	122	28.4	7.7	21	74.6	79.2	3261	994
CO	Conejos	4.98	123	17.2	4.7	18.9	76.8	81.4	8951	2728
FL	Broward	4.98	124	25.3	8.3	22.5	76.5	82	11	3
OR	Columbia	4.98	125	27.9	7.7	18.9	75.5	80.8	761	232
CA	Yuba	4.97	126	31	7.3	24.8	72.1	78.9	1073	327
NM	Eddy	4.97	127	31.2	9.9	26.9	73.8	80.1	3739	1140
NV	Nye	4.97	128	31	7.9	28.7	72.2	78.8	5823	1775
OR	Clatsop	4.97	129	25.7	7.6	18.7	76.6	80.5	862	263
CO	Costilla	4.96	130	20.4	5.7	18.8	74.5	80.1	8861	2701
UT	Summit	4.96	131	15.7	4.5	13	78.7	82.8	8472	2582
CO	Gunnison	4.94	132	15.7	4.8	15.3	80	84.2	9548	2910
WA	Skagit	4.94	133	27.4	6.8	17.3	76.9	81.1	2403	732
AZ	Coconino	4.93	134	24.9	7.5	17	75.8	80.8	5914	1803
UT	Utah	4.93	135	25.5	7.3	16.4	78.5	81.7	6264	1909
UT	Wasatch	4.92	136	23.5	6.3	15.5	77.5	80.5	8034	2449
CO	Saguache	4.91	137	20.7	4.8	18.2	74.9	79.9	9206	2806
WY	Albany	4.91	138	22	5.7	19.4	77.2	81.1	7464	2275
AZ	Maricopa	4.87	139	23.6	7.6	19.3	76.8	81.6	1677	511
NV	Clark	4.86	140	26	8.8	25.6	74.1	79.7	3305	1008
WA	Pacific	4.85	141	32.6	10.2	22.1	74.8	80.3	581	177
CA	Kern	4.84	142	28.6	8.1	23.7	73.5	78.7	2377	724
CO	Fremont	4.82	143	22.2	6.8	19.6	74.9	79.9	7525	2294
FL	Sarasota	4.78	144	21.3	7.3	18.1	77.8	83.8	21	6
CA	San Joaquin	4.77	145	29.6	8.5	21.4	74.9	80.1	158	48
NM	Dona Ana	4.77	146	25.6	6.9	17.5	76.3	80.9	4463	1360
FL	Indian River	4.72	147	22.2	8.4	22.6	77	82.6	25	8
TX	Kendall	4.72	148	23.8	7.8	23.9	76.5	81.2	1558	475

HEALTHIEST PLACES TO LIVE

ST	COUNTY	USDA	AMEN	OBES	DIAB	INACT	M AGE	W AGE	ALT ft	ALT m
FL	Okeechobee	4.70	149	31.7	9.4	31	72.2	78.7	44	13
MT	Glacier	4.69	150	30.9	11.5	30.8	74.4	80.2	4812	1467
WA	Snohomish	4.68	151	28.1	7.8	19.1	77.3	81.1	2135	651
FL	Manatee	4.66	152	25.9	8.9	24	75.9	82.8	55	17
WA	Pierce	4.62	153	30.7	9.2	20.2	75.5	80.4	2244	684
ID	Valley	4.59	154	27	6.8	23.3	76.7	81	6466	1971
TX	Brewster	4.58	155	27.2	8	25.1	75	80.8	3614	1102
CO	Eagle	4.57	156	13.9	4.2	11.8	79.1	83.1	9074	2766
ID	Bonner	4.57	157	22.2	6.6	19	76.1	80.7	3168	966
OR	Hood River	4.54	158	22.3	7.4	16.8	76.3	81.5	3018	920
WA	Cowlitz	4.54	159	37	8.8	22.3	74.6	79.3	1345	410
WA	King	4.53	160	22.3	6.6	16.7	78.6	82.8	1842	561
TX	Kerr	4.52	161	29.5	9.2	22.1	75.5	81.5	2005	611
CA	Merced	4.51	162	31.8	7.6	20.3	75	79.9	368	112
FL	Osceola	4.50	163	29.2	9.3	26	76	80.8	60	18
OR	Jackson	4.50	164	22.8	6.6	13.9	76.2	81.5	3182	970
TX	El Paso	4.46	165	23.7	8.3	21.7	76.3	82	4069	1240
UT	Sanpete	4.44	166	26.7	7.3	23.3	75.4	80.2	7311	2228
CO	Montezuma	4.41	167	18.9	5.7	19.8	75.6	80.9	6813	2077
TX	Pecos	4.40	168	29.4	8.9	28.1	73.2	78.7	3133	955
CA	Glenn	4.38	169	26.9	7.3	18.5	73.6	79.2	1263	385
CO	Dolores	4.38	170	20.3	5.2	20.8	75.6	80.9	8330	2539
TX	Burnet	4.36	171	28.5	8.4	25.7	76.9	82.3	1159	353
WA	San Juan	4.35	172	19.2	4.9	13.1	77.3	81.1	180	55
CA	Colusa	4.34	173	24.4	7.4	17.2	74.2	80.3	767	234
OR	Multnomah	4.33	174	24.1	7.5	16.4	75.3	80.2	1025	313
FL	Hillsborough	4.32	175	26	9.6	24.1	74.7	80.4	63	19
UT	Daggett	4.30	176	27.7	7	19.4	75	79.8	7536	2297
OR	Lane	4.29	177	27	7.1	16.6	76.1	81.1	2146	654
NM	Lincoln	4.26	178	20.8	5.5	20	76.3	81.8	5852	1784
OR	Josephine	4.26	179	25	8.1	20.7	73.9	80.3	2418	737
TX	Uvalde	4.26	180	30	9.1	27	73.7	79.9	1190	363
WA	Clark	4.25	181	28.8	8.2	18.8	77.3	81.4	727	221
AZ	La Paz	4.24	182	32.6	9.2	31.2	73.9	81	1370	418
AZ	Yuma	4.24	183	30.2	8.7	23.2	78	83.8	878	268
NV	Pershing	4.23	184	29	7.7	26	74.7	80.1	4891	1491
FL	Hendry	4.22	185	34.6	10.7	31.2	71.8	77.8	21	6
MT	Carbon	4.22	186	27	6.1	24.8	74.6	80.3	5572	1698
UT	Salt Lake	4.21	187	24.4	7.5	18.4	77.1	81.3	5577	1700
OR	Lake	4.19	188	25.5	7.7	19.8	74.4	78.7	5132	1564
NM	Taos	4.16	189	18.8	5.9	15.7	75.4	81.8	8533	2601
CO	Moffat	4.14	190	23.2	6	26.1	74.8	80.3	6733	2052
FL	Highlands	4.14	191	30.2	9.8	26.6	75.5	81.6	74	23
NV	Esmeralda	4.12	192	28.6	7.4	23.2	72.2	78.8	5670	1728
WY	Platte	4.10	193	24.6	8.6	26.8	75.9	81.2	5155	1571
CA	Trinity	4.07	194	23.6	7.3	20.6	74.6	80.7	3805	1160

ST	COUNTY	USDA	AMEN	OBES	DIAB	INACT	M AGE	W AGE	ALT ft	ALT m
TX	Blanco	4.05	195	28.3	8.6	25.1	76.6	81.3	1334	407
AZ	Pima	4.04	196	25.9	7.1	19.3	75.8	81.7	2647	807
NM	Torrance	4.02	197	25.2	6.5	23.8	74.3	79.4	6455	1967
NM	Otero	4.00	198	25.9	7.8	22	75.6	79.7	5301	1616
TX	Hudspeth	4.00	199	28.2	8.8	29.2	76.3	82	4437	1352
UT	Garfield	4.00	200	24.8	7	23.2	75.2	79.9	6778	2066
FL	Polk	3.98	201	33.5	10.9	25.3	74.3	80	117	36
WY	Park	3.96	202	21.7	6	21.2	76.1	81.5	7529	2295
WA	Grays Harbor	3.94	203	32.7	10.3	23.7	73.7	79	515	157
FL	Brevard	3.93	204	28.8	9.7	23.7	75.9	81.2	16	5
MT	Broadwater	3.93	205	25.8	6.2	23.2	75.9	80.9	5015	1529
MT	Teton	3.88	206	24.8	6.2	25.1	74.4	80.2	4502	1372
NM	Chaves	3.87	207	29.6	7.5	25.9	73	79.7	4233	1290
NV	Humboldt	3.87	208	29.4	7	24.4	74.7	80.1	5085	1550
UT	Piute	3.87	209	24.3	6.9	24.4	75.2	79.9	7786	2373
MT	Gallatin	3.86	210	17.4	4.4	17.3	78.3	82.4	6274	1912
NV	Lincoln	3.86	211	26.3	8.7	22.9	74.1	79.7	5266	1605
ID	Adams	3.83	212	27.3	7.6	22	76.7	81	4804	1464
MT	Lake	3.82	213	27.8	7	21.9	75.9	80.6	3973	1211
CO	Garfield	3.81	214	17.3	5.4	15.5	76.7	81.5	7893	2406
TX	Kinney	3.80	215	29.5	8.6	27	74.2	80.1	1240	378
NM	Bernalillo	3.77	216	19.9	6	15.9	74.8	81.1	5967	1819
TX	Llano	3.75	217	27.4	9.1	26.9	76.6	81.3	1230	375
NM	San Miguel	3.73	218	22.7	6.4	19	72.7	79.8	5930	1807
TX	Coke	3.73	219	31.7	8.4	29.9	73.2	78.8	2127	648
UT	Duchesne	3.73	220	27.6	8.6	24.5	75	79.8	7792	2375
UT	Morgan	3.72	221	22.3	6.8	18.2	78.8	81.8	6736	2053
FL	Hernando	3.71	222	29.2	8.6	24.8	74.3	81.1	73	22
TX	Aransas	3.71	223	27.8	8.6	26.5	73.9	81.3	8	2
UT	Weber	3.71	224	27.1	8	19.3	76.3	80.5	5649	1722
WY	Fremont	3.71	225	24.6	7.3	24.6	73.3	79.7	7037	2145
NM	Colfax	3.70	226	21.1	6.2	23.7	75.4	80.3	7214	2199
NV	Lander	3.67	227	26.9	7.6	24.3	74.9	80.3	6000	1829
NM	Sandoval	3.66	228	24.3	6.4	19.1	76.4	81.1	6720	2048
UT	Sevier	3.66	229	26	8	21.9	75.5	79.8	7550	2301
CA	Sacramento	3.65	230	28	8.3	19	75.6	81	103	32
OR	Linn	3.65	231	29.1	7.7	20.1	75.2	80.1	2071	631
CO	Delta	3.64	232	20.3	5.6	22.7	75.9	81.5	6982	2128
ID	Shoshone	3.64	233	29.6	7.8	26.9	74.6	80.2	4239	1292
OR	Clackamas	3.64	234	26.1	7.9	16.9	77.8	81.4	2160	658
ID	Bear Lake	3.62	235	25	7.5	28.9	76.2	80.9	6769	2063
TX	Culberson	3.62	236	28.1	8.8	26.2	76.3	82	4130	1259
MT	Park	3.61	237	21.2	5.2	21.4	78.3	82.4	6960	2122
CO	Las Animas	3.60	238	21.9	6.2	23.3	75	80.5	5947	1813
UT	San Juan	3.60	239	28.3	8.7	29	74.9	80.2	5658	1725
CO	Rio Blanco	3.59	240	20	5.4	18.9	74.8	80.3	7231	2204

HEALTHIEST PLACES TO LIVE

ST	COUNTY	USDA	AMEN	OBES	DIAB	INACT	M AGE	W AGE	ALT ft	ALT m
CA	San Bernardino	3.57	241	27.8	8.1	21.7	74.3	79.5	2666	813
SC	Oconee	3.55	242	31.1	10	24.5	74	79.9	1094	333
UT	Uintah	3.53	243	28.6	8.6	27.2	75	80.6	6258	1908
OR	Marion	3.51	244	30.3	8.1	19	75.8	80.6	1553	473
ID	Kootenai	3.50	245	25.4	7.5	19.6	77.5	81.8	2940	896
MT	Beaverhead	3.50	246	23	7.1	20	76.6	79.8	7078	2157
CA	Kings	3.48	247	27.5	7.6	22.4	74.6	79.6	343	105
TX	Real	3.48	248	29.4	9	26.9	73.7	79.9	2043	623
AZ	Apache	3.45	249	33.1	13.1	27.5	70.8	80	6554	1998
FL	Volusia	3.45	250	25.9	9.6	24.6	74.3	80.6	28	9
MT	Pondera	3.45	251	29	7	28.2	74.4	80.2	4062	1238
OR	Harney	3.45	252	26.2	7.7	19.5	75.9	80.4	4848	1478
FL	Citrus	3.43	253	29.8	9.6	25.1	73.1	80.8	53	16
NM	De Baca	3.43	254	23	6.7	26.4	72.9	79.6	4435	1352
WA	Island	3.41	255	26.3	7.8	15.5	79.8	83.1	157	48
FL	Lake	3.40	256	27.1	9.1	22.2	76.8	82.9	83	25
ID	Boise	3.40	257	27.9	7.3	19	75.8	80.4	5531	1686
WA	Lewis	3.40	258	34.7	9	21.2	75.1	79.8	1900	579
NM	McKinley	3.39	259	35.9	12.4	25.9	71.5	79.5	6942	2116
OR	Wasco	3.38	260	32.9	7.6	19.4	75.9	80.8	2497	761
FL	Pasco	3.37	261	28.9	8.8	27.4	73.7	80.6	72	22
NM	Hidalgo	3.37	262	24.1	6.1	23.5	73.2	79.8	4735	1443
AZ	Pinal	3.36	263	29.8	9	23.6	75.3	80.7	2340	713
CA	Siskiyou	3.36	264	25	7	18.7	74.6	80.7	4254	1297
OR	Morrow	3.34	265	26	8.3	24.1	75.6	80.5	2355	718
NC	Macon	3.33	266	26.3	8.1	23	74.5	80.8	3085	940
TX	Nueces	3.33	267	30.2	9.8	23.7	74.3	80.5	55	17
WA	Kittitas	3.33	268	26.4	7.1	18.5	77.2	81.3	3169	966
WA	Pend Oreille	3.33	269	30.7	7.7	19.7	74.5	80	3454	1053
WA	Thurston	3.32	270	28.4	8.2	18.5	77	81.3	492	150
WY	Uinta	3.32	271	30.3	7	23.1	75.7	80.9	7249	2210
TX	Loving	3.31	272	28.1	8.5	25.4	72.2	78	2954	900
UT	Box Elder	3.29	273	26.8	7.6	22	76.8	81	4839	1475
OR	Polk	3.28	274	29.7	7.6	18.9	77.7	82.2	862	263
OR	Yamhill	3.25	275	27.2	6.9	18.7	76.6	80.6	678	207
TX	Comal	3.25	276	25.7	8.3	25	76.8	81.8	1026	313
WA	Wahkiakum	3.25	277	29.3	9.1	20.1	74.8	80.3	676	206
CA	Tehama	3.24	278	25.2	8.3	16.7	74.1	79.1	2144	653
TX	Travis	3.24	279	24.7	8	19.2	77.6	81.4	726	221
MT	Madison	3.22	280	24.2	6	26.3	74.6	79.8	6657	2029
OK	Atoka	3.20	281	32.1	11.3	28.9	71.3	77.3	660	201
MT	Sweet Grass	3.19	282	20.8	6.2	27.9	75.8	80.9	5623	1714
GA	Towns	3.18	283	27.4	9.4	26.2	75.1	81	2551	778
ID	Idaho	3.17	284	29.3	7.6	24	75.8	80.6	5119	1560
TX	Terrell	3.17	285	26.7	8.6	29.5	75	80.8	2398	731
MT	Lewis and Clark	3.16	286	23.2	6.2	19	76.7	80.5	5337	1627
TX	Edwards	3.15	287	29.3	8.9	27.4	73.7	79.9	2129	649

ST	COUNTY	USDA	AMEN	OBES	DIAB	INACT	M AGE	W AGE	ALT ft	ALT m
TX	Kleberg	3.15	288	30	8.7	26.8	73.6	79.6	48	15
FL	Seminole	3.14	289	25	10.1	20.2	77.1	81.5	37	11
NC	Graham	3.14	290	28.2	10.1	25.9	72	78.6	2801	854
TX	Kenedy	3.14	291	29.2	8.8	26.8	73.8	78.4	28	8
NM	Socorro	3.13	292	26.9	7.3	21.8	74.3	79.4	5989	1825
UT	Carbon	3.13	293	24.1	7.8	25.1	74.6	80.2	7129	2173
GA	Rabun	3.11	294	27.1	9.4	23.1	75.1	81	2289	698
ID	Benewah	3.10	295	29.1	8.7	28.1	74.6	80.2	3123	952
OR	Benton	3.10	296	22.4	6.8	14.8	78.7	81.9	787	240
ID	Caribou	3.08	297	23.9	7	26.2	76.2	80.9	6494	1979
MT	Wheatland	3.07	298	25.4	6.6	29.9	75.8	80.9	4859	1481
TX	Presidio	3.06	299	24.8	8.2	25.5	75	80.8	4287	1307
NC	Clay	3.05	300	25.8	8.1	22.3	73.4	79.7	2683	818
WY	Laramie	3.05	301	25.1	7.9	23.4	74.9	79.8	5987	1825
NM	Cibola	3.04	302	32.3	11.2	26	73.4	80.4	7096	2163
NM	Los Alamos	3.04	303	18.8	5.3	14.4	80.1	83	7655	2333
NM	Valencia	3.04	304	27.5	7	24.1	73.4	79.6	5424	1653
NV	White Pine	3.04	305	30	7.5	24	74.9	80.3	6825	2080
NM	Santa Fe	3.02	306	14.1	3.9	12	78.1	82.9	6924	2110
SC	Pickens	3.02	307	28.3	9.5	26.6	74.2	79.7	1122	342
NC	Cherokee	3.00	308	27.4	9.7	25.5	73.4	79.7	2133	650
MN	Cook	2.99	309	26.9	7.3	18.3	76.3	81.7	1617	493
FL	St. Johns	2.98	310	21.5	7.4	17.7	77.6	82.8	22	7
NC	Swain	2.97	311	32.5	12.1	28.5	72	78.6	3171	966
UT	Kane	2.97	312	24.1	7.5	21.6	74.9	80.2	5736	1748
FL	Orange	2.96	313	26.6	9.6	24.1	75.5	80.9	77	23
ID	Fremont	2.95	314	23.4	7.9	22.3	76.2	80.4	6163	1879
CO	Montrose	2.94	315	18.6	4.9	18.9	75.3	81	6943	2116
GA	Union	2.94	316	27.8	9.7	23	74.9	80.1	2362	720
ID	Blaine	2.94	317	17.2	5.3	13.3	79.3	83.6	6103	1860
ID	Elmore	2.94	318	28.5	8.5	23.9	75.5	79.9	4737	1444
TN	Carter	2.93	319	34.7	10.8	31.7	72.4	78.6	2655	809
TX	San Saba	2.92	320	29.3	8.9	29.8	76.4	81.6	1445	440
MA	Dukes	2.89	321	18.2	7.8	18.1	78.2	82.9	58	18
MA	Nantucket	2.89	322	22.6	7.6	19.8	78.1	82.9	26	8
CO	Denver	2.88	323	18.2	6.1	16.3	74.4	80.9	5335	1626
NM	Luna	2.87	324	27.6	7.1	21.4	73.2	79.8	4514	1376
WY	Converse	2.86	325	28.4	6.7	23.7	75.9	81.2	5426	1654
FL	Sumter	2.84	326	29.4	9.4	19.5	74.4	80.2	74	23
TX	Reeves	2.84	327	30.4	9.5	27.3	73.2	78.7	2981	909
MT	Meagher	2.83	328	25	6.5	27.3	75.9	80.9	5861	1786
NM	San Juan	2.83	329	29.6	8.5	24.1	73.9	80.1	6047	1843
UT	Tooele	2.83	330	29.5	9.6	22.1	76.1	79.5	4788	1459
TX	Lampasas	2.81	331	30.5	8.4	25.5	75.4	79.8	1231	375
MT	Flathead	2.80	332	21.8	5.6	19.2	75.5	80.5	4908	1496
OR	Wheeler	2.79	333	25.8	7.7	18.8	75.6	80.5	3742	1141

ST	COUNTY	USDA	AMEN	OBES	DIAB	INACT	M AGE	W AGE	ALT ft	ALT m
GA	Fannin	2.78	334	29	9.9	23.5	72.9	79.3	2109	643
WY	Johnson	2.78	335	23.3	7.2	21.9	76.6	81.5	5557	1694
AR	Marion	2.74	336	33.3	10.4	25.9	75.1	79.4	849	259
FL	DeSoto	2.74	337	34.6	11.2	30.7	74.2	80.1	55	17
TX	Henderson	2.72	338	25.6	9.2	28.4	73	79.2	410	125
FL	Flagler	2.70	339	29	9	22.4	76.7	83.1	21	6
ID	Camas	2.70	340	25.9	7.6	20.9	74.3	80	6320	1926
ME	Washington	2.69	341	30.9	9.5	29.8	73.1	80.1	277	84
UT	Millard	2.69	342	28.5	6.6	21	75.2	79.9	5412	1650
OR	Wallowa	2.68	343	25.4	6.9	19.3	75.7	80.2	4447	1355
TX	Live Oak	2.67	344	28.6	8.7	28.1	74.6	80.4	246	75
FL	Franklin	2.66	345	27.5	9.1	28.9	72.4	78.5	13	4
NM	Guadalupe	2.66	346	25	6.3	22.9	72.9	79.6	5179	1578
OR	Washington	2.65	347	23.9	6.1	16.5	78.9	82.5	743	227
AR	Baxter	2.64	348	29.8	8	30.3	73.4	79.8	746	227
RI	Washington	2.64	349	20.9	5.8	18.7	78.1	82	156	48
MT	Fergus	2.63	350	23.7	6	22.7	75.3	80.8	3779	1152
MT	Stillwater	2.63	351	26.6	6.3	22.3	75.8	80.9	5036	1535
TX	Bexar	2.63	352	28.2	8.7	22.5	74.9	80.7	818	249
UT	Cache	2.63	353	23.8	6.5	17.9	78.8	81.8	6306	1922
WY	Sweetwater	2.63	354	29.1	7.1	24.4	74.8	80.5	6869	2094
NC	Jackson	2.62	355	33.4	11.1	24.1	74.6	79.6	3365	1026
TX	Tom Green	2.62	356	29.5	9.1	25.5	74.3	79.9	2080	634
ID	Boundary	2.61	357	23.2	7.1	25.9	76.1	80.7	4068	1240
WA	Kitsap	2.61	358	29.3	7.3	18	77.7	80.9	295	90
CO	Crowley	2.60	359	22.5	6.4	22.9	74.1	80	4539	1383
TX	Potter	2.60	360	33.9	9.4	30.8	71.7	77.4	3389	1033
FL	Marion	2.59	361	32.7	9.9	26.9	73.9	80.9	81	25
TX	Gillespie	2.59	362	28	8.2	25.7	76.4	81.6	1832	558
WA	Stevens	2.58	363	27.1	7.7	22.3	74.5	80	2738	835
UT	Washington	2.57	364	24	6.5	17.1	78.8	83.5	5072	1546
WY	Crook	2.57	365	22.7	6.1	22.2	75.9	81.5	4270	1301
TX	Refugio	2.56	366	29.3	9.1	28.2	73.3	79.8	42	13
OK	Sequoyah	2.55	367	36.4	12.6	38.1	71.7	78.8	695	212
OK	Marshall	2.54	368	34.9	9.7	31	73	78.8	741	226
CT	New Haven	2.52	369	26.7	8.2	26	76.3	81.3	319	97
TX	Ector	2.50	370	32	9.5	27.8	72.2	78	3018	920
WY	Big Horn	2.49	371	27.6	7	25.7	75	80.6	5422	1653
WY	Natrona	2.49	372	27.2	7.1	23.6	74.9	81.1	6069	1850
CO	Adams	2.48	373	24.6	6.9	21.3	77.6	81.4	5088	1551
GA	Dawson	2.48	374	26.6	9.2	22.9	74.6	80.2	1469	448
FL	Levy	2.47	375	34.2	10.6	31.4	71.5	78.7	40	12
TX	Mitchell	2.47	376	31.4	9.7	28.5	72.1	78	2180	665
TX	Cameron	2.46	377	27.2	8.5	22.8	76.9	83	26	8
TX	Moore	2.46	378	31.4	8.9	30.3	73.7	78.9	3503	1068
CO	Bent	2.45	379	24.5	6	22.6	74.2	79.3	4130	1259

ST	COUNTY	USDA	AMEN	OBES	DIAB	INACT	M AGE	W AGE	ALT ft	ALT m
ID	Gem	2.45	380	30.5	7.1	25.2	75.8	80.4	3598	1097
TX	Crosby	2.45	381	27.9	8.9	29.6	72.9	78.7	2925	892
TX	Shelby	2.45	382	32.6	10	31.6	71.3	77.6	296	90
FL	Alachua	2.44	383	25.1	8.3	22.6	75.1	79.8	103	31
CT	New London	2.43	384	23.3	7.4	22.1	76.4	81.5	248	76
FL	Dixie	2.42	385	34.9	10.6	33.2	71.3	78.8	27	8
OR	Baker	2.42	386	26.3	7.9	18.8	75.7	80.2	4359	1329
AR	Van Buren	2.41	387	31.9	9.1	33	73.5	79.7	978	298
NC	Transylvania	2.40	388	24.5	7.4	22.8	75.5	82.1	2824	861
AR	Benton	2.39	389	28	7.2	27.8	76.8	81.8	1230	375
OK	Cherokee	2.39	390	36.4	10.6	31.2	73.2	78.6	855	261
TX	Borden	2.39	391	28.1	8.7	27	72.4	77.8	2542	775
UT	Beaver	2.39	392	26.5	7.5	22.3	75.2	79.9	6359	1938
AR	Johnson	2.37	393	35.6	9.8	30.7	72.5	78.7	1035	316
UT	Iron	2.37	394	25.2	7.1	19.5	76.2	80.3	6376	1943
TX	McCulloch	2.36	395	28.4	8.9	29.3	73.6	78.3	1681	512
TX	Randall	2.36	396	25.8	8.9	21.4	75.6	80.2	3623	1104
TX	Zapata	2.36	397	30.2	8	27.9	74.1	80	436	133
CO	Arapahoe	2.35	398	19.4	5.8	17.2	78.4	82.3	5468	1667
FL	Putnam	2.35	399	35.6	11.8	30.9	70.9	78	54	16
FL	Escambia	2.34	400	29.4	10.5	25.5	73.6	79	150	46
GA	Greene	2.34	401	32.4	11.6	25.8	73.2	78.5	568	173
GA	Putnam	2.34	402	29.3	11.3	24.2	73	78.7	490	149
GA	Gilmer	2.33	403	30.3	10.2	24.4	72.6	78.5	1839	560
ID	Clearwater	2.33	404	31.6	7.6	24.9	75.8	80.6	3881	1183
MT	Lincoln	2.33	405	25.4	7.2	23.2	74.7	79.8	4259	1298
MT	Sanders	2.33	406	23.1	7.1	25.5	74.7	79.8	4102	1250
CT	Middlesex	2.32	407	22.9	6.3	20.2	77.8	82.5	286	87
FL	Taylor	2.32	408	35.4	11	30.7	72.5	78.3	41	12
CO	Kiowa	2.31	409	23.9	5.5	19.8	74.4	80.6	4157	1267
FL	Duval	2.31	410	27.8	11	26.2	72.5	78	36	11
WA	Ferry	2.31	411	25.4	6.4	23.5	75.7	80.4	3275	998
WA	Garfield	2.31	412	34.6	10.7	24.5	77.1	80.8	2721	829
TX	Concho	2.30	413	30.4	8.7	25.6	73.6	78.3	1859	566
AR	Pope	2.29	414	32	9	25.3	75.1	79	857	261
MO	Perry	2.29	415	33.6	9.4	25.8	74.8	80	553	169
OK	Comanche	2.29	416	32.8	9.8	31.3	73.2	78.4	1309	399
NC	Ashe	2.28	417	23.3	7.4	24.7	73.7	79.2	3198	975
MT	Granite	2.27	418	22.7	5.8	24.3	75.5	80.5	6118	1865
MT	Jefferson	2.27	419	20.9	6.6	19.9	75.9	80.9	5869	1789
CO	Mesa	2.26	420	22.2	5.4	17.8	75.9	81.2	6846	2087
CT	Fairfield	2.25	421	18	5.8	19.2	78.9	83.3	378	115
FL	Gulf	2.25	422	29.8	10.3	27.1	72	77.7	17	5
FL	Hardee	2.25	423	37.6	12.2	31.2	73.2	78.9	87	26
TX	Jasper	2.25	424	30.1	10.1	33.7	72.9	78.2	155	47
CO	Otero	2.24	425	25.5	6.4	22.1	74.4	80.6	4448	1356

HEALTHIEST PLACES TO LIVE

ST	COUNTY	USDA	AMEN	OBES	DIAB	INACT	M AGE	W AGE	ALT ft	ALT m
MO	Stone	2.24	426	30.4	8.9	26.7	75.1	81.2	1138	347
NC	Haywood	2.23	427	28.8	8.5	22.7	74	80.2	3581	1092
TX	Howard	2.23	428	31.5	9.1	28.9	72.4	77.8	2525	769
WA	Whitman	2.23	429	28	8.2	21	77.1	80.8	2076	633
NC	McDowell	2.21	430	33.6	10.6	29.4	73.2	79.2	1811	552
MT	Cascade	2.20	431	25.5	7.6	23.4	75.6	81.2	4273	1302
AL	Tallapoosa	2.19	432	37.7	12	30	71.7	78.2	631	192
AR	Cleburne	2.19	433	27.4	10.4	30.4	74.4	79.5	714	218
VA	Bath	2.19	434	27.7	9	25.3	75.1	80.6	2213	674
FL	Walton	2.18	435	26.4	9.4	25.7	73.7	79.7	165	50
MO	Wayne	2.18	436	29.5	9.2	30.1	71.8	78.2	578	176
NC	Buncombe	2.18	437	24	7.9	19.6	74.6	80.5	2684	818
TX	Hays	2.18	438	29.4	8.6	26.3	77	80.8	978	298
TX	San Jacinto	2.18	439	29.7	9.4	29.6	71.7	78.4	214	65
ID	Washington	2.17	440	27.7	8.7	24.9	76.7	81	3698	1127
WY	Sheridan	2.17	441	24.5	7.5	19.1	76.6	81.5	5151	1570
FL	Bay	2.15	442	26.8	8.9	23.5	73.7	79.2	55	17
MT	Silver Bow	2.15	443	25.2	7.1	24.6	74.6	79.8	6456	1968
NE	Garden	2.14	444	27.9	7.8	29.8	76.1	80.2	3804	1159
RI	Newport	2.14	445	21.4	6.1	18.6	77.9	81.7	102	31
TX	Coleman	2.14	446	27.7	8.3	31.8	73.1	79.5	1705	520
TX	Sabine	2.13	447	31.3	8.8	28.1	71.8	78.2	243	74
TX	Nacogdoches	2.12	448	29.7	9.3	26.5	72.6	78.8	330	101
AL	Elmore	2.11	449	31.3	11.8	31.5	73.1	78.8	382	117
CO	Pueblo	2.11	450	23.6	6.9	19.3	74.1	80	5212	1589
TX	Nolan	2.11	451	30.4	9.3	28.3	72.1	78	2353	717
ID	Owyhee	2.10	452	29.9	8.7	28.4	75.5	79.9	4773	1455
GA	Baldwin	2.09	453	31.2	11.6	27.8	72.1	77.7	388	118
OK	McCurtain	2.08	454	33.7	10.1	37.5	70.2	77.5	632	193
UT	Grand	2.08	455	19.9	5.8	18.2	75.7	80	5752	1753
GA	Glynn	2.06	456	27	9.3	24.6	73	79	13	4
ME	Knox	2.06	457	25.8	7.6	20.7	76.7	81.4	235	72
MO	Ste. Genevieve	2.06	458	30.6	9.1	33	74.8	80.2	679	207
AR	Franklin	2.05	459	34.8	10	29.5	73.3	79.3	852	260
NV	Elko	2.05	460	30.6	7.2	24.7	75	79.7	6144	1873
FL	Nassau	2.04	461	28.5	8.6	23.6	74.6	79.4	39	12
ID	Power	2.04	462	30	7.5	24.1	75.6	80.5	5178	1578
TX	Haskell	2.04	463	29	8.7	26.6	72.6	79	1535	468
TX	Taylor	2.04	464	28.6	8.9	32.9	73.6	79	2008	612
OK	Bryan	2.03	465	33	10.2	31	72.7	78	615	188
FL	Clay	2.01	466	29.2	10	24.1	74.8	79.1	89	27
FL	Okaloosa	2.01	467	29.4	8.9	22.2	75.6	80.2	172	52
OK	Texas	2.01	468	29.8	8.6	30.6	74.4	79.8	3171	966
FL	Jefferson	2.00	469	34.2	11.6	27.9	72.5	78.3	88	27
GA	McIntosh	2.00	470	31.3	11.4	28.8	70.6	77.8	14	4
ID	Bonneville	2.00	471	26.6	8.3	20.4	76.4	80	6090	1856

ST	COUNTY	USDA	AMEN	OBES	DIAB	INACT	M AGE	W AGE	ALT ft	ALT m
NE	Sheridan	2.00	472	27	7.8	29.7	74.4	80.9	3829	1167
OK	Haskell	2.00	473	33	10	33.9	72.3	78.8	617	188
WY	Goshen	2.00	474	26.8	6.7	29.2	76.3	80.9	4650	1417
NC	Henderson	1.99	475	24.3	7.9	22.1	75.6	80.8	2413	736
OK	Kiowa	1.99	476	32.6	10.5	34.5	72.4	78.7	1502	458
TX	Starr	1.99	477	29.2	8.5	28.9	74.1	80	359	109
AR	Boone	1.98	478	29.7	9.9	30.6	74.1	79.6	1169	356
TX	San Patricio	1.97	479	29.6	9.9	27.8	73.7	79.9	60	18
WA	Klickitat	1.97	480	27.4	7.3	21.4	76.3	81	2020	616
GA	McDuffie	1.96	481	29.9	11.6	26.9	70.1	76.3	441	134
TX	San Augustine	1.96	482	30.4	10.3	29.7	71.8	78.2	272	83
FL	Wakulla	1.95	483	34.8	10.5	27.3	74.5	79.8	33	10
FL	Washington	1.95	484	35.6	12.3	29.6	71.3	77.6	103	32
MO	Barry	1.95	485	30.2	8.7	31.6	72.7	79.2	1319	402
NC	Avery	1.95	486	30.2	9.1	20.7	73.1	79.5	3536	1078
FL	Santa Rosa	1.94	487	28	10	24.6	75.6	79.8	146	45
GA	Cherokee	1.93	488	27.2	7.8	22.3	76	79.7	1072	327
TX	Parmer	1.93	489	30.7	8.6	28.2	73.7	79.3	4052	1235
NC	Madison	1.92	490	28.8	8.7	21.4	73.9	79	2649	807
NV	Eureka	1.92	491	26.8	7.2	25.6	74.9	80.3	6211	1893
TX	Angelina	1.92	492	32.1	9.5	28.8	73.1	78.7	230	70
VA	Franklin	1.92	493	29.6	9.4	24.4	74.6	80.2	1198	365
AZ	Navajo	1.91	494	31.6	12.3	24.9	71.4	79.5	6016	1834
ID	Bingham	1.91	495	33.5	10.8	22.8	75.4	80.4	5125	1562
UT	Juab	1.91	496	29.1	7.2	21.2	75.4	80.2	5528	1685
ID	Teton	1.90	497	24.7	7.7	17.4	76.7	80.4	6512	1985
TX	Hutchinson	1.90	498	31.3	8.9	26.2	73.8	79.3	3060	933
MT	Judith Basin	1.89	499	24.7	5.8	28	75.6	81.2	5039	1536
SD	Fall River	1.89	500	32.3	8.3	21.5	71.1	78.5	3596	1096
GA	Camden	1.88	501	29.1	11.2	24.1	74.2	79.5	15	5
NC	Wilkes	1.88	502	30.2	10	30.7	72.9	79	1490	454
TX	Rusk	1.88	503	31.4	9.8	27.6	73	78.9	403	123
ID	Ada	1.87	504	23.2	7	15.1	77.8	81.9	3074	937
ME	Hancock	1.87	505	25.1	7.2	19.6	76	81.3	293	89
TN	Campbell	1.87	506	34.9	11.4	34.5	70.9	77.4	1561	476
TX	Galveston	1.87	507	29.2	9.5	24.6	73.4	78.7	12	4
GA	Butts	1.86	508	30.8	11.8	25.7	71.9	76.9	630	192
MT	Petroleum	1.86	509	23.7	6.6	24.5	76.1	81	2958	901
TX	Calhoun	1.86	510	29.5	8.8	24.9	73.8	78.9	12	4
TX	Willacy	1.85	511	29.5	8.8	28.1	73.8	78.4	23	7
NC	Polk	1.84	512	22.8	7	23	74.9	80.8	1220	372
TX	Polk	1.84	513	32.8	9.4	29.2	69.8	78.6	237	72
WA	Columbia	1.84	514	29.1	9	17.4	77.1	80.8	2805	855
SC	Greenville	1.83	515	28	9.4	24.3	74.1	79.9	1081	329
AL	Baldwin	1.82	516	25.7	9.9	24.2	74.4	80.3	121	37
ID	Canyon	1.82	517	29.4	8.5	22.6	75.1	80.3	2490	759
NC	Burke	1.82	518	28.5	10.1	27.2	73.3	79.3	1492	455

ST	COUNTY	USDA	AMEN	OBES	DIAB	INACT	M AGE	W AGE	ALT ft	ALT m
NC	Watauga	1.82	519	24.9	8.8	20.8	76.7	80.8	3298	1005
GA	Bibb	1.81	520	30	11.8	28.2	70	76.9	383	117
ID	Cassia	1.81	521	28.6	8.5	22.8	75.6	80.5	5375	1638
MT	Mineral	1.80	522	28.4	6.9	28.3	76.7	81	4712	1436
ID	Payette	1.79	523	26.6	8.1	24.6	75	79.6	2596	791
MT	Powell	1.79	524	24.4	7	25.5	75.5	80.5	5676	1730
NM	Lea	1.79	525	31.7	7.8	29.8	73.2	78.9	3784	1153
MS	Grenada	1.78	526	37.6	12.3	35	68.8	76.7	253	77
VA	Alleghany	1.77	527	26	8.4	23.8	72.8	79	2000	610
VA	Covington	1.77	528	28.8	9.5	24.9	72.8	79	1397	426
FL	Jackson	1.76	529	33	12.3	31	72.5	77.9	124	38
GA	Chatham	1.76	530	29	10.9	23.4	73	78.4	11	3
SD	Lawrence	1.76	531	22.8	5.7	23.6	77	81.3	4968	1514
TN	Sevier	1.76	532	30.3	10.5	28.2	73.6	79.6	1978	603
TX	Briscoe	1.76	533	28.5	8.7	25.3	74.6	79.8	2791	851
TX	McMullen	1.76	534	29.9	8.9	27	72.9	78.7	330	101
AR	Carroll	1.75	535	26.6	9.1	26.8	74.3	79.4	1330	405
AR	Logan	1.75	536	29.2	10.1	30.2	72.5	78.7	666	203
FL	Leon	1.75	537	28.1	9.8	21.2	76.1	80.4	102	31
OK	Pushmataha	1.75	538	31	10.9	33.8	70.2	77.5	808	246
MT	Missoula	1.74	539	20.5	5.3	16.7	76.7	81	4954	1510
ID	Bannock	1.73	540	29.6	8.8	20.3	75.9	80.3	5633	1717
CA	Sutter	1.72	541	26.4	7.8	21.9	75	80.4	77	23
TX	Colorado	1.72	542	29.1	9.3	29	73.5	79.3	237	72
CO	Weld	1.70	543	25	6.2	18.5	77.6	81.4	4964	1513
MO	St. Francois	1.70	544	31.4	9.4	27.2	72.1	77.6	922	281
TX	Baylor	1.70	545	27.7	8.8	26.6	72.6	79	1254	382
ID	Franklin	1.68	546	30	8.2	23.3	76.2	80.9	5829	1777
MO	Camden	1.68	547	27.1	8.3	30.7	75	81	864	263
OR	Malheur	1.68	548	26.4	7.7	21	74.2	80	4291	1308
TN	Franklin	1.68	549	34.2	9.4	33	73.5	78.9	1158	353
OK	Johnston	1.67	550	30.3	10.7	33	71.1	78.1	847	258
TN	Pickett	1.67	551	32.1	10.3	31.6	71.2	77.1	1055	321
TN	Polk	1.67	552	33.4	11.2	33.2	70.9	77.7	1365	416
MS	Tishomingo	1.66	553	29	10.3	29.5	70.8	77.8	527	161
NM	Quay	1.66	554	24.7	6.1	27.3	72.9	79.6	4323	1318
SC	Beaufort	1.66	555	21.4	7	17.2	78	83.3	10	3
FL	Gadsden	1.65	556	35.7	12.6	31.1	70.1	77.9	202	62
AR	Garland	1.64	557	28.4	8.6	26.7	72.5	79.6	704	215
OK	Pittsburg	1.64	558	32.6	11	33.8	72.2	78.4	739	225
OR	Umatilla	1.64	559	34.1	8.7	24.2	75.6	80.5	2632	802
TX	Crockett	1.64	560	29.9	8.7	26.2	73.4	78.5	2438	743
AR	Yell	1.63	561	36.3	12.2	28.6	71.6	78.3	608	185
LA	Sabine	1.63	562	36.2	12.5	31.6	72.8	78.9	254	77
MO	Taney	1.63	563	32.4	8.8	29.3	74.5	79.9	966	295
NC	Dare	1.63	564	28.5	8.4	23.7	75.9	80.4	4	1
NE	Morrill	1.63	565	28.3	9.8	26.6	74.4	80.9	4004	1220

ST	COUNTY	USDA	AMEN	OBES	DIAB	INACT	M AGE	W AGE	ALT ft	ALT m
OR	Sherman	1.61	566	25.3	7.6	17.8	75.9	80.8	1846	563
TX	Goliad	1.61	567	29.2	9	25.6	73.3	79.8	199	61
FL	Union	1.60	568	35.7	12.9	31.7	68.1	77.7	124	38
MO	Ozark	1.60	569	27.7	8.2	29	72.5	79.3	904	276
AL	Coosa	1.59	570	34	12.8	33.7	70.4	77.3	647	197
CO	Alamosa	1.59	571	20.4	6.2	19.9	74.5	80.1	7744	2360
MT	Ravalli	1.59	572	20.8	5.3	20	77.1	81.3	5918	1804
AL	Wilcox	1.58	573	43.6	15.5	34.4	69.9	76.3	198	60
TX	Montgomery	1.58	574	26.3	8.6	22.3	75.6	80.2	208	63
WA	Benton	1.58	575	31.1	8.7	19.8	77.4	80.6	958	292
KS	Norton	1.57	576	30.4	8.2	24.8	76.3	81.5	2342	714
TN	Claiborne	1.57	577	30.6	10.3	34.4	71.1	77.7	1478	451
TX	Chambers	1.57	578	28.2	8.7	29.8	74.1	79.8	15	5
GA	Pickens	1.56	579	26.4	10	22.5	74.5	79.7	1417	432
OK	Cimarron	1.56	580	31.8	9.1	34.7	74.4	79.8	4139	1262
WA	Chelan	1.56	581	24.2	7.3	19.1	77.8	81.9	3944	1202
AR	Stone	1.55	582	32.6	9.3	33.8	73.5	79.7	885	270
GA	White	1.55	583	29.3	9.2	23	74.6	79.7	1737	529
ME	Lincoln	1.55	584	23.8	6.7	19.4	77.3	81	158	48
NC	Mitchell	1.55	585	28.7	9	24.4	72.8	79.1	3130	954
TX	Jones	1.55	586	31	9.6	29.3	72.9	78.9	1690	515
GA	Wilkinson	1.54	587	32	11.8	27.2	70.6	76.1	345	105
TX	Mason	1.54	588	27.6	8.4	27	76.4	81.6	1631	497
TX	Matagorda	1.54	589	28.3	9.8	27	73.4	77.9	26	8
AL	Mobile	1.52	590	31.7	11.6	30.2	70.7	77.8	123	38
GA	Hancock	1.52	591	36.8	14.5	28.5	68.4	75.4	486	148
MA	Barnstable	1.52	592	18.1	6.1	16.6	78.1	82.9	55	17
NY	Suffolk	1.52	593	25.3	7.1	22.2	77.6	81.7	76	23
TN	Hamblen	1.52	594	32.9	11.7	32.7	72.4	78.3	1247	380
KY	Lyon	1.51	595	34.3	10.1	29.8	72.3	77.9	433	132
MT	Deer Lodge	1.51	596	27	6.7	22.9	76.6	79.8	6664	2031
NC	Caldwell	1.51	597	30.6	9.1	26.7	72.9	78.7	1503	458
TN	Monroe	1.51	598	34	10.4	31	72.5	78.7	1439	438
NE	Keith	1.50	599	28.4	6.9	21.7	76.1	80.2	3353	1022
NC	Lincoln	1.49	600	27.2	10	22.9	73.3	78.9	879	268
SC	Georgetown	1.49	601	35.9	11	29.6	73.7	79	21	6
CT	Tolland	1.48	602	22.2	6.9	19.1	78.3	82.5	581	177
NC	Hyde	1.48	603	32.2	11.3	30.1	71.6	77.6	5	2
WA	Yakima	1.48	604	32.3	8.9	24	75	80.1	2834	864
MO	Benton	1.47	605	33	9.4	29.7	73	78.8	856	261
NC	Alleghany	1.47	606	25.5	8.6	28.2	73.7	79.2	2868	874
TX	Sutton	1.47	607	28.1	8.5	26	75.5	81	2252	686
GA	Jasper	1.46	608	28.7	10.8	27.6	73	78.7	545	166
GA	Liberty	1.46	609	31.8	13.1	27	73	78.1	35	11
TX	Ward	1.46	610	28.6	8.9	29.6	73.4	78.5	2612	796
WV	Grant	1.46	611	34.9	12.1	28.9	73.9	79.3	2076	633
GA	Newton	1.45	612	31.1	10.8	26	72.6	78.1	700	213

HEALTHIEST PLACES TO LIVE

ST	COUNTY	USDA	AMEN	OBES	DIAB	INACT	M AGE	W AGE	ALT ft	ALT m
SC	Charleston	1.45	613	27.5	9.7	23.6	73.8	80	13	4
TN	Grainger	1.45	614	32	10.4	32.9	71.2	77.2	1289	393
TX	Jim Wells	1.45	615	31.5	8.7	26	72.8	79.8	215	66
TX	Palo Pinto	1.45	616	29.6	9.2	26.2	72.6	79.1	1042	318
TX	Trinity	1.45	617	32.3	9.8	31.4	71.7	78.4	248	76
AR	Crawford	1.44	618	33.3	8.2	29.4	72.7	78.6	930	284
AR	Izard	1.44	619	30	8.4	30.4	72.5	78.7	654	199
NM	Roosevelt	1.44	620	27.2	5.9	28	73.6	79.3	4240	1292
TX	Newton	1.44	621	31.3	10	30.4	71.1	77.4	167	51
TX	Scurry	1.44	622	29.2	8.3	29.1	73.2	79.3	2357	718
AL	Hale	1.43	623	43.5	14	35.2	69.3	75.5	211	64
CO	Morgan	1.43	624	25.9	6.6	23	75	80.7	4492	1369
MA	Essex	1.43	625	23.2	8.3	21.7	77.4	81.7	86	26
TX	Washington	1.43	626	29.2	8.8	27.1	73.7	80.2	304	93
ID	Minidoka	1.42	627	30.1	9.5	25.6	74.2	79.6	4374	1333
TX	Midland	1.42	628	26.5	7.7	29.5	75.9	81.1	2765	843
ID	Nez Perce	1.41	629	30.5	9.6	22.8	76.1	80.7	2558	780
MO	Reynolds	1.41	630	33.4	9.2	32.8	70.4	77.3	950	290
ID	Jefferson	1.40	631	25.3	8.4	23.8	75.4	80.4	4879	1487
TX	Burleson	1.40	632	32.5	9.8	30.8	74.7	79.4	319	97
TX	Denton	1.40	633	29.4	9.4	24.6	77.3	80.9	643	196
TX	Marion	1.40	634	30.9	10.3	28.9	71.7	78.4	266	81
AL	St. Clair	1.39	635	35.5	12.5	34.7	71.8	77.7	699	213
TN	Jefferson	1.39	636	32.3	10.5	31.4	73	78.7	1151	351
TX	Rockwall	1.39	637	26.5	8.4	27.3	76.9	80.8	523	159
VA	Bedford	1.39	638	25.3	7.7	28.3	75.8	80.9	1050	320
VA	Bedford City	1.39	639	30.5	10	23.8	75.8	80.9	973	297
MT	Big Horn	1.38	640	36.3	11.8	27.1	74.6	80.3	3982	1214
OR	Union	1.38	641	27.5	7.4	18.1	76.3	80.5	4331	1320
TX	Austin	1.38	642	29.5	9	25.9	74.5	80.2	240	73
TX	Karnes	1.38	643	30.4	9.3	28.4	72.1	79.1	353	108
TX	Stephens	1.38	644	28.3	8.4	27.7	72.6	79.1	1282	391
GA	Upson	1.37	645	30.3	11.3	26.7	70.5	76.3	660	201
NC	Montgomery	1.37	646	32.6	10.7	27.5	71.8	78	522	159
NC	Yancey	1.37	647	27.9	7.8	26.5	74.5	79.8	3365	1026
TX	Wood	1.37	648	30.1	9	28.8	73.3	80.3	442	135
RI	Bristol	1.36	649	20.5	5.2	19	77	82.6	32	10
TN	Anderson	1.36	650	31.2	10.5	31.5	73.7	79.2	1299	396
WA	Okanogan	1.36	651	27.5	7.9	22	75.4	81.1	3741	1140
TN	Union	1.35	652	31.9	9.9	31.6	71.1	77.9	1227	374
TX	Hood	1.35	653	30.4	8.6	23.9	75.7	80	872	266
TX	Panola	1.35	654	30.2	9.7	26.3	72.1	78.9	287	88
AL	Talladega	1.34	655	36.9	13.3	34.6	70.5	77.2	613	187
FL	Bradford	1.34	656	35.1	12.1	29.8	71.8	78.9	144	44
GA	Clay	1.34	657	33	14.2	28.8	69.6	75.8	300	91
OK	Love	1.34	658	29.3	11.2	31.7	73	78.8	804	245
OK	Murray	1.34	659	34.2	10.1	31.2	71.6	78.1	1046	319

ST	COUNTY	USDA	AMEN	OBES	DIAB	INACT	M AGE	W AGE	ALT ft	ALT m
TX	Crane	1.34	660	29.8	9.4	28	73.4	78.5	2566	782
KY	Russell	1.33	661	33.8	11	32.6	72.5	78.5	902	275
NC	Person	1.33	662	33.1	11	27	72.2	78.3	565	172
TN	Rhea	1.33	663	34.2	10.2	30.6	71.1	78	1146	349
VA	Lancaster	1.33	664	31.6	9.9	28.6	72.5	78.7	44	13
WA	Spokane	1.33	665	27.8	7.9	20.2	76.2	80.5	2388	728
AR	Montgomery	1.32	666	28.7	9.1	27	73.2	78.7	906	276
NC	Catawba	1.32	667	26.4	8.2	26.1	74	79.1	981	299
NC	Iredell	1.32	668	28.2	8.1	24.7	73.9	80.2	895	273
TX	Lynn	1.32	669	29.4	9.2	27.7	72.9	78.7	3083	940
MS	Lauderdale	1.31	670	35.4	13.2	29.8	70	77.1	383	117
OK	Le Flore	1.31	671	31.9	10.4	36.9	71.3	78.1	830	253
TN	Cocke	1.31	672	36.9	11.4	33.4	69.9	76.7	1725	526
TX	Brazoria	1.31	673	26.9	9.9	25.9	75.3	78.8	26	8
TX	Lamb	1.31	674	31.7	8.5	26.5	72.1	78.6	3636	1108
TX	Winkler	1.31	675	30.8	9.4	27.4	72.2	78	2914	888
FL	Madison	1.30	676	36.3	12.2	31.1	70.2	76.5	104	32
NJ	Morris	1.30	677	21.4	6.6	20.5	79.5	82.2	636	194
NJ	Passaic	1.30	678	24.2	8.2	27.4	76.3	81.1	587	179
NJ	Sussex	1.30	679	26.4	7.4	21.8	77.2	80.6	806	246
RI	Kent	1.30	680	26.7	7.8	24.5	75.9	81	286	87
TN	Meigs	1.30	681	34.3	11.5	33.6	71.1	78	812	248
CO	Logan	1.29	682	23.1	5.5	22.1	75.8	80.2	4193	1278
OK	Jefferson	1.29	683	34.1	10.2	34.4	71.7	78.1	900	274
TN	Clay	1.29	684	32.7	10.5	28.6	71.2	77.1	783	239
VA	Northampton	1.29	685	30.2	11.3	28.7	71.5	77.6	18	6
VA	Pulaski	1.29	686	26.9	9.8	23.5	72.9	78.8	2178	664
CT	Windham	1.28	687	29.7	8.3	25.2	75.4	80.7	471	143
GA	Lumpkin	1.28	688	27.5	8.6	20.3	73.6	79	1658	505
ME	Oxford	1.28	689	27.4	8.3	24.1	74.5	80	1175	358
NM	Harding	1.28	690	28.3	6.2	20.5	75.4	80.3	5044	1537
TX	Waller	1.28	691	31.4	9.8	30.1	73.8	78.8	203	62
AL	Monroe	1.27	692	35.7	12.2	31.2	71.1	77.2	269	82
SD	Pennington	1.27	693	26.2	7.3	22.1	76.6	81.5	3562	1086
TN	Sullivan	1.27	694	35.3	12	29.4	72.6	79	1688	515
TX	Hemphill	1.27	695	27.5	8.5	28.4	73.8	79.3	2523	769
VA	Gloucester	1.27	696	28.6	8.5	24.3	75	80.7	44	13
VA	Hampton	1.27	697	36.7	11.8	27.6	74.4	79.1	4	1
VA	Middlesex	1.27	698	28.6	9.2	28.1	72.4	79.2	54	16
VA	Newport News	1.27	699	33.5	11.2	29.2	73.1	79.1	10	3
VA	Patrick	1.27	700	30.4	9.7	24.9	73.4	78.9	1577	481
VA	Poquoson	1.27	701	28.3	8.5	21.9	78.3	81.3	3	1
VA	York	1.27	702	27.8	9.1	22.1	78.3	81.3	33	10
AL	Clarke	1.26	703	35.7	12.9	37.1	72.1	77.6	228	69
AR	Searcy	1.26	704	31.7	10.1	31.9	73.1	79.2	1137	346
MD	Allegany	1.26	705	30.7	12.3	31	74	79.7	1252	382

HEALTHIEST PLACES TO LIVE

ST	COUNTY	USDA	AMEN	OBES	DIAB	INACT	M AGE	W AGE	ALT ft	ALT m
PA	Pike	1.26	706	30.8	9	23.9	77.3	82.3	1234	376
TX	Bell	1.26	707	28.7	10.4	28.3	74.5	79.7	668	203
AL	Jackson	1.25	708	30.8	12	29.3	71.2	77.6	1051	320
KY	Laurel	1.25	709	37	12.9	35.7	72	77.7	1138	347
NC	New Hanover	1.25	710	25.5	10.2	20.6	75.5	80.8	22	7
TN	Blount	1.25	711	33.3	9.5	26.4	74.1	79.6	1420	433
TX	Cherokee	1.25	712	33	10.3	29.6	71.9	79	391	119
VA	Harrisonburg	1.25	713	29.1	9.2	25.5	75.6	80.5	1357	414
VA	Rockingham	1.25	714	26.6	8	20.1	75.8	81	1706	520
MO	Cedar	1.24	715	31.3	9.1	27.8	73.9	80	907	276
NC	Surry	1.24	716	31.9	11.2	26.7	72.8	79	1231	375
MO	Carter	1.23	717	30.5	9.3	29.7	70.4	77.3	726	221
TN	DeKalb	1.23	718	32.1	10	29	71.5	78.4	872	266
TX	Castro	1.23	719	29.6	8.8	29.1	73.7	79.3	3770	1149
AR	Washington	1.22	720	29.6	9.1	24.9	74.9	80.1	1399	426
GA	Habersham	1.22	721	26.7	9	25.5	74.6	80	1527	465
MO	Hickory	1.22	722	32.7	8.6	26.4	72.8	79	947	289
MO	Morgan	1.22	723	29.1	8.6	35	73.5	79.6	884	269
MT	Musselshell	1.22	724	21.5	6.6	26.7	75.8	80.9	3510	1070
NC	Carteret	1.22	725	28.5	8.4	27.2	74.6	79.8	13	4
TN	Roane	1.22	726	35.4	11.3	33.9	73.2	79.4	909	277
WA	Asotin	1.22	727	29.2	9	22.8	75.4	81.6	2773	845
FL	Gilchrist	1.21	728	32.8	10	28	71.3	78.8	58	18
OK	McIntosh	1.21	729	36.9	9.7	34.8	72.2	79.4	660	201
TN	Hawkins	1.21	730	34.6	11.3	31.5	72.6	78.6	1416	432
TX	Carson	1.21	731	31.1	9.2	25.5	74.6	79.8	3349	1021
ME	Piscataquis	1.20	732	33.7	8.6	23.5	74.3	80.5	1073	327
NJ	Bergen	1.20	733	21.6	6.8	23.3	79.3	83.5	192	59
VA	Grayson	1.20	734	28.9	9.6	26.3	72.3	77.9	3015	919
TX	Oldham	1.19	735	30.3	9	28.4	72.4	79.1	3697	1127
VA	Northumberland	1.19	736	34.6	9.7	26.7	73	79.5	54	16
OK	Carter	1.18	737	34.7	9.1	34.8	71.7	77.7	914	279
TX	Runnels	1.18	738	34	8.8	26.5	73.2	78.8	1828	557
TX	Tyler	1.18	739	28.7	9.8	28.8	72.4	78.4	203	62
VA	Virginia Beach	1.18	740	26.5	8.7	24.6	76.8	81	9	3
GA	Bartow	1.17	741	25.3	9.3	24.8	71.9	78.2	856	261
NC	Alexander	1.17	742	28.3	8.9	24	73.9	78.9	1197	365
OK	Osage	1.17	743	31.7	10.1	34.1	74.4	80	932	284
TX	Somervell	1.17	744	28.7	8.7	27.2	73.9	79.6	817	249
GA	Murray	1.16	745	29.3	10.4	31.4	70.8	77.8	1107	338
TN	Hamilton	1.16	746	30.5	9.5	26.7	73.4	79.5	978	298
VA	Accomack	1.16	747	33.6	10.5	29.2	71.5	77.6	19	6
AR	Clark	1.15	748	34.1	10.7	30.5	72.9	78.5	317	97
AR	Pike	1.15	749	31.4	9.7	27.6	73.1	79.3	586	179
KY	Whitley	1.15	750	33.1	12.9	34.1	70.7	77	1194	364
SC	Clarendon	1.15	751	37	12.3	32	70.8	77.4	103	31

ST	COUNTY	USDA	AMEN	OBES	DIAB	INACT	M AGE	W AGE	ALT ft	ALT m
VA	Botetourt	1.15	752	28.8	9	20.7	75.7	80.4	1483	452
VA	James City	1.15	753	27	8	20.1	78.1	82.5	65	20
VA	Williamsburg	1.15	754	29.4	9.8	23.7	78.1	82.5	55	17
TN	Loudon	1.14	755	31.3	10.7	28.7	74.2	80	911	278
TX	Lubbock	1.14	756	27.4	8.3	26.2	74	79.2	3232	985
CO	Prowers	1.13	757	22.3	6.1	26.9	74.2	79.3	3801	1159
GA	Lincoln	1.13	758	32.6	11.4	28.7	70.8	76.8	394	120
GA	Monroe	1.13	759	30.6	10.6	26	73.1	78.1	542	165
ID	Latah	1.13	760	26.3	7.8	17.7	77.6	81.6	2944	897
OK	Stephens	1.13	761	31	8.6	28.7	73.4	78.8	1101	336
TN	Benton	1.13	762	34.1	11.2	30.3	70.6	77.8	470	143
AL	Shelby	1.12	763	27.6	8.3	23.5	75.6	80	578	176
FL	Calhoun	1.12	764	34.4	11.6	29.7	72	77.7	97	29
NC	Brunswick	1.12	765	29.9	8.6	25.6	74.4	80	40	12
TX	Limestone	1.12	766	28.6	9.7	26.6	71	77.7	495	151
TX	Webb	1.12	767	29.2	9.1	27.7	75.3	81.8	588	179
LA	Red River	1.11	768	34.8	11.3	32.4	70	76.1	161	49
MO	St. Clair	1.11	769	31.7	9	30.7	72.8	79	816	249
NE	Scotts Bluff	1.11	770	32.5	8.7	27	74.4	80.9	4149	1265
OK	Ellis	1.11	771	30.8	9.4	32.8	74.4	79.8	2298	700
TX	Garza	1.11	772	32.1	9.1	28.6	73.2	79.3	2518	768
TX	Terry	1.11	773	30.5	9.4	30.9	73.1	78.8	3337	1017
VA	Mathews	1.11	774	29.1	9	24.4	75	80.7	4	1
AR	Sebastian	1.10	775	30	9.7	33.9	73.6	79.3	633	193
GA	Talbot	1.10	776	34.7	13	28.6	69.4	76	620	189
WY	Washakie	1.10	777	24	7.2	23.8	75	80.6	5211	1588
AL	Morgan	1.09	778	33	10.2	26.6	72.9	78.9	703	214
MA	Plymouth	1.09	779	22.8	7.4	20.5	76.3	81.3	80	24
AR	Polk	1.08	780	38.5	9.4	30.9	73.1	79.3	1180	360
MT	Yellowstone	1.08	781	27.6	7.3	23.5	76.1	81	3482	1061
WY	Hot Springs	1.08	782	24.2	7.3	22.9	76.1	81.5	6124	1867
PA	Dauphin	1.07	783	31.9	9.3	27.2	74.8	80.1	681	208
TX	Anderson	1.07	784	32.7	10.7	32	69.8	77.8	378	115
TX	Walker	1.07	785	32.5	9.6	27.9	73.9	78.8	277	84
VA	Warren	1.07	786	28.4	9.7	23.9	75.2	79.8	860	262
OK	Cleveland	1.06	787	29.5	9.4	26.1	75	79.8	1144	349
WA	Walla Walla	1.06	788	28.7	8.5	16.3	76.4	80.9	1198	365
CO	Lincoln	1.05	789	21.6	6.4	23.1	74.4	80.6	5122	1561
CT	Hartford	1.05	790	23.8	7.3	22.5	76.6	81.7	316	96
GA	Quitman	1.05	791	32.8	12.3	30.7	69.6	75.8	331	101
IL	Williamson	1.05	792	30.4	7.4	31.1	73.2	79.2	466	142
ME	Cumberland	1.05	793	21.6	6.8	16.3	77.1	81.7	282	86
ME	Sagadahoc	1.05	794	25.7	7.6	19.8	76.5	80.5	139	42
TX	Hunt	1.05	795	31.1	10.3	30.4	73.1	78.7	541	165
CT	Litchfield	1.04	796	19.7	6.1	18.5	77.3	82.5	914	279
GA	Decatur	1.04	797	33.7	12.5	31.8	70.7	77.8	168	51
GA	Warren	1.04	798	35	12.3	27.3	68.4	75.4	502	153

HEALTHIEST PLACES TO LIVE

ST	COUNTY	USDA	AMEN	OBES	DIAB	INACT	M AGE	W AGE	ALT ft	ALT m
NY	Bronx	1.04	799	27.3	9.6	30.1	73.9	80.5	77	24
OK	Pontotoc	1.04	800	37	10.4	34.7	72.9	78.2	971	296
TX	Fayette	1.04	801	29	8.6	26	74.1	79.9	362	110
TX	Hardin	1.04	802	30.2	10.6	29.2	73.5	78.3	71	22
TX	Jefferson	1.04	803	31.5	10.7	30.2	72.4	78.4	12	4
AR	Scott	1.02	804	32.3	9.4	32	73.2	78.7	933	284
TX	Childress	1.02	805	29.6	9.4	25.9	72.2	77.9	1765	538
TX	Kimble	1.02	806	27.1	8.3	25.4	75.5	81	2031	619
TX	Tarrant	1.02	807	27.6	8.7	22.8	75.3	79.9	656	200
TX	Upton	1.02	808	28.9	8.7	27.6	73.4	78.5	2743	836
MO	Madison	1.01	809	34.7	9.4	28.6	72.7	78.7	809	247
MS	Itawamba	1.01	810	35.1	12.2	35.6	71.6	77.3	394	120
TX	Collin	1.01	811	24.3	7.6	22.1	79.7	82.5	613	187
TX	Coryell	1.01	812	29.8	10.8	28.2	74.9	79.8	953	291
MS	Harrison	1.00	813	36	11.3	29.5	71	78.6	77	23
NC	Pamlico	1.00	814	28	9.8	25.2	73	78.5	13	4
OK	Adair	1.00	815	36.5	13.1	32.5	71.3	77.7	1068	325
AR	Howard	0.99	816	34.7	11.6	32.8	72	78	584	178
GA	Forsyth	0.99	817	23	9.2	20.2	77.2	81.8	1156	352
ID	Lewis	0.99	818	30.5	8	24.1	75.8	80.6	3403	1037
KY	Trigg	0.99	819	34.2	9.7	33.5	73	79.3	484	147
NM	Union	0.99	820	24.3	5.9	24.6	75.4	80.3	5423	1653
SC	Lexington	0.99	821	31.2	9.1	25.4	74.5	80	389	119
GA	Jones	0.98	822	29.3	10.4	29.4	73.1	79.3	468	143
TN	Stewart	0.98	823	33	10.2	32.6	72.4	78.3	509	155
GA	Crawford	0.97	824	29.7	10.5	27.5	70.6	76.6	473	144
KY	Rowan	0.97	825	35.4	10.3	30.6	72.4	79	992	302
MT	Toole	0.97	826	28.6	7.6	26.6	74.6	80.7	3508	1069
RI	Providence	0.97	827	27	8.3	27.1	75.7	81.4	362	110
SD	Custer	0.97	828	25.9	6.6	24	71.1	78.5	4234	1290
AL	Etowah	0.96	829	32.5	11.8	33.3	70.5	77.2	766	233
GA	Hall	0.96	830	27.9	10.5	21.9	74.7	79.7	1136	346
ID	Twin Falls	0.96	831	26.1	8.2	23.1	75.4	79.9	4795	1461
MO	Cole	0.96	832	27.9	8.8	26.1	75.7	80.5	696	212
MO	Jefferson	0.96	833	34.9	10.1	30.9	74.1	78.4	614	187
OK	Washington	0.96	834	31.3	9	29	75.1	80.3	729	222
TX	Duval	0.96	835	30.3	8.8	26.3	73.4	78.6	487	148
IL	Alexander	0.95	836	31	9.3	29.8	69.9	77	392	119
MO	Dade	0.95	837	29.5	8.8	26.4	73.7	79	1024	312
NJ	Warren	0.95	838	27.1	7.5	25.4	76.7	80.7	604	184
OK	Caddo	0.95	839	33.6	10.4	32.6	72	78.5	1416	432
GA	Lanier	0.94	840	31	11.7	29.4	69.4	76.5	200	61
MI	Charlevoix	0.94	841	28	8.9	21.2	76.8	81.4	798	243
NM	Curry	0.94	842	27.1	8.6	27.4	74.2	79.1	4437	1352
PA	Monroe	0.94	843	29.2	9	25.6	75.6	80.4	1241	378
TX	Bastrop	0.94	844	30.8	9.5	26.3	74	79.3	465	142
TX	Deaf Smith	0.94	845	30.4	8.6	28	72.4	79.1	4046	1233

ST	COUNTY	USDA	AMEN	OBES	DIAB	INACT	M AGE	W AGE	ALT ft	ALT m
VA	Page	0.94	846	32.2	8.9	26.4	73.9	80	1402	427
GA	Troup	0.93	847	32.7	11.9	28.9	71.4	77.1	725	221
MI	Emmet	0.93	848	31.7	7.9	21.5	77.7	81.6	794	242
NH	Carroll	0.93	849	24.7	7.3	20	77.1	82.4	1033	315
AL	Choctaw	0.92	850	38.8	14.3	34.1	70.4	77	197	60
CO	Sedgwick	0.92	851	24.3	5.2	19.4	75.8	80.2	3761	1146
ID	Madison	0.92	852	27.4	8	22.9	76.7	80.4	5579	1700
UT	Wayne	0.92	853	24.6	6.8	20.3	75.5	79.8	6110	1862
MO	Cape Girardeau	0.91	854	27.4	9	27.2	75	80.2	462	141
TX	Bailey	0.91	855	28.8	8.9	28.2	73.1	78.8	3874	1181
TX	Martin	0.91	856	29.1	8.6	26.4	72.4	77.8	2779	847
TX	Williamson	0.91	857	26.8	7.3	19.7	79.3	82.7	751	229
AL	Lauderdale	0.90	858	33	12.2	32	73.3	79.7	639	195
CO	Elbert	0.90	859	21.2	4.5	18.9	77.9	81.9	5965	1818
TX	Atascosa	0.90	860	29.6	8.5	28	74.6	80.4	434	132
AR	Perry	0.89	861	32.8	10	33.1	72.5	78.1	557	170
FL	Holmes	0.89	862	30.4	12.9	32.7	71.8	78	131	40
KY	Wayne	0.89	863	33.3	11.3	40.6	71.6	77.8	1049	320
MI	Manistee	0.89	864	27.5	8.5	27.2	75.3	80.8	790	241
NC	Richmond	0.89	865	31.7	10.7	29.8	70.7	77.1	335	102
OK	Latimer	0.89	866	34.5	10.7	34.3	72.3	78.8	876	267
AL	Winston	0.88	867	36.5	10.3	32.4	70.9	77.6	722	220
NC	Currituck	0.88	868	32.3	9.1	23.5	73.7	79.6	6	2
OK	Coal	0.88	869	32.8	10.3	31.9	71.1	78.1	684	208
OK	Cotton	0.88	870	34	9.7	35.7	71.7	78.1	1005	306
PA	Westmoreland	0.88	871	28	8.6	26.9	75.8	80.9	1312	400
SC	Horry	0.88	872	29.1	10.2	24.4	73.7	79.8	50	15
TX	Lee	0.88	873	31	9.4	28.7	74.6	80.2	409	125
TX	Wilbarger	0.88	874	30.4	9.2	25.9	73.2	78.7	1231	375
GA	Seminole	0.87	875	32.9	11.7	25.8	70.1	77.2	137	42
MO	Wright	0.87	876	33.5	8	34	72.1	78.8	1320	402
TN	Smith	0.87	877	32.4	10.8	31.5	71.3	77.6	692	211
TX	Wise	0.87	878	31.3	8.6	29.1	73.8	79	879	268
ID	Custer	0.86	879	27.2	7.3	22.7	75.8	80.4	7615	2321
ME	York	0.86	880	25.7	7.2	20.4	77	81.5	309	94
MO	St. Charles	0.86	881	29.3	8	24.4	77.5	81.1	531	162
MO	Washington	0.86	882	29.7	9	27.8	70.4	77.3	933	284
MS	Monroe	0.86	883	35.5	12.1	35.7	71.2	78.3	283	86
TN	Jackson	0.86	884	35	11.6	32.5	71.3	77.6	756	231
TX	Donley	0.86	885	30.4	9.3	27.5	74.6	79.8	2672	814
TX	Floyd	0.86	886	28.6	9.6	28.7	73.8	79	3140	957
AR	Pulaski	0.85	887	32.1	10	28.6	72.1	78.9	335	102
LA	St. Mary	0.85	888	37.9	11.6	32.2	70.3	78	4	1
MD	Washington	0.85	889	29.9	9.8	27.7	74.6	79.7	639	195
MS	Jackson	0.85	890	32.8	11.3	28.7	72.1	77.7	45	14
AL	Perry	0.84	891	40.5	17.8	34.1	69.3	75.5	277	84
FL	Lafayette	0.84	892	32.9	11.5	29.9	72.4	78.2	65	20

ST	COUNTY	USDA	AMEN	OBES	DIAB	INACT	M AGE	W AGE	ALT ft	ALT m
TX	Bosque	0.84	893	27.4	8.2	24.8	73.8	79.5	830	253
TX	Gaines	0.84	894	30.7	9.2	29.2	73.9	78.9	3320	1012
TX	Titus	0.84	895	33	9	27.1	72.5	78.1	358	109
MA	Suffolk	0.83	896	22.1	8.6	22.1	75.8	81.9	57	17
MO	Miller	0.83	897	30.2	8.4	30	73.6	78.9	787	240
NJ	Hunterdon	0.83	898	20.5	6.2	18.4	79.4	82.7	400	122
TN	Marion	0.83	899	31.7	9.4	35.6	71.2	77.8	1321	403
TX	Hill	0.83	900	32.8	9.3	31.2	72.7	79.1	631	192
UT	Emery	0.83	901	28.5	7.3	20.8	75.7	80	5846	1782
VA	Amherst	0.83	902	29.9	10.4	24.9	73.2	79.4	1129	344
NC	Mecklenburg	0.82	903	25.6	8.5	20.4	75.6	80.7	687	209
TN	Henderson	0.82	904	32.3	9.1	31.5	71.3	77.3	500	152
WV	Hardy	0.82	905	32.8	11.2	26.8	73.9	79.3	1742	531
WV	Pendleton	0.82	906	34.8	10.8	30.8	73.3	78.6	2567	783
KS	Trego	0.81	907	33.1	7.6	28.7	76.3	81.5	2346	715
MA	Berkshire	0.81	908	23.5	7.5	21.1	76.9	81.1	1404	428
MO	Iron	0.81	909	33.6	9.1	28	70.4	77.3	1078	328
PA	Clearfield	0.81	910	29.1	9	23.7	74.8	80.8	1636	499
SC	McCormick	0.81	911	35.2	11.9	25.3	72	78.1	411	125
NH	Belknap	0.80	912	26.4	8	21.7	76	82	755	230
NY	Westchester	0.80	913	17	6.7	18.6	79.2	83.3	340	104
TX	Wichita	0.80	914	31.1	10.6	30.3	72.5	78.7	1046	319
GA	Columbia	0.79	915	25.4	9.3	22.2	75.4	80.2	357	109
TX	Bowie	0.79	916	32.8	9.7	29.4	72.4	78.4	316	96
TX	Gray	0.79	917	31.1	10.3	37.6	73.2	78.9	3006	916
VA	Surry	0.79	918	34.5	11.7	26.2	72	77.8	77	24
WY	Campbell	0.79	919	31.3	7.9	27.5	75.9	81.5	4501	1372
AL	Autauga	0.78	920	33.9	11.7	31.9	72.9	78	365	111
KY	Lewis	0.78	921	35	12.2	34.8	69.8	77.2	867	264
TX	Grayson	0.78	922	26.5	8.6	25.6	73.6	79.1	707	216
TX	Rains	0.78	923	30.1	9	27.1	73.6	78.9	454	138
LA	Cameron	0.77	924	32.1	10.2	25	72.6	78	3	1
NY	Rockland	0.77	925	25.2	8.7	24.3	78.7	82.8	422	129
ID	Gooding	0.76	926	28.9	7.8	26.2	74.3	80	3867	1179
KY	Meade	0.76	927	35.6	11.6	31.8	74.4	79.6	640	195
LA	St. Tammany	0.76	928	27.2	8.9	23.9	74.1	79.6	48	14
NC	Cleveland	0.76	929	32.5	11.6	29.2	71.8	78.2	889	271
NY	Nassau	0.76	930	20.8	7.3	22.3	79.4	83.3	94	29
TX	Franklin	0.76	931	27.2	8.8	30.1	73.8	80	404	123
TX	McLennan	0.76	932	30	9.3	24.9	73.4	79.2	572	174
KY	Livingston	0.75	933	33.8	12.5	34.6	73.8	79.6	428	130
MI	Benzie	0.75	934	29.5	8.8	23	75.7	80.9	777	237
NC	Onslow	0.74	935	30.2	9.9	24	74.5	79.6	42	13
OK	Greer	0.74	936	32.8	10.2	33.9	72.4	78.7	1653	504
TN	Johnson	0.74	937	32	10.8	31.2	70.8	77.4	2915	888
TX	Grimes	0.74	938	33.4	9.4	25.7	73.1	78.5	299	91
GA	Echols	0.73	939	28.9	10.2	24.9	72.2	77.9	142	43

ST	COUNTY	USDA	AMEN	OBES	DIAB	INACT	M AGE	W AGE	ALT ft	ALT m
KY	McCreary	0.73	940	32.3	12.4	40.8	69	76.2	1159	353
MI	Leelanau	0.73	941	31.3	8.5	26.6	78.6	82.8	731	223
PA	Cameron	0.73	942	28.8	8.8	25.9	75.2	80	1671	509
KY	Union	0.72	943	35.8	10.4	33.2	72.8	78.8	401	122
MS	Leake	0.72	944	35.9	13	38.7	68.4	76.2	406	124
OK	Delaware	0.72	945	31.9	11.1	34.9	73.3	79	945	288
PA	Northumberland	0.72	946	31.7	8.1	29.6	74.3	80.2	774	236
TX	Milam	0.72	947	32.2	9.8	30.1	73.3	78.2	406	124
TX	Smith	0.72	948	28.5	8.7	25.7	75	81	445	136
AL	Randolph	0.71	949	32.5	12.6	33.8	70.8	77.4	916	279
IL	Jackson	0.71	950	27.5	8.3	27.7	75.3	80.1	449	137
LA	Webster	0.71	951	35.7	11.7	30.8	70.7	77.1	228	70
MD	Anne Arundel	0.71	952	27.4	8.5	20.1	75.7	80.2	88	27
SC	Anderson	0.71	953	30.1	10.7	28.8	71.8	79	756	231
SC	Berkeley	0.71	954	37.7	12.3	30.1	73.9	79.2	45	14
TX	Camp	0.71	955	31.2	10.4	26.6	71.3	78.3	353	107
TX	La Salle	0.71	956	29.6	8.6	26.8	72.9	78.7	429	131
AL	Colbert	0.70	957	33.4	11.7	33.7	71.9	78.3	589	180
FL	Suwannee	0.70	958	30.7	9.8	29.1	72.4	78.2	96	29
GA	Bryan	0.70	959	28	9.6	24.6	73.7	78.9	43	13
GA	Cook	0.70	960	32.9	11.5	27.8	70	76.4	246	75
NY	Ulster	0.70	961	26.5	7.5	22.9	76.6	80.9	1134	346
OK	Beaver	0.70	962	32.6	8.8	31.2	74.4	79.8	2568	783
WV	Hampshire	0.69	963	35.1	9.9	30.3	73.3	79.2	1201	366
NC	Stanly	0.68	964	26.6	9.6	30.8	73.2	79.4	515	157
PA	Wyoming	0.68	965	30.4	8.5	24.3	74.8	80.7	1256	383
TX	Andrews	0.68	966	29.6	8.9	27.1	73.9	78.9	3177	968
TX	Gonzales	0.68	967	31.6	9.5	28.2	72.1	79.1	342	104
TX	Medina	0.68	968	29.6	9.2	24.9	75.3	79.8	960	292
WV	Mineral	0.68	969	34	10.8	30.8	73.8	79.3	1281	390
NC	Tyrrell	0.67	970	32	11.1	28	71.6	77.6	5	1
PA	Carbon	0.67	971	29.7	9.3	26.3	73.6	79.5	1244	379
SC	Colleton	0.67	972	34.1	12	32.6	69.7	77.4	50	15
SC	Fairfield	0.67	973	39.1	14	35.1	69	76.8	406	124
TN	Washington	0.67	974	29.5	10.2	28.6	72.5	79.6	1700	518
VA	Carroll	0.67	975	31	10	28.5	73	79	2470	753
VA	Galax	0.67	976	29.8	8.8	24.4	72.3	77.9	2487	758
WV	Summers	0.67	977	34.7	11	33.1	72.6	79.2	2147	654
KS	Greenwood	0.66	978	34.3	7.8	30.4	74.7	80.4	1175	358
NJ	Ocean	0.66	979	26.7	8.6	24	76	81.8	85	26
FL	Baker	0.65	980	34.8	12.7	32.6	68.1	77.7	126	38
GA	Wilkes	0.65	981	31	12.3	28.4	70.8	76.8	500	153
KY	Cumberland	0.65	982	33.7	11	32.1	70.2	77.3	762	232
LA	Caddo	0.65	983	32.1	11.5	30.4	70.8	77.6	212	65
MD	Calvert	0.65	984	27.8	8.8	23.1	75	79.7	79	24
MT	Garfield	0.65	985	25.8	6.2	26.8	75.7	81	2810	856
AL	Cherokee	0.64	986	31.1	11.2	34.6	71.3	77.9	756	231

ST	COUNTY	USDA	AMEN	OBES	DIAB	INACT	M AGE	W AGE	ALT ft	ALT m
AL	Cullman	0.64	987	32.2	11.9	28.7	71.9	78.4	750	229
KY	Johnson	0.64	988	38.2	11.7	34.5	69.7	77.4	891	272
MO	St. Louis	0.64	989	28.8	8	23.8	76.1	80.8	542	165
NJ	Monmouth	0.64	990	21.3	7.5	21.2	77.3	81.6	111	34
OK	McClain	0.64	991	33.7	9.8	27.8	74.6	79.8	1114	340
PA	Beaver	0.64	992	31.1	9.2	26.6	74.6	80.4	1053	321
TX	Dallas	0.64	993	30.5	10.2	25.3	75.1	80.3	511	156
VA	Buena Vista	0.64	994	29.1	8.8	23.7	74.3	80.4	999	304
VA	Lexington	0.64	995	29.2	9.5	23.7	74.3	80.4	1055	322
VA	Richmond	0.64	996	32.5	9.9	29.2	72.5	78.7	82	25
VA	Rockbridge	0.64	997	29	8.7	27.4	74.3	80.4	1606	489
ID	Jerome	0.63	998	31.6	8.2	19.5	74.7	80.3	3996	1218
IL	Randolph	0.63	999	29.2	7.4	25.3	73.8	79.2	464	141
KY	Gallatin	0.63	1000	32.8	11.1	37.2	72.6	78.7	644	196
OH	Noble	0.63	1001	33.1	9.4	27.5	74.4	79.8	964	294
TX	Cass	0.63	1002	30.6	9.9	32.3	71.7	78.4	319	97
TX	Cooke	0.63	1003	33	9.8	27.2	74.8	80.6	839	256
TX	Kaufman	0.63	1004	35.8	9.3	31.8	72.7	77.6	430	131
TX	Robertson	0.63	1005	31.6	10.1	28.2	72.8	78.4	379	116
GA	Hart	0.62	1006	30.4	9.6	24.4	72	78.4	742	226
KY	Clinton	0.62	1007	32.8	10.2	36.1	70.2	77.3	961	293
KY	Edmonson	0.62	1008	33.5	12.5	28.1	72.8	77.8	627	191
KY	Greenup	0.62	1009	35.3	13.3	31.7	73.3	78.5	758	231
MO	Greene	0.62	1010	30.2	8.5	25.2	74.7	80.7	1226	374
SD	Dewey	0.62	1011	42.3	15.5	33.9	72.9	79.9	2004	611
TN	Knox	0.62	1012	30.5	10.3	27.3	74.3	79.5	1009	307
TX	Knox	0.62	1013	28.2	9.4	26.3	72.6	79	1453	443
WA	Grant	0.62	1014	32.4	8.7	22.9	75.5	79.7	1400	427
KY	Pulaski	0.61	1015	30.5	10.2	32.2	72.5	78.9	1012	308
MO	Dent	0.61	1016	31.7	8.6	29.6	72.8	78.6	1189	362
MS	Neshoba	0.61	1017	35	13.6	33.7	71.1	77.3	455	139
TN	Humphreys	0.61	1018	31.6	11.4	30.7	72.1	78.5	565	172
TX	Stonewall	0.61	1019	29.2	9	28	72.9	78.9	1750	533
VA	Dickenson	0.61	1020	31.4	9.6	29	70.2	77.4	1896	578
MI	Mason	0.60	1021	32	8.6	26.7	75.5	80.5	693	211
TX	Reagan	0.60	1022	28.6	8.9	28.7	75.9	81.1	2650	808
FL	Columbia	0.59	1023	33.8	10.9	28.4	71.8	77.8	109	33
SC	Jasper	0.59	1024	39.7	12.9	30.2	71.1	77	31	9
TX	Brazos	0.59	1025	30.2	9.1	22.9	77.1	80.4	284	87
VA	Charles City	0.59	1026	33.6	11.3	30.2	72	77.8	63	19
CO	Washington	0.58	1027	21.1	5.6	24.3	75	80.7	4604	1403
FL	Hamilton	0.58	1028	38.3	13.3	33.3	70.2	76.5	108	33
KS	Butler	0.58	1029	32.5	8.3	23.5	75.8	80.3	1396	425
MI	Antrim	0.58	1030	30.6	8.1	22.6	76.2	80.9	895	273
OK	Creek	0.58	1031	33.9	10.1	32.4	72.1	78.2	832	254
OK	Seminole	0.58	1032	37	10.3	34.6	71.3	78.2	927	283
TX	Guadalupe	0.58	1033	29.8	8.2	23.9	76.5	81.1	564	172

ST	COUNTY	USDA	AMEN	OBES	DIAB	INACT	M AGE	W AGE	ALT ft	ALT m
IL	Union	0.57	1034	30.4	7.7	31.5	72.9	79.7	503	153
TX	Navarro	0.57	1035	32.5	9.1	30.3	72.3	78.9	402	122
NE	Dawson	0.56	1036	32.1	8.4	26.4	75.6	80.9	2519	768
SC	Richland	0.56	1037	30.6	11.2	26.4	73.1	78.8	256	78
TN	Houston	0.56	1038	34	10.4	29.3	72.4	78.3	564	172
WA	Lincoln	0.56	1039	32.3	7.2	21.5	75.7	80.4	2148	655
KY	Estill	0.55	1040	34.6	11.7	36.8	70.3	76.9	900	274
MD	Charles	0.55	1041	32.3	10	24.7	74.7	79.2	113	34
OH	Guernsey	0.55	1042	30.1	9.7	30.8	73.4	79.4	962	293
AL	Lawrence	0.54	1043	38	12.4	35.3	71.5	77.7	678	207
GA	Tattnall	0.54	1044	28.9	10.9	28.1	70.6	77.1	162	49
MA	Bristol	0.54	1045	28.8	9.9	28.1	75.8	81.4	100	30
MO	Pulaski	0.54	1046	32.4	9.5	27.5	74.6	79.5	984	300
TN	Cumberland	0.54	1047	28.2	9.5	25.6	74.7	80.6	1784	544
GA	Stephens	0.53	1048	32.7	10.4	27.1	71.7	78.1	910	277
KY	Lee	0.53	1049	33.4	11.1	35.5	68.2	76.2	946	288
MD	St. Mary's	0.53	1050	28.6	9.6	23.4	75.5	80.3	75	23
MS	Yalobusha	0.53	1051	38.8	13.4	34.5	68.6	76.3	327	100
VA	Halifax	0.53	1052	33.9	11.8	31.3	70.6	78	461	140
MT	McCone	0.52	1053	26	6	26.2	75.7	81	2483	757
NC	Pender	0.52	1054	32.2	10.7	23.7	74.3	79.5	37	11
SC	Spartanburg	0.52	1055	30	9.9	27.5	72	78.4	769	234
TX	Harrison	0.52	1056	33.9	10.2	32.9	72.3	78.3	312	95
TX	Maverick	0.52	1057	29.8	9	29	74.2	80.1	794	242
AL	Jefferson	0.51	1058	31.9	11.7	28.8	71	77.8	575	175
AL	Walker	0.51	1059	35	13	36.9	68.3	75.9	472	144
AR	Fulton	0.51	1060	31.7	9.3	28.1	72.5	78.7	737	225
LA	Ouachita	0.51	1061	31.8	12.3	29.5	72.1	77.8	102	31
NC	Chowan	0.51	1062	30.4	10.8	28.1	73	78.8	18	5
OK	Harper	0.51	1063	30.9	10	34.6	74.4	79.8	1982	604
TX	Caldwell	0.51	1064	32.3	8.8	24.8	73.5	79.4	497	151
TX	Hartley	0.51	1065	30.7	9.8	27.8	73.7	78.9	3947	1203
TX	Menard	0.51	1066	30.5	8.6	26.3	76.4	81.6	2101	640
TX	Young	0.51	1067	29.9	9.6	26.6	73.3	78.8	1179	359
VA	Isle of Wight	0.51	1068	31	11.4	26.9	72.8	78.9	53	16
AL	Tuscaloosa	0.50	1069	34.4	11.8	28.8	71.9	77.8	361	110
KY	Bracken	0.50	1070	33.3	11.1	30.3	72.3	78.5	798	243
LA	Terrebonne	0.50	1071	38.9	12.4	32.5	71.8	78.6	3	1
MS	Lafayette	0.50	1072	32.3	10.3	28.9	72.5	79.4	389	119
NC	Perquimans	0.50	1073	34	9.7	26.6	73	78.8	12	4
SD	Bennett	0.50	1074	36.9	11.7	28.7	71	78.3	3168	966
TX	DeWitt	0.50	1075	28.4	9.1	25.2	73.3	79.2	283	86
AR	Hot Spring	0.49	1076	34.7	10.2	33.9	72.7	78.4	455	139
AR	Saline	0.49	1077	31.1	10	25.2	74.7	79.8	537	164
AR	Sharp	0.49	1078	29.2	8.9	32.1	72.7	79.4	560	171
MO	Bollinger	0.49	1079	35.1	8.9	31.5	72.7	78.7	596	182
MS	Winston	0.49	1080	36.8	14.2	34.1	70.4	78.6	456	139

HEALTHIEST PLACES TO LIVE

ST	COUNTY	USDA	AMEN	OBES	DIAB	INACT	M AGE	W AGE	ALT ft	ALT m
NJ	Hudson	0.49	1081	23.9	8.3	28.6	75.8	81.3	37	11
PA	Schuylkill	0.49	1082	31.8	8.8	31.7	73.2	79.5	1052	321
TX	Zavala	0.49	1083	29.6	8.7	27.4	72.2	78.1	691	211
CO	Baca	0.48	1084	22.7	5.7	22.3	74.2	79.3	4292	1308
KY	Hancock	0.48	1085	34.5	9.7	30.8	72.8	78.9	504	154
LA	Iberia	0.48	1086	33.7	11.3	31	72	78	7	2
MO	Ripley	0.48	1087	31.6	8.9	34.4	70.7	77.8	519	158
TX	Dimmit	0.48	1088	28.9	9	26.3	72.2	78.1	609	186
VA	Chesapeake	0.48	1089	27.2	9.1	22	74.6	79.6	13	4
VA	Essex	0.48	1090	32.7	10.8	27.4	72.4	79.2	87	26
VA	Norfolk	0.48	1091	32.9	10.9	26.6	70.9	77.5	9	3
VA	Portsmouth	0.48	1092	39.1	12	29	70.7	76.9	8	2
ME	Somerset	0.47	1093	35.1	9.8	26.4	74.8	79.8	1180	360
MO	Gasconade	0.47	1094	32.4	8.5	31.1	73.7	79.1	774	236
PA	Allegheny	0.47	1095	28.4	8.4	24.6	74.7	80.2	1043	318
PA	Clinton	0.47	1096	31.9	8	28.4	74.3	79.8	1438	438
KY	Crittenden	0.46	1097	33	9.9	37.8	72.3	77.9	477	145
KY	Menifee	0.46	1098	35.9	11.9	31.6	70.8	77.6	1059	323
MO	Pike	0.46	1099	32.7	10.2	31.5	73.8	78.8	668	204
OK	Custer	0.46	1100	31.3	9.6	34.6	73.3	79.7	1729	527
TX	Hidalgo	0.46	1101	30	10.2	23.8	77.8	83.4	129	39
KY	Taylor	0.45	1102	33.2	10.5	26.8	73.2	78.7	837	255
MO	Texas	0.45	1103	35.6	8.2	31.9	72	78.5	1253	382
MT	Liberty	0.45	1104	26.2	5.9	32.5	74.6	80.7	3372	1028
NC	Caswell	0.45	1105	30.9	12.1	27.9	71.7	78.1	577	176
NC	Rutherford	0.45	1106	31.2	9.9	29.8	71.4	78	1114	340
OK	Muskogee	0.45	1107	32.3	11	35.4	71.9	78.3	597	182
OR	Gilliam	0.45	1108	27.2	7.5	17.8	75.9	80.8	1934	590
PA	Lancaster	0.45	1109	29.3	8.1	21.3	76.8	81.4	462	141
SC	Sumter	0.45	1110	36.7	12.8	31.7	71.6	78.5	162	49
SC	York	0.45	1111	29.4	9	25.5	74	79.2	618	188
TX	Kent	0.45	1112	28.9	8.5	26.6	72.9	78.9	2113	644
GA	Paulding	0.44	1113	26	10.9	25.7	74.1	78.4	1026	313
LA	Vermilion	0.44	1114	33.3	10.4	27.6	71.9	78.5	6	2
MI	Keweenaw	0.44	1115	31.9	8.9	25.1	75.2	80.1	847	258
OR	Grant	0.44	1116	24.2	7.6	18.4	75.9	80.4	4696	1431
PA	Wayne	0.44	1117	27.4	8.9	23.9	74.3	80	1463	446
TN	Hardin	0.44	1118	30.3	9.4	33.9	71.5	78.1	507	154
TX	Orange	0.44	1119	29.7	10	33.9	71.5	78	12	4
TX	Wilson	0.44	1120	29.3	9.6	26.4	74.3	79.6	458	140
ID	Lemhi	0.43	1121	23	7.3	16.4	76.2	80.4	6928	2112
NC	Pasquotank	0.43	1122	33.4	10.9	25.9	73.7	78.3	8	3
SD	Butte	0.43	1123	31	7	30.5	74.8	80.5	3019	920
TN	Perry	0.43	1124	31.3	9.7	30.2	70.6	78.2	602	183
MO	Osage	0.42	1125	29.7	8.7	26.8	74.3	79.8	715	218
MS	Clarke	0.42	1126	33.8	10.9	37.7	71.2	77.6	325	99
NC	Camden	0.42	1127	32	9.8	25.4	72.9	78.2	10	3

ST	COUNTY	USDA	AMEN	OBES	DIAB	INACT	M AGE	W AGE	ALT ft	ALT m
NC	Gaston	0.42	1128	26.2	9	28.4	71.9	78.1	763	233
OH	Muskingum	0.42	1129	28.5	11	30.3	73.9	79.3	891	272
OK	Payne	0.42	1130	31.1	9.6	28.1	76.2	79.9	938	286
TX	Swisher	0.42	1131	29.4	9.1	29	74.6	79.8	3452	1052
TX	Van Zandt	0.42	1132	29.4	9.5	29.5	73.6	79.2	466	142
WA	Douglas	0.42	1133	27.7	7.8	20	76.3	81.1	2237	682
NC	Chatham	0.41	1134	24.8	8	21.7	75.4	80.5	424	129
OK	Tillman	0.41	1135	33.1	10.9	32.5	71.7	78.1	1189	362
TX	Morris	0.41	1136	31.8	10.7	29.4	71.3	78.3	350	107
WV	Morgan	0.41	1137	31.4	11	29.2	74.1	80	888	271
KS	Wabaunsee	0.40	1138	31.7	7.7	24.8	75.3	80.4	1253	382
KY	Mason	0.40	1139	31.5	10.5	29.8	72.9	79.1	831	253
PA	Indiana	0.40	1140	29.3	8.5	29.3	76.2	81	1426	435
PA	Washington	0.40	1141	29	9.3	24.5	75.1	80.6	1139	347
TX	Freestone	0.40	1142	31.7	9.5	28.1	73.4	79.1	385	117
TX	Frio	0.40	1143	28.6	8.5	29.7	72.9	78.7	581	177
TX	King	0.40	1144	28.5	8.7	26.3	73.2	78.7	1805	550
GA	Candler	0.39	1145	31	10.3	27.5	70.1	77.7	214	65
KS	Geary	0.39	1146	29.3	9.1	29.9	74.4	80.2	1272	388
KY	Campbell	0.39	1147	27.9	9.6	26.3	73.7	79.6	679	207
KY	Morgan	0.39	1148	35.1	12.6	34.4	70.8	76.9	976	297
KY	Spencer	0.39	1149	36.2	10.3	29.9	75	79	654	199
LA	Natchitoches	0.39	1150	35.7	11.6	33.1	70.9	77.2	166	51
MO	Moniteau	0.39	1151	29.6	9.2	32	74.4	79.9	802	244
MS	Noxubee	0.39	1152	39.9	13.7	33.4	68.9	76.5	230	70
TX	Ochiltree	0.39	1153	28.5	8.3	26.4	74.2	79.8	2920	890
WV	Hancock	0.39	1154	32.6	11.7	27.3	73.9	79	998	304
AL	Chilton	0.38	1155	35.3	11.1	30.4	70.4	77.3	528	161
MO	Franklin	0.38	1156	30.7	8.3	26.7	74.2	79.4	667	203
NJ	Cumberland	0.38	1157	33.2	10.2	30.7	72.7	78.6	47	14
OK	Garvin	0.38	1158	29.4	9.9	33.7	71.6	78.1	1004	306
TN	Hancock	0.38	1159	31.3	10.9	34.9	71.2	77.2	1515	462
TX	Dickens	0.38	1160	30.5	9.1	27	73.2	78.7	2395	730
WV	Brooke	0.38	1161	36.3	13	34.1	73.8	78.8	1003	306
AL	Marshall	0.37	1162	29.2	10.9	31.5	71.5	77.5	880	268
GA	Morgan	0.37	1163	29	11.1	24.5	73.2	78.5	609	186
KY	Carroll	0.37	1164	31.9	10.5	34.4	72.8	78.6	645	196
KY	Harlan	0.37	1165	32.3	13.8	34.8	68.4	76.2	2095	638
LA	De Soto	0.37	1166	36.6	11.8	30.9	70.5	77.3	240	73
LA	St. Bernard	0.37	1167	32.3	10.8	31.7	70.6	76.1	3	1
MI	Grand Traverse	0.37	1168	30.2	7.5	19.5	77.7	82	905	276
MO	Lincoln	0.37	1169	35.4	10.1	26.8	73.7	79	607	185
NY	Putnam	0.37	1170	27.9	7	22.5	78.6	82.6	649	198
TN	Moore	0.37	1171	30.9	9.8	28.6	72.8	79	988	301
TX	Hockley	0.37	1172	29.6	8.6	30.6	72.9	78.7	3485	1062
FL	Liberty	0.36	1173	35.8	11.5	31.7	72.4	78.5	75	23
GA	Crisp	0.36	1174	34.1	11.4	31.3	69.8	76.6	326	99

HEALTHIEST PLACES TO LIVE

ST	COUNTY	USDA	AMEN	OBES	DIAB	INACT	M AGE	W AGE	ALT ft	ALT m
KS	Douglas	0.36	1175	26.5	7	19.6	78.1	81.9	966	295
PA	Armstrong	0.36	1176	33.9	8.6	26	74.8	79.7	1208	368
TN	Unicoi	0.36	1177	33.2	10.4	30.3	71.4	78.6	2735	834
TX	Armstrong	0.36	1178	29	8.6	26.9	74.6	79.8	3125	952
TX	Comanche	0.36	1179	28.2	8.6	27.1	72.9	79.5	1360	415
TX	Lamar	0.36	1180	25.8	9.4	31	72.5	78.2	492	150
TX	Leon	0.36	1181	31.1	9.7	30.3	73.8	79.3	346	105
VA	Nelson	0.36	1182	26.4	9.1	22.7	73.1	79.7	1150	350
GA	Brooks	0.35	1183	30.8	12.6	30.3	70.1	76.7	191	58
KY	Breckinridge	0.35	1184	33.4	11.2	31.3	72.8	78.9	618	188
LA	Caldwell	0.35	1185	37.5	11.1	31.4	70.1	76.8	119	36
MD	Garrett	0.35	1186	30	10.1	29.5	75	80.2	2460	750
MI	Alcona	0.35	1187	30.5	9.3	24	75.2	79.6	853	260
NY	Delaware	0.35	1188	27.4	7.6	26.3	75	80	1824	556
TX	Brown	0.35	1189	31	8.9	27.2	72.4	78.9	1522	464
TX	Jack	0.35	1190	30.4	9.5	27.3	74.9	81.1	1091	332
MD	Worcester	0.34	1191	30.2	8.3	23.2	75.3	80.7	23	7
MS	Newton	0.34	1192	33.4	11.4	33	71.8	77.9	426	130
NH	Rockingham	0.34	1193	25.3	6.8	20.1	77.8	81.7	266	81
OK	Okfuskee	0.34	1194	33.3	11.1	36.3	71.6	77.3	837	255
TN	Decatur	0.34	1195	31	10.5	34.4	70.6	78.2	474	144
TX	Falls	0.34	1196	30.6	10.6	29.6	70.9	76.7	430	131
GA	Floyd	0.33	1197	28.9	9.2	28.7	72.1	78.2	755	230
GA	Tift	0.33	1198	33.2	12.1	28.9	72.1	78.2	328	100
PA	Lycoming	0.33	1199	30.1	8.5	27.5	74.9	80	1290	393
TN	Davidson	0.33	1200	29.8	9.5	26.9	73.3	79.2	579	177
TX	Callahan	0.33	1201	30.7	8.4	24	73.1	79.5	1801	549
GA	Berrien	0.32	1202	30.4	10.5	29.1	71.1	77.6	256	78
KS	Mitchell	0.32	1203	28	8.5	24.3	75.5	80.1	1509	460
KY	Bath	0.32	1204	33	12.1	34.6	71	77.5	844	257
KY	Jefferson	0.32	1205	33.6	10.5	28.5	73.4	79.2	556	169
NH	Grafton	0.32	1206	23.7	7.1	19	78.8	82	1492	455
GA	Clinch	0.31	1207	32.7	11.1	29.9	72.2	77.9	150	46
KY	Trimble	0.31	1208	33.6	11	34.1	73	78.9	728	222
MO	Howell	0.31	1209	30.6	10.1	29	72.2	79	1058	322
NC	Washington	0.31	1210	34.9	12	28.4	71.6	77.6	15	4
NY	Greene	0.31	1211	28.2	8.2	25.1	73.8	80	1420	433
TX	Wheeler	0.31	1212	29.4	9.1	28	73.2	78.9	2454	748
CO	Yuma	0.30	1213	23.7	5.3	21.1	75.2	79.9	3934	1199
LA	Plaquemines	0.30	1214	34	12.3	30.9	72.8	79.1	4	1
NE	Howard	0.30	1215	29.4	6.4	28.9	76.2	80.7	1917	584
NY	Albany	0.30	1216	24.2	7.1	22.4	76.1	80.8	770	235
PA	Luzerne	0.30	1217	29.7	8.8	29.7	73.3	79.8	1268	386
TX	Fisher	0.30	1218	30.5	8.5	28.3	72.9	78.9	1997	609
VA	Highland	0.30	1219	27.2	8.4	21.8	75.1	80.6	2850	869
GA	Thomas	0.29	1220	34.1	12.2	28.4	72	78.8	210	64
IN	Monroe	0.29	1221	25.8	9.6	22.3	76.6	81.6	733	224

ST	COUNTY	USDA	AMEN	OBES	DIAB	INACT	M AGE	W AGE	ALT ft	ALT m
KY	Boone	0.29	1222	30.8	9.4	28.3	75.4	79.6	751	229
KY	Elliott	0.29	1223	37.6	10.6	37.5	70.2	77.3	914	279
MO	Howard	0.29	1224	31.1	8.4	31.5	75.2	79.9	712	217
MT	Phillips	0.29	1225	26.4	6.2	30.4	75.3	80.8	2666	813
NE	Frontier	0.29	1226	33.3	7	30.7	76	81	2645	806
OK	Choctaw	0.29	1227	34.2	11.1	33.4	71.3	77.3	492	150
PA	Bradford	0.29	1228	34	8.1	27.7	75.2	80.6	1368	417
GA	Evans	0.28	1229	31.8	12.2	28.6	70.1	77.7	141	43
GA	Pulaski	0.28	1230	30.2	10.7	30.4	70.9	77.1	278	85
IL	Johnson	0.28	1231	28.9	8.2	29.5	72.8	78.8	506	154
KY	Boyd	0.28	1232	35.9	13.1	32.6	72.5	78.2	727	221
OH	Morgan	0.28	1233	35.2	10.4	29.7	73.2	79.8	885	270
SC	Darlington	0.28	1234	35.7	12.6	33.4	69.9	76.8	176	54
TN	Scott	0.28	1235	31.8	10.2	36.4	70.7	77.1	1514	461
TX	Upshur	0.28	1236	30.4	10.3	34.9	72.3	78.4	383	117
GA	Lowndes	0.27	1237	33.9	11.9	27.6	72.2	77.9	192	59
PA	Fayette	0.27	1238	35.2	11.4	32.9	73.4	80	1488	453
SC	Kershaw	0.27	1239	31.6	9.7	27.1	73	78.9	297	90
SC	Marlboro	0.27	1240	42.7	12.7	33.1	68.1	75.3	147	45
TX	Hall	0.27	1241	28.5	9	26.2	72.2	77.9	2059	628
TX	Sterling	0.27	1242	28.8	8.5	27.5	73.2	78.8	2482	756
VA	Montgomery	0.27	1243	28.5	7.7	22.3	75.8	79.6	2022	616
VA	Radford	0.27	1244	27.8	9.3	22.8	74.5	79.7	1861	567
GA	Colquitt	0.26	1245	31.4	11	28.2	70.9	77.2	282	86
MI	Oceana	0.26	1246	35.2	9.6	24.9	75.4	80.9	763	233
NE	Sherman	0.26	1247	31.4	6.7	29.3	76.2	80.7	2157	657
NH	Cheshire	0.26	1248	28.2	7.8	21.3	77.4	81.4	1041	317
OK	Pottawatomie	0.26	1249	34.5	9.8	34.5	72.7	77.9	1024	312
VA	Hopewell	0.26	1250	33.5	11	29.1	71.7	77.5	98	30
VA	Prince George	0.26	1251	33.9	11.8	28.4	74.9	79.3	88	27
LA	Bossier	0.25	1252	31	11.7	26.4	73.4	79.1	209	64
MS	Hancock	0.25	1253	35.4	10.9	28.9	73.9	79.7	59	18
NE	Lincoln	0.25	1254	31.8	8	27.4	76.1	81.4	2983	909
PA	Susquehanna	0.25	1255	26.8	9.9	25.5	74.7	80.1	1424	434
SC	Orangeburg	0.25	1256	41	13.5	32.2	69.4	76.9	183	56
TN	Sumner	0.25	1257	30	10	28.1	74.9	79.4	691	211
VA	Norton	0.25	1258	28	9	24	71.1	77.1	2246	684
VA	Westmoreland	0.25	1259	29.3	10.4	28.9	73	79.5	68	21
VA	Wise	0.25	1260	35.4	10.2	37.5	71.1	77.1	2296	700
GA	Atkinson	0.24	1261	29.1	10.1	29.5	69.4	76.5	212	65
GA	Toombs	0.24	1262	31.5	11.8	31.6	70.6	77.5	197	60
KY	Adair	0.24	1263	36.5	12.1	37.5	72.6	78.1	848	258
MA	Worcester	0.24	1264	25.2	8	22.6	76.4	81.2	709	216
MN	Lake	0.24	1265	29.2	7.4	22.2	76.3	81.7	1560	475
NY	Hamilton	0.24	1266	24.7	8.6	21.4	75.6	80.7	1985	605
OK	Oklahoma	0.24	1267	29.7	9.9	30.1	73.2	78.8	1143	348
PA	Lawrence	0.24	1268	29.6	9.5	27.7	74.5	80.6	1093	333

HEALTHIEST PLACES TO LIVE

ST	COUNTY	USDA	AMEN	OBES	DIAB	INACT	M AGE	W AGE	ALT ft	ALT m
TN	Putnam	0.24	1269	32.7	9.5	28.1	73.4	79	1182	360
TX	Eastland	0.24	1270	29.4	9.1	27.2	72.9	79.5	1514	462
TX	Ellis	0.24	1271	29.7	8.9	25.2	75	78.9	533	162
VA	New Kent	0.24	1272	28.6	9.8	21.2	78.1	82.5	89	27
AL	Blount	0.23	1273	32.1	11.5	35.1	72.5	78.8	788	240
GA	Irwin	0.23	1274	31.1	10.9	25.4	70.8	76.6	314	96
GA	Sumter	0.23	1275	34.7	13	29.7	70.9	77	385	117
KS	Chautauqua	0.23	1276	29.5	7.7	24.7	73	79.9	958	292
MS	Calhoun	0.23	1277	33	12.2	36	70.6	77.9	346	105
NC	Wake	0.23	1278	25.7	7.8	18.5	77.6	82	324	99
NY	Richmond	0.23	1279	27.3	8.7	28.8	76.6	81.4	87	27
OK	Rogers	0.23	1280	32.2	10.3	30.8	75	79.2	674	205
TX	Glasscock	0.23	1281	28.6	8.8	27.5	75.9	81.1	2654	809
AL	Calhoun	0.22	1282	33.8	12.9	33.3	70.5	77.3	760	232
GA	Heard	0.22	1283	28.1	9.9	27.3	71.4	77.1	794	242
GA	Lee	0.22	1284	27.6	9.7	24.3	74.9	80	271	83
KS	Clark	0.22	1285	32.4	7.9	27.8	75.4	80	2162	659
LA	Union	0.22	1286	35.7	12.2	34.7	71.7	77.6	148	45
PA	Greene	0.22	1287	28	9.1	33.6	74.7	79.8	1196	365
TX	Dallam	0.22	1288	27.4	8.9	28.8	73.7	78.9	4150	1265
TX	Fannin	0.22	1289	29.8	9.2	30.9	72.9	78.4	595	181
TX	Madison	0.22	1290	31.5	10	27	72.8	78.4	278	85
WV	Barbour	0.22	1291	34.1	10.8	28.1	72.8	79.2	1668	508
AL	Clay	0.21	1292	34.8	12.7	36.2	71.8	78	1023	312
AL	Cleburne	0.21	1293	30.1	11.1	32.8	71.8	78	1050	320
GA	Calhoun	0.21	1294	33.8	12.6	27.4	67.6	74.7	238	73
GA	Polk	0.21	1295	29.1	11.1	26.4	70.4	76.9	914	279
IN	Orange	0.21	1296	32.7	10.4	35.4	73.5	78.9	675	206
KY	Grayson	0.21	1297	30.9	11.7	32.8	71.9	77.8	638	194
KY	Muhlenberg	0.21	1298	31.8	9.9	31.9	71.6	77.8	481	146
OH	Washington	0.21	1299	33.1	9.9	22.5	74.7	79.5	822	251
OK	Mayes	0.21	1300	34.9	10.8	37	73.1	79.7	712	217
TX	Gregg	0.21	1301	32.3	10.2	29.6	71.8	78.7	332	101
TX	Yoakum	0.21	1302	29.9	8.5	28	73.9	78.9	3661	1116
LA	Jackson	0.20	1303	30.6	9.3	32.4	71.5	77.1	230	70
LA	Vernon	0.20	1304	36.4	11.3	28.9	73.8	79.3	251	77
MD	Dorchester	0.20	1305	35.6	11.1	29.8	72.5	78.7	12	4
ME	Waldo	0.20	1306	27.8	8.1	22.2	75.4	80.8	357	109
MO	Maries	0.20	1307	31.1	9.2	29.4	74.3	79.8	885	270
NC	Yadkin	0.20	1308	30.1	9.4	27.6	73.5	79.3	934	285
ND	Dunn	0.20	1309	30.6	8.8	31.3	75.7	82.2	2259	689
OH	Perry	0.20	1310	33.2	9.9	31.9	72.8	79.6	944	288
SC	Calhoun	0.20	1311	39.6	12.9	32.8	71.9	78.1	214	65
SD	Sully	0.20	1312	35.3	6.4	27	76.6	81.5	1799	548
TN	Overton	0.20	1313	33.2	9.6	33.8	71.2	77.1	1187	362
AL	Barbour	0.19	1314	37.1	13.2	33.8	71	76.9	374	114

ST	COUNTY	USDA	AMEN	OBES	DIAB	INACT	M AGE	W AGE	ALT ft	ALT m
GA	Bulloch	0.19	1315	31.1	12.2	26.1	73.2	78.9	158	48
MT	Blaine	0.19	1316	35.3	10.9	32.4	74.4	80.2	3070	936
NC	Craven	0.19	1317	33.9	10.5	26.3	74.4	79.2	27	8
GA	Harris	0.18	1318	27	10.5	20	74.9	80.1	696	212
LA	Jefferson	0.18	1319	31.9	11.1	28.6	72.4	79.5	4	1
MI	Presque Isle	0.18	1320	32.8	9.1	23.3	74.7	80.4	746	228
SC	Newberry	0.18	1321	36.8	10.7	30.4	71.7	78.5	433	132
ID	Oneida	0.17	1322	28.7	7.1	25.7	75.6	80.5	5531	1686
LA	Pointe Coupee	0.17	1323	31.9	10.9	29.9	71.7	78.1	24	7
ME	Franklin	0.17	1324	28.7	7.1	21.4	76.1	80.3	1552	473
TX	Hopkins	0.17	1325	32.7	10.2	28.8	73.6	78.9	477	145
VA	Suffolk	0.17	1326	31.9	11.2	26.4	72.6	78	42	13
WI	Kewaunee	0.17	1327	33.8	7.9	24	76.3	81.6	732	223
AL	Franklin	0.16	1328	31.4	13.3	36.4	70.7	77.1	744	227
GA	Early	0.16	1329	30.1	12.2	29.5	69.6	75.8	225	69
GA	Grady	0.16	1330	32.9	11.5	29.5	70.8	78	229	70
MS	Rankin	0.16	1331	34.7	10.7	27.9	74.8	80.9	360	110
OK	Dewey	0.16	1332	32.6	10	32.7	73.3	79.7	1873	571
PA	Lackawanna	0.16	1333	25.6	8.1	28.3	74	80.3	1456	444
GA	Bleckley	0.15	1334	28.7	10.6	27.2	70.5	77.1	328	100
KS	Phillips	0.15	1335	34.3	8.3	24.6	76.3	81.5	2024	617
MO	Clay	0.15	1336	27.6	8.5	26.5	76.1	80.3	883	269
PA	Huntingdon	0.15	1337	30.6	9.3	30.6	74.6	79.8	1136	346
GA	Rockdale	0.14	1338	32.1	10.9	27.2	74.4	78.9	785	239
LA	Orleans	0.14	1339	29.7	11.7	28.8	68.4	79.5	3	1
MO	Warren	0.14	1340	31.7	8.9	28.2	75.3	80.2	706	215
NJ	Union	0.14	1341	22	8.2	25.2	77.2	81.1	127	39
NY	Sullivan	0.14	1342	26.2	8.6	23.8	74.6	79.9	1428	435
TN	Greene	0.14	1343	32.5	10.1	33	72.6	77.8	1548	472
TX	Hardeman	0.14	1344	29.8	8.8	26.9	72.2	77.9	1518	463
TX	Parker	0.14	1345	31.2	9.8	29.7	74.4	79.3	974	297
VT	Windsor	0.14	1346	24.2	6.4	19.1	77.2	81.7	1273	388
AL	Pickens	0.13	1347	36.9	13.9	32.5	70.3	76.7	273	83
KS	Elk	0.13	1348	32.3	9.8	26.5	73	79.9	1109	338
OH	Belmont	0.13	1349	30.6	9.9	28.5	73.5	79.4	1107	337
OK	Lincoln	0.13	1350	30.9	10.4	39.8	72.4	78.5	935	285
KS	Russell	0.12	1351	32.5	8	27.3	75.2	80.7	1751	534
KY	Bell	0.12	1352	35.9	13.9	32.3	69.3	75.9	1659	506
KY	Carter	0.12	1353	34.5	11.4	42.8	70.8	77.5	860	262
MO	Platte	0.12	1354	28	8.8	28.1	76.8	81.5	889	271
MS	Adams	0.12	1355	37.8	12.5	38.8	70.8	77.6	170	52
NC	Moore	0.12	1356	27.2	7.8	22.5	75.3	80.9	426	130
TX	Johnson	0.12	1357	31.1	10.1	29.1	74.2	78.8	791	241
GA	Turner	0.11	1358	34.1	12.4	32.4	70.8	76.6	356	109
LA	Lafourche	0.11	1359	35.7	12	31	73.1	79.3	4	1
NY	Saratoga	0.11	1360	25.8	7.1	23.4	78	82.3	730	222

HEALTHIEST PLACES TO LIVE

ST	COUNTY	USDA	AMEN	OBES	DIAB	INACT	M AGE	W AGE	ALT ft	ALT m
PA	Montour	0.11	1361	29.2	9.4	28.1	75.4	80.5	688	210
TX	Houston	0.11	1362	31	10.1	26.3	72.3	77.8	302	92
TX	Irion	0.11	1363	28.6	8.8	27.8	74.3	79.9	2406	733
VA	Wythe	0.11	1364	29.3	9.2	24.5	73.2	78.6	2474	754
WV	Cabell	0.11	1365	33	12.9	30.4	71.3	78.2	751	229
MD	Cecil	0.10	1366	31.2	8.9	27.9	73.8	79.4	181	55
MD	Frederick	0.10	1367	26.2	8.2	21.8	76.8	81.2	599	183
MD	Talbot	0.10	1368	26.3	7.5	20.9	76.4	81.7	26	8
NC	Rockingham	0.10	1369	33.3	10	29.6	71.7	77.9	703	214
AR	Independence	0.09	1370	30.1	10.1	32.3	73.5	78.9	433	132
NY	Orange	0.09	1371	25.9	8.1	25.9	76.3	80.9	634	193
SC	Lancaster	0.09	1372	32.5	11	31.4	72.9	79.1	519	158
VA	Giles	0.09	1373	28.8	9.7	27.4	72.5	78.8	2479	756
VT	Chittenden	0.09	1374	20.1	5.2	15	77.5	82.1	685	209
VT	Orleans	0.09	1375	28.5	6.9	24.5	75.4	80.3	1319	402
GA	Muscogee	0.08	1376	35	12.4	27.8	70.9	77.5	389	119
LA	Catahoula	0.08	1377	34	11.3	33.6	70.1	76.8	67	21
LA	Claiborne	0.08	1378	34.2	12.3	32.7	71.1	76.7	265	81
MI	Cheboygan	0.08	1379	39.1	9.1	26.7	75.8	80.6	744	227
MO	Christian	0.08	1380	27.1	7.7	26.2	75.1	80.1	1246	380
TX	Liberty	0.08	1381	30.5	9.1	31.3	71	77.3	71	22
TX	Schleicher	0.08	1382	29.4	8.6	26.5	73.6	78.3	2370	722
AL	Henry	0.07	1383	34	12.8	30.1	70.5	77.2	328	100
GA	Montgomery	0.07	1384	31.2	10.5	26.7	71.3	76.5	227	69
GA	Wheeler	0.07	1385	30.1	10.9	26.3	71.3	76.5	179	55
ID	Butte	0.07	1386	29	8	23.2	76.2	80.4	5977	1822
IL	Hardin	0.07	1387	30.1	8	26	73	79.5	482	147
KY	Knott	0.07	1388	33.7	13.2	36.5	69.7	77.6	1332	406
LA	Livingston	0.07	1389	30.8	9.7	30	72.3	78.6	32	10
MI	Alpena	0.07	1390	31.2	8	21	75.4	81.2	745	227
NH	Hillsborough	0.07	1391	26.7	7.9	21.8	77.3	81.4	652	199
NJ	Cape May	0.07	1392	24.9	8.4	22.3	74.2	80.2	13	4
PA	Elk	0.07	1393	31.5	9.4	28.4	74.9	80.7	1769	539
SD	Hughes	0.07	1394	29.6	8.4	21.3	76.2	81.5	1718	524
GA	Appling	0.06	1395	32.5	11.1	31.4	70.8	76.9	174	53
GA	Worth	0.06	1396	29.5	10.2	26.4	71.8	78.3	331	101
MO	Chariton	0.06	1397	31.2	9.7	28.8	75.2	79.9	695	212
MT	Golden Valley	0.06	1398	27.2	6.5	24.2	75.8	80.9	4220	1286
NC	Anson	0.06	1399	35.5	12.3	29.5	70.9	77.1	336	102
TN	Henry	0.06	1400	34.7	10.6	32.3	71.6	77.9	469	143
DE	Sussex	0.05	1401	29.2	9.3	24.8	74.8	80.8	31	9
GA	Brantley	0.05	1402	28.9	9.5	28	70.6	77.2	66	20
MS	Montgomery	0.05	1403	36.4	13.7	36.1	70.7	77.9	379	115
NC	Vance	0.05	1404	32.8	12.1	32	69.5	76.5	384	117
OK	Kay	0.05	1405	36.9	10.9	31.3	73	78.7	1069	326
OK	Wagoner	0.05	1406	30.6	11.2	33.8	74.8	80	599	183

ST	COUNTY	USDA	AMEN	OBES	DIAB	INACT	M AGE	W AGE	ALT ft	ALT m
TN	Lauderdale	0.05	1407	36	10.9	34.8	69.8	76.4	304	93
TX	Hansford	0.05	1408	28.2	8.8	28.5	74.2	79.8	3137	956
KY	Floyd	0.04	1409	36.8	14.6	39.9	69.7	76.2	1031	314
MD	Harford	0.04	1410	27.8	8.3	24.5	75.6	80.6	320	98
MS	Marion	0.04	1411	36.3	12	28.9	68.7	76.2	246	75
NE	Buffalo	0.04	1412	29.6	7	23.1	76.7	81.7	2185	666
VT	Windham	0.04	1413	23.1	5.6	15.8	76.7	81.9	1353	412
OK	Ottawa	0.03	1414	34.7	11.2	34.8	72.2	78.4	839	256
TX	Erath	0.03	1415	28	9.2	25.5	73.9	79.6	1251	381
TX	Foard	0.03	1416	29.5	9.6	28.3	73.2	78.7	1497	456
GA	Richmond	0.02	1417	32.4	11.2	27.3	69.7	77.2	290	89
GA	Treutlen	0.02	1418	34.9	10.7	28.3	71.3	76.5	269	82
MS	Attala	0.02	1419	38.6	12.7	35.2	68.2	77.3	403	123
MS	Greene	0.02	1420	39.7	12.1	32.7	70.7	76.6	170	52
NC	Beaufort	0.02	1421	36.2	10.4	28.4	73	78.5	23	7
NC	Stokes	0.02	1422	27.9	8.3	25	73.1	79.5	976	297
NH	Merrimack	0.02	1423	25.3	6.9	20	77.1	81.4	729	222
SC	Saluda	0.02	1424	33.2	11	31.7	72.6	78.2	484	147
TN	Grundy	0.02	1425	30.7	9.9	31.8	68.8	77.9	1706	520
WV	Nicholas	0.02	1426	36.2	11.2	32.9	73	78.5	2051	625
DE	New Castle	0.01	1427	26.8	7.2	21.9	75.2	80.1	90	27
GA	Laurens	0.01	1428	35.9	11.3	28.4	71.4	77.2	284	87
GA	Stewart	0.01	1429	35.3	13.7	29	69.6	75.8	417	127
NY	Queens	0.01	1430	22.2	9	28	79	83.7	54	17
OH	Carroll	0.01	1431	30	9.1	23.6	75	80.2	1128	344
OK	Pawnee	0.01	1432	35.1	12.4	37.2	74	79	888	271
PA	Bucks	0.01	1433	23.9	8	22.1	77.1	81.4	337	103
PA	Somerset	0.01	1434	31.4	9	26.8	74.6	80.8	2193	668
PA	Sullivan	0.01	1435	33.6	9.2	27.4	74.8	80.7	1774	541
TX	Collingsworth	0.01	1436	30	9	27.6	73.2	78.9	2137	651
VA	Roanoke	0.01	1437	27	9.2	22.8	76	80.5	1680	512
VA	Roanoke City	0.01	1438	34.4	10.5	26.5	71.2	78.8	1038	316
VA	Salem	0.01	1439	27.9	9	22.4	75	80.6	1087	331
MA	Franklin	0.00	1440	24.2	6.7	18.7	77.1	81.3	853	260
NY	Warren	0.00	1441	29.3	8.2	19.8	76.7	81.4	1285	392
CO	Kit Carson	-0.01	1442	27	5.5	26.4	75.2	79.9	4418	1347
GA	Johnson	-0.01	1443	34.8	12.8	29.4	70.6	76.1	332	101
LA	W Baton Rouge	-0.01	1444	31.8	11.5	29.3	71.7	77.2	15	5
MA	Hampshire	-0.01	1445	22.1	6.6	16.9	77.5	81.6	739	225
MS	Madison	-0.01	1446	28.5	10.8	25.9	69.9	75.9	283	86
NC	Randolph	-0.01	1447	29.6	9.6	29.5	73.6	79.7	649	198
OH	Athens	-0.01	1448	32.2	11.4	28.7	73.7	79.3	806	246
OH	Harrison	-0.01	1449	31.6	11.6	28.8	73.7	79	1102	336
WV	Taylor	-0.01	1450	32.4	11	35.2	73.8	78.8	1341	409
WY	Niobrara	-0.01	1451	23.7	6.3	28.5	76.3	80.9	4532	1381
GA	Screven	-0.02	1452	30.7	11.9	29.5	70.1	76.4	149	45

HEALTHIEST PLACES TO LIVE

ST	COUNTY	USDA	AMEN	OBES	DIAB	INACT	M AGE	W AGE	ALT ft	ALT m
LA	La Salle	-0.02	1453	32.7	10.9	30.9	71.8	77.4	126	38
MO	Boone	-0.02	1454	27.4	7.5	21.6	76.5	80.5	765	233
MT	Treasure	-0.02	1455	24.6	6.2	26.8	76.1	81	3032	924
NE	Box Butte	-0.02	1456	31.7	8.2	25.4	75.4	80.3	4169	1271
NJ	Essex	-0.02	1457	25.8	9.2	27.5	73.8	79.8	234	71
TX	Jackson	-0.02	1458	30.4	8.9	26.1	73.7	79.7	57	17
VA	Albemarle	-0.02	1459	27.1	8.7	19.1	77.8	81.7	741	226
VA	Charlottesville	-0.02	1460	26.9	9.2	26.8	75.6	81.5	453	138
AL	Escambia	-0.03	1461	35.9	12.1	37	71.5	77.6	242	74
KY	Mercer	-0.03	1462	33.8	10.5	33.8	73.2	79.1	846	258
LA	Bienville	-0.03	1463	39.1	11.2	29	70	76.1	241	73
MS	Forrest	-0.03	1464	36.4	12	32.7	71.9	77.5	217	66
MT	Valley	-0.03	1465	27.2	7.8	28.7	75.7	81	2581	787
NY	Schuyler	-0.03	1466	27.3	7.1	28.8	76.2	80.5	1312	400
NY	Yates	-0.03	1467	24.4	7.5	26.1	76	81.5	1035	315
VA	Mecklenburg	-0.03	1468	32.4	10.8	27.8	70.9	78	360	110
AL	Greene	-0.04	1469	47.9	16.2	37.3	67.9	76.6	167	51
CO	Cheyenne	-0.04	1470	20.9	5.4	19.6	74.4	80.6	4350	1326
GA	Houston	-0.04	1471	28.7	10.5	25.6	74.2	79.6	347	106
GA	Long	-0.04	1472	30.1	11.2	25.3	70.6	77.8	63	19
LA	Winn	-0.04	1473	32.6	10.3	36.8	69.7	76.8	165	50
MD	Somerset	-0.04	1474	39.7	11.4	32	72	77.4	11	3
MI	Ottawa	-0.04	1475	25.2	8.2	21.3	78.8	82.4	655	200
NJ	Atlantic	-0.04	1476	28	8.8	24.6	73.6	79.8	48	15
OK	Noble	-0.04	1477	34.2	9.9	31.3	74.7	80.3	1015	309
PA	Northampton	-0.04	1478	29.7	7.1	23.7	76.5	81.8	578	176
SC	Aiken	-0.04	1479	32.8	10	25.1	73.6	79.2	363	111
SC	Chester	-0.04	1480	31.8	11.3	33	70.2	77.9	490	149
TX	Harris	-0.04	1481	28.5	9	23.3	75.8	80.5	85	26
WA	Skamania	-0.04	1482	32	7.4	20.4	76.3	81	2892	881
ND	McKenzie	-0.05	1483	33.5	8.3	28.6	75.7	82.2	2249	685
OK	Hughes	-0.05	1484	32.9	11.7	31.2	71.6	77.3	825	251
OK	Jackson	-0.05	1485	34.5	11.4	32.7	73.7	78.1	1393	425
PA	Columbia	-0.05	1486	35.7	8.6	27.4	74.9	80.8	972	296
TN	Fentress	-0.05	1487	35.6	11.7	32.7	69.5	77.1	1484	452
WV	Mason	-0.05	1488	36.8	10.7	32.3	71.9	78.6	721	220
AR	Little River	-0.06	1489	33.1	10.4	31	72	78	315	96
ID	Clark	-0.06	1490	28.2	8.1	22.8	76.2	80.4	6414	1955
IL	Monroe	-0.06	1491	27.9	7.8	29.2	76.8	80.7	510	156
KY	Butler	-0.06	1492	33.2	11.5	30.6	72.8	77.8	515	157
MO	Callaway	-0.06	1493	35.4	10.4	28.7	73.9	80.1	765	233
MS	Panola	-0.06	1494	35.9	12.6	36.7	68.8	75.7	287	88
NE	Valley	-0.06	1495	29.5	8	28.6	76.2	80.7	2202	671
OH	Clermont	-0.06	1496	29.5	9	24.4	75.6	79.5	819	249
VA	King William	-0.06	1497	29.7	9.4	28.1	73.3	79	89	27
DE	Kent	-0.07	1498	32.5	11	27.9	73.5	79.5	33	10

ST	COUNTY	USDA	AMEN	OBES	DIAB	INACT	M AGE	W AGE	ALT ft	ALT m
GA	Baker	-0.07	1499	32.6	13	27.5	70.1	77.2	176	54
KY	Hart	-0.07	1500	34	10	35.6	72.4	78.2	707	216
MS	Lowndes	-0.07	1501	37.3	13	33.5	72.5	78.4	222	68
NY	Dutchess	-0.07	1502	27.3	9	22.5	77.4	81.6	537	164
TX	Hale	-0.07	1503	29.4	8.6	28.5	73.8	79	3407	1038
WV	Monongalia	-0.07	1504	27.8	9.6	24.9	75.4	80.1	1280	390
AR	Faulkner	-0.08	1505	32.2	10.8	28.8	73.5	79.8	428	130
GA	Dodge	-0.08	1506	35.8	12.6	30.1	70.7	76.4	300	92
IL	Carroll	-0.08	1507	26.7	8.6	30.3	75.6	81.1	765	233
MA	Hampden	-0.08	1508	28.4	9.3	25.7	75.2	80.5	629	192
MD	Queen Anne's	-0.08	1509	26.8	7.8	23.4	76.1	81.8	42	13
MO	Cooper	-0.08	1510	30.4	9.1	25.7	74.4	79.9	743	227
MS	Lawrence	-0.08	1511	36.5	14.2	34	69.9	76.9	311	95
NE	Grant	-0.08	1512	25.4	6.9	29.8	76.1	80.2	3773	1150
NE	Kimball	-0.08	1513	28.7	7.6	24.3	75.8	80.7	4933	1504
OH	Brown	-0.08	1514	33.8	10.2	32.4	73.5	78.7	879	268
TX	Lavaca	-0.08	1515	27.8	8.7	26.5	74.2	80.6	252	77
WV	Jackson	-0.08	1516	35.8	11.7	28.7	74.2	79	806	246
KS	Pottawatomie	-0.09	1517	30.8	8.7	24.2	75.8	80.8	1223	373
MS	Wilkinson	-0.09	1518	39.7	14.9	35.3	69.3	76.1	214	65
NC	Davidson	-0.09	1519	29.3	8.9	29.1	73	78.8	761	232
NH	Coos	-0.09	1520	30.8	8	27.8	74.3	80.4	1857	566
TX	Shackelford	-0.09	1521	28.4	8.5	26.7	72.6	79.1	1545	471
AR	Lawrence	-0.10	1522	34.6	10.7	32.5	71.6	78.6	311	95
GA	Ben Hill	-0.10	1523	32.6	12	29.9	70.1	76	297	90
GA	Effingham	-0.10	1524	31.4	10.5	25.7	74.4	78.8	70	21
KY	Madison	-0.10	1525	30.2	9.7	30.3	73.8	79.5	888	271
KY	Monroe	-0.10	1526	35.5	10.5	32.4	71.5	77.9	833	254
LA	St. Charles	-0.10	1527	32.2	10.1	28.8	73.6	79.3	4	1
NC	Rowan	-0.10	1528	31.6	10.8	29.2	73.4	79.3	746	227
NH	Strafford	-0.10	1529	29.3	8.3	22.9	76.5	81	423	129
OK	Canadian	-0.10	1530	32.1	10.6	29.2	75.7	79.9	1350	412
SD	Shannon	-0.10	1531	40.9	16.8	32.4	71.1	78.5	3101	945
GA	Carroll	-0.11	1532	30.7	12.7	24.7	72.6	77.8	1035	315
GA	Twiggs	-0.11	1533	32	12.2	29.4	70.5	77.1	390	119
KS	Riley	-0.11	1534	26.5	8	19.6	78.1	81.9	1244	379
MO	Laclede	-0.11	1535	31.9	8.8	33.8	73.4	78.8	1138	347
SC	Greenwood	-0.11	1536	34.7	10.1	30.4	72.5	78.5	535	163
TX	Red River	-0.11	1537	31.3	10	31.3	72.5	78.1	400	122
GA	Dooly	-0.12	1538	34	11.5	29.4	69.2	76.2	333	101
GA	Wayne	-0.12	1539	32.2	9.6	31.3	70.9	77.3	85	26
TX	Cochran	-0.12	1540	30.1	9.1	27.9	73.1	78.8	3784	1153
VA	Augusta	-0.12	1541	26.5	8.7	25.1	75.1	80.6	1870	570
VA	Stafford	-0.12	1542	29.2	8.4	20.4	76.2	79.5	212	65
VA	Staunton	-0.12	1543	29	9.1	24.2	73.7	79.7	1527	465
VA	Waynesboro	-0.12	1544	28.9	9.1	25.3	74	80.9	1356	413

ST	COUNTY	USDA	AMEN	OBES	DIAB	INACT	M AGE	W AGE	ALT ft	ALT m
WV	Kanawha	-0.12	1545	31.8	11.3	30.4	72	78.3	1015	309
WV	Pleasants	-0.12	1546	31.2	11	29.7	73.3	79	860	262
AR	Sevier	-0.13	1547	32.2	12	32.7	71.8	77.9	435	132
GA	Taliaferro	-0.13	1548	34.8	12.7	30.1	70.8	76.8	535	163
PA	Adams	-0.13	1549	26.1	8.9	27.1	76.1	80.5	758	231
VA	King & Queen	-0.13	1550	34.1	10.6	27.7	73.3	79	87	26
WV	Fayette	-0.13	1551	33.9	12.1	33.4	71.1	77.8	1957	596
WV	Ohio	-0.13	1552	30.3	10.8	28.9	74.2	79.8	1084	331
WV	Raleigh	-0.13	1553	34	11.9	34.4	72.4	78.6	2241	683
KS	Cheyenne	-0.14	1554	32.8	7.6	20.4	76	80.6	3450	1052
ME	Aroostook	-0.14	1555	31.8	10.5	32.4	74.6	80.1	855	261
ME	Kennebec	-0.14	1556	30.1	8.2	22.5	75.7	80.4	287	87
MO	Carroll	-0.14	1557	31.7	7.9	25.6	74.5	80.4	737	225
MS	Warren	-0.14	1558	39.1	12	30.9	71.1	77.3	156	48
AL	Bibb	-0.15	1559	34.1	11.2	36.8	69.8	77.1	413	126
MO	Holt	-0.15	1560	30.6	8.8	26.9	76.2	80.7	939	286
SC	Marion	-0.15	1561	38.4	13.3	33.6	68.8	76	55	17
SD	Stanley	-0.15	1562	33.1	7.5	30.6	76.6	81.5	1868	570
WI	Door	-0.15	1563	31.7	6.7	19.8	78.2	82.7	676	206
GA	Emanuel	-0.16	1564	30.9	11.2	26.8	69.3	75.6	260	79
KS	Meade	-0.16	1565	30.9	8.4	23.9	75.4	80	2527	770
MO	Phelps	-0.16	1566	31.3	8.4	27.5	74.4	79.2	990	302
MS	Choctaw	-0.16	1567	34.3	12	29	71.1	77.3	475	145
VT	Grand Isle	-0.16	1568	26.2	5.5	18.1	76.4	81.1	106	32
AL	Covington	-0.17	1569	37.2	10.9	36	71.4	77.9	299	91
GA	Cobb	-0.17	1570	23.3	9.1	21.3	77.6	81.3	981	299
GA	Ware	-0.17	1571	31.2	12.1	33.7	69.7	76.6	139	42
KS	Wyandotte	-0.17	1572	37.9	11.7	32.5	71.1	77.5	882	269
MI	Iosco	-0.17	1573	34.3	8.3	22.9	73.5	79.5	737	225
NH	Sullivan	-0.17	1574	28.8	7.8	25	75.6	81.2	1179	359
NY	Kings	-0.17	1575	24.5	9.5	27.6	76.8	82.3	40	12
OH	Fairfield	-0.17	1576	30.7	9.7	27.3	75.6	79.8	938	286
OK	Alfalfa	-0.17	1577	31.8	9.7	32.1	74.4	79.7	1267	386
TN	Bradley	-0.17	1578	29.5	11.6	30.2	73.3	79.2	848	258
VA	King George	-0.17	1579	28	9.5	21.5	74.7	79.7	88	27
WI	Dane	-0.17	1580	23.9	6.1	17.7	78.7	82.5	957	292
AL	Dallas	-0.18	1581	41.9	14.2	33.3	68.5	75.3	195	59
KY	Pike	-0.18	1582	36.9	13.9	38.1	68.7	76.3	1297	395
LA	Concordia	-0.18	1583	33.1	10.7	32.2	69.9	76.7	44	14
IL	Gallatin	-0.19	1584	28.2	7.7	27	73	79.5	391	119
IN	Martin	-0.19	1585	29.2	8.6	30	74.2	79.8	571	174
KS	Ellsworth	-0.19	1586	35.5	8.7	24.2	75.2	80.7	1675	511
KY	Lawrence	-0.19	1587	36.1	12	35.7	70.2	77.3	812	247
KY	Perry	-0.19	1588	38.8	13.1	39.2	68.4	76.6	1261	384
PA	Mifflin	-0.19	1589	30.6	9.3	28.3	74.7	80.3	1072	327
TN	Maury	-0.19	1590	33	10.6	30	72.8	78.5	730	222

ST	COUNTY	USDA	AMEN	OBES	DIAB	INACT	M AGE	W AGE	ALT ft	ALT m
TX	Cottle	-0.19	1591	29.8	9	28.5	73.2	78.7	1808	551
WV	Wayne	-0.19	1592	35.5	11.8	31	72.3	77.9	856	261
WV	Wood	-0.19	1593	32	11.7	31	74.9	79.5	794	242
IN	Crawford	-0.20	1594	36	9.8	30.2	73.5	78.9	638	195
IN	Switzerland	-0.20	1595	27.5	9.7	27.1	74.7	79.5	749	228
KS	Jewell	-0.20	1596	34.2	8.6	24.7	75.7	82	1664	507
LA	Grant	-0.20	1597	31.6	10.8	32.1	71.3	78.1	139	42
MO	Dallas	-0.20	1598	32	8.1	28.6	73.1	78.7	1093	333
MO	McDonald	-0.20	1599	31.8	8.6	31.2	71.9	77.8	1100	335
NJ	Salem	-0.20	1600	33.8	9.3	30.6	73.4	78.7	44	13
OK	Blaine	-0.20	1601	33.4	9.8	30.8	73.6	79.4	1486	453
WV	Greenbrier	-0.20	1602	29	10.2	29.7	73.3	78.7	2627	801
GA	Terrell	-0.21	1603	37.3	12.5	29.7	67.6	74.7	336	102
GA	Washington	-0.21	1604	34.5	12.7	27.3	70.1	77	371	113
KS	Seward	-0.21	1605	35.8	7.7	29.6	73.3	79.2	2809	856
KY	Hopkins	-0.21	1606	35.4	10.7	33.4	72.3	78.1	445	136
KY	Ohio	-0.21	1607	32.6	12.2	35.3	72.8	78.3	489	149
LA	Rapides	-0.21	1608	32.6	12.4	30.5	72	77.5	119	36
OH	Monroe	-0.21	1609	33.7	9.8	30.9	74.4	79.8	1033	315
SC	Barnwell	-0.21	1610	37.2	11.8	31	70.4	76.5	232	71
GA	Jenkins	-0.22	1611	32.4	11.5	26.7	70.1	76.4	208	63
IL	Pope	-0.22	1612	29.8	7.9	28	72.4	78.7	507	155
LA	Assumption	-0.22	1613	32.8	10.9	30	71.1	77.8	5	2
MO	Randolph	-0.22	1614	34.8	10.3	31.6	73.7	79.9	794	242
MT	Richland	-0.22	1615	30.9	6	28.9	75.3	80.5	2283	696
TX	Motley	-0.22	1616	29.1	8.9	27.3	73.2	78.7	2330	710
WV	Tyler	-0.22	1617	33.2	10.9	28.1	73	78.9	938	286
KY	Boyle	-0.23	1618	31.3	11.1	29.9	73.9	79	958	292
MD	Kent	-0.23	1619	28.1	8.8	25.8	74.5	80.6	39	12
MO	Shannon	-0.23	1620	34.7	10.1	30.9	71.9	78.7	981	299
NY	Oswego	-0.23	1621	33.7	9.2	26.1	74.9	79.3	575	175
PA	Cambria	-0.23	1622	36.3	11.5	29.7	74.3	80.1	1931	588
TN	Cheatham	-0.23	1623	31.5	9.3	32.1	73.5	78.8	588	179
VA	Bristol	-0.23	1624	28.1	9	24.7	72.8	79.4	1771	540
VA	Washington	-0.23	1625	27.6	9.8	28.4	73.3	78.9	2170	662
AL	Lee	-0.24	1626	29.8	11.3	27.9	73.9	78.6	615	187
AL	Russell	-0.24	1627	39.5	12.5	36.5	69.3	76.3	339	103
GA	Fayette	-0.24	1628	23.6	9.8	20.3	77.8	82	865	264
GA	Fulton	-0.24	1629	23.8	9.2	19.8	75	80.2	940	287
KY	Marshall	-0.24	1630	37.1	9.5	25.8	73.8	79.6	414	126
MS	DeSoto	-0.24	1631	32.4	10	30.3	73.9	78.8	293	89
NY	Fulton	-0.24	1632	28.5	7.9	25.9	75.2	81.1	1222	372
TX	Dawson	-0.24	1633	31.1	9.8	28.8	73.1	78.8	2954	900
NC	Warren	-0.25	1634	36.8	12.6	29.8	70.4	76.9	301	92
NE	Arthur	-0.25	1635	27.4	7.3	26.8	76.1	80.2	3671	1119
OH	Columbiana	-0.25	1636	35.6	11.4	28.1	74.2	79.4	1136	346

HEALTHIEST PLACES TO LIVE

ST	COUNTY	USDA	AMEN	OBES	DIAB	INACT	M AGE	W AGE	ALT ft	ALT m
OK	Grady	-0.25	1637	37.4	8.4	28	73.1	78.9	1220	372
PA	Butler	-0.25	1638	26.5	8.6	22.5	75.9	80.8	1241	378
PA	Tioga	-0.25	1639	31.5	8.6	25.9	75.8	80.4	1709	521
SC	Edgefield	-0.25	1640	35.6	10.1	25.6	72	77.6	432	132
AR	Newton	-0.26	1641	35.9	11	31.5	73.1	79.2	1557	475
MS	Lamar	-0.26	1642	31.4	9.2	28.8	74	78.9	307	93
NC	Durham	-0.26	1643	30.1	9.4	20.8	74.4	80.1	369	112
NY	Chautauqua	-0.26	1644	28.1	7.6	24.6	75.7	80.4	1376	419
NY	Essex	-0.26	1645	27.4	7.9	22.4	75.6	80.7	1541	470
IA	Allamakee	-0.27	1646	28.9	7.7	22.1	76	80.2	974	297
LA	West Feliciana	-0.27	1647	32.3	12	29.8	71.7	77.2	137	42
OK	Logan	-0.27	1648	32.5	10.2	29.8	74.5	79.8	1036	316
SC	Allendale	-0.27	1649	34.7	14	34.7	68.7	76.2	148	45
AL	Montgomery	-0.28	1650	34.1	13.5	29.5	71.7	78	270	82
GA	Coweta	-0.28	1651	29.3	9.9	23.7	74.1	79.1	839	256
LA	Tangipahoa	-0.28	1652	35.3	10.6	31.4	70.2	76	118	36
MO	Crawford	-0.28	1653	32.3	8	28.4	73.1	79.2	928	283
MS	Perry	-0.28	1654	35.5	12.4	35.8	70.7	76.6	175	53
NY	Tompkins	-0.28	1655	23.1	7	21.7	77.7	81.4	1200	366
OK	Roger Mills	-0.28	1656	33.8	9.5	34.2	73.3	79.7	2149	655
VA	Henry	-0.28	1657	28.7	10.4	31.3	71.2	78.3	913	278
VA	Martinsville	-0.28	1658	33.5	10.8	27.6	71.2	78.3	897	274
VT	Addison	-0.28	1659	22.8	5.6	18.5	77.1	82.3	849	259
GA	Wilcox	-0.29	1660	32.9	11	31.9	70.9	77.1	302	92
IN	Brown	-0.29	1661	29	9.6	24.8	75.8	81	756	230
MS	Pike	-0.29	1662	39.9	13.7	35.2	69.9	76.5	347	106
WV	Tucker	-0.29	1663	32.8	10.5	35.5	72.8	79.2	2776	846
AR	Miller	-0.30	1664	37.9	12.3	35	73.3	79	261	80
GA	DeKalb	-0.30	1665	26.1	9.9	21.2	75.9	81.4	915	279
IL	Lake	-0.30	1666	24	7.1	18.9	78.5	81.7	740	226
MI	Berrien	-0.30	1667	32.9	9.4	27.6	74.8	79.8	680	207
NC	Bertie	-0.30	1668	37.7	13	29.9	68.8	76.2	38	12
NY	Schoharie	-0.30	1669	27.5	7.9	26.8	75.7	81.2	1503	458
OK	Tulsa	-0.30	1670	28.9	9.3	28.3	73.3	78.2	682	208
OK	Washita	-0.30	1671	28.3	9	28.5	72	78.5	1632	497
PA	Clarion	-0.30	1672	32.4	9.9	28.5	74.9	80.3	1396	426
SD	Haakon	-0.30	1673	30	7.1	27.5	76.6	81.5	2287	697
TN	Trousdale	-0.30	1674	32.8	10.4	34.7	71	77.4	640	195
VA	Danville	-0.30	1675	31.1	10.1	28.7	70.2	76.9	516	157
VA	Pittsylvania	-0.30	1676	29.4	10.2	26.8	72.5	79.3	703	214
VT	Franklin	-0.30	1677	27.9	7.2	24.4	76.4	81.1	671	205
AL	Marion	-0.31	1678	33.2	10.6	34.5	71	77.7	635	193
GA	Dougherty	-0.31	1679	34.7	13	27.5	70.8	77.6	203	62
MO	Montgomery	-0.31	1680	31.6	9.3	28.5	73.7	79.1	732	223
NC	Bladen	-0.31	1681	37.1	12.2	30	69.3	76.7	86	26
NY	New York	-0.31	1682	15.2	7.2	16.4	78.7	83.7	48	15

ST	COUNTY	USDA	AMEN	OBES	DIAB	INACT	M AGE	W AGE	ALT ft	ALT m
SC	Cherokee	-0.31	1683	30.6	11	30.7	70.1	76.7	690	210
VA	Buckingham	-0.31	1684	32.6	10.9	28.1	71.3	76.9	500	152
AR	Randolph	-0.32	1685	35.7	11.1	31.7	72.6	79.1	407	124
GA	Clayton	-0.32	1686	34.7	12.4	29.9	73.5	78.8	886	270
ME	Androscoggin	-0.32	1687	32.1	8.7	26.5	75.2	79.9	345	105
MS	Webster	-0.32	1688	33.9	11.5	34	71.1	77.3	418	127
NY	Cattaraugus	-0.32	1689	28.8	9.1	26	74.5	80	1700	518
GA	Spalding	-0.33	1690	31.6	10.9	27.6	71.2	77	818	249
NY	Columbia	-0.33	1691	25.3	6.7	21.1	75.9	80.6	620	189
OH	Lorain	-0.33	1692	31.6	10.4	27.5	75.6	80.3	774	236
OH	Tuscarawas	-0.33	1693	33.4	9.8	28.4	75.3	80.3	1019	311
TX	Archer	-0.33	1694	28.1	10	27.4	74.9	81.1	1071	327
AL	Chambers	-0.34	1695	35.5	14.2	35	70.2	77.2	750	228
GA	Elbert	-0.34	1696	36.3	12.2	30	71.7	78.1	553	169
IN	Dubois	-0.34	1697	31.5	8.3	24	75.5	80.9	534	163
KY	Franklin	-0.34	1698	33	10.1	31.1	74.3	78.7	730	223
LA	St. John Baptist	-0.34	1699	38.5	11.5	32	71.3	76.8	4	1
LA	St. Martin	-0.34	1700	35.5	11.7	29.7	71.6	77.5	8	2
MT	Rosebud	-0.34	1701	35.1	9.1	29.3	76.1	81	3092	943
NC	Union	-0.34	1702	27.9	8.3	22.4	75.2	79.8	566	173
NY	Clinton	-0.34	1703	28.9	7.6	24	75.8	80.5	918	280
PA	Juniata	-0.34	1704	30.4	9.4	26.6	74.6	80.8	865	264
TX	Brooks	-0.34	1705	28.7	8.7	28.3	73.4	78.6	187	57
WV	Marshall	-0.34	1706	33.1	10.2	34.7	73.8	80.2	1108	338
WV	Wirt	-0.34	1707	37.3	12.7	28.1	72	78	866	264
GA	Chattahoochee	-0.35	1708	32.7	12	27.2	71.9	78.2	409	125
GA	Gwinnett	-0.35	1709	25.2	8.7	20.7	77.2	80.9	997	304
IN	Lawrence	-0.35	1710	28.1	11.2	28.8	74	79.5	653	199
KS	Finney	-0.35	1711	32.8	9.1	25.8	75.3	80.2	2834	864
KS	Leavenworth	-0.35	1712	31.2	9.1	24.8	75.2	80	938	286
KY	Rockcastle	-0.35	1713	36.5	10.7	37.3	71.1	77.2	1154	352
MS	Claiborne	-0.35	1714	41.6	14.5	39.9	67.8	74.5	177	54
SC	Laurens	-0.35	1715	37.2	10.9	31.8	71.2	77.7	605	184
TN	McMinn	-0.35	1716	33.8	10.7	32.6	71.9	78.3	913	278
VT	Rutland	-0.35	1717	28	6.9	22.2	76.1	81.5	1256	383
GA	Charlton	-0.36	1718	30.8	10.8	29.8	70.6	77.2	96	29
GA	Telfair	-0.36	1719	29.6	11.5	27	70.1	76	205	62
GA	Whitfield	-0.36	1720	29	10.7	27.9	72.5	78.6	842	257
KS	Kearny	-0.36	1721	31.2	8.7	24.9	74.6	79.4	3161	963
KS	Woodson	-0.36	1722	31.4	9.1	31.1	74	79.6	1037	316
MO	Newton	-0.36	1723	32.3	10.2	30.5	74.7	80	1135	346
MS	Clay	-0.36	1724	38.1	12.9	36.8	71	77.8	242	74
OK	Nowata	-0.36	1725	33	10.3	29	73.2	79	760	232
TN	Lake	-0.36	1726	35.2	11.9	37.3	71.8	77.9	277	84
TX	Bee	-0.36	1727	28.4	9.7	25.9	74.2	79.4	240	73
TX	Clay	-0.36	1728	29.4	8.7	31.5	73.2	79.6	954	291

HEALTHIEST PLACES TO LIVE

ST	COUNTY	USDA	AMEN	OBES	DIAB	INACT	M AGE	W AGE	ALT ft	ALT m
MD	Baltimore	-0.37	1729	31	11.7	30.6	66.7	75.6	436	133
MD	Baltimore City	-0.37	1730	27.2	8.6	27.1	75.1	80.3	202	62
WI	Manitowoc	-0.37	1731	31.1	7	22.2	77	81.6	775	236
WI	Sheboygan	-0.37	1732	28.6	7.7	22.4	76.7	81.2	845	257
AL	Fayette	-0.38	1733	36.9	12.2	31.8	70.5	78	487	148
IN	Perry	-0.38	1734	32.4	8.6	29	74	79.5	548	167
MS	Jones	-0.38	1735	37.6	12.3	32	71.8	77.9	247	75
SC	Chesterfield	-0.38	1736	34.9	11.4	32.5	69.7	76.8	326	99
TN	Tipton	-0.38	1737	35.6	11	32.4	72.2	78	320	98
VA	Campbell	-0.38	1738	31.8	9.5	23.5	74.7	80.1	692	211
VA	Frederick	-0.38	1739	28.2	8.5	26	75.3	80.5	916	279
VA	Lynchburg	-0.38	1740	31.8	10.7	29.3	74.3	79.2	743	226
VA	Russell	-0.38	1741	30.2	10.4	33.4	71.3	77.5	2239	682
VA	Winchester	-0.38	1742	29.5	9.3	24.5	73.9	80.6	748	228
GA	Dade	-0.39	1743	27.9	10	23.2	71.7	78.3	1293	394
GA	Haralson	-0.39	1744	30.7	10.4	27.8	71.4	77.7	1166	355
MT	Prairie	-0.39	1745	27.5	6.6	27.8	75.7	81	2724	830
NC	Columbus	-0.39	1746	33.9	11.3	27.8	69.4	76.8	70	21
NE	Dawes	-0.39	1747	28.4	7.1	24.3	75.4	80.3	3827	1166
TN	Dyer	-0.39	1748	36	10.8	34.2	71.2	77.7	292	89
WA	Franklin	-0.39	1749	30.7	9.5	20.5	75.4	79.2	931	284
WI	Ozaukee	-0.39	1750	25.7	6.9	17.5	78.6	82.7	777	237
GA	Walker	-0.40	1751	30.5	10	34.9	71.3	78	1078	329
IL	Jo Daviess	-0.40	1752	28.9	7.5	22.9	76.5	81.6	838	255
KS	Morris	-0.40	1753	33.6	8.9	24.7	74.7	80.4	1410	430
MI	Muskegon	-0.40	1754	34.7	9.9	25.8	74.3	79.3	667	203
MO	Lewis	-0.40	1755	33.9	8.6	29	74	80.2	631	192
MS	Tunica	-0.40	1756	40.2	14.2	39.1	66	74.1	181	55
OK	Beckham	-0.40	1757	34.8	9.9	33.3	72	77.9	1953	595
PA	Centre	-0.40	1758	26.8	8.4	20.4	77.8	81.3	1472	449
PA	Lehigh	-0.40	1759	28.9	9.3	24.1	76.2	81.8	589	179
WI	Milwaukee	-0.40	1760	32.1	9.9	26.6	73.9	79.7	700	213
AL	Lowndes	-0.41	1761	44.7	16.4	37.5	69.9	76.4	251	76
ID	Lincoln	-0.41	1762	24.7	7.4	23.2	74.3	80	4370	1332
IL	Saline	-0.41	1763	29.2	8.3	31.6	72.4	78.7	421	128
KY	Leslie	-0.41	1764	36.2	14	37.5	69.2	76.1	1419	433
NE	Harlan	-0.41	1765	26.9	6.7	27.9	75.6	80.3	2133	650
TX	Roberts	-0.41	1766	28.5	8.6	27.7	73.8	79.3	2830	863
AL	Limestone	-0.42	1767	31.3	10	30.9	73	79	690	210
AR	Conway	-0.42	1768	33.2	10.3	29.1	72.5	78.1	492	150
AR	Lee	-0.42	1769	36.7	12	37.1	69.5	76.3	194	59
KS	Reno	-0.42	1770	33.1	9.4	22.2	75.4	80.6	1602	488
NE	Nance	-0.42	1771	28	8	29.5	75.6	80.5	1736	529
OH	Lake	-0.42	1772	28.5	10.6	24.6	76.1	81	765	233
WV	Pocahontas	-0.42	1773	30.9	10.8	27.4	73.3	78.6	3215	980
AR	Madison	-0.43	1774	30.9	9.8	28.2	73	79.4	1651	503

ST	COUNTY	USDA	AMEN	OBES	DIAB	INACT	M AGE	W AGE	ALT ft	ALT m
TX	Lipscomb	-0.43	1775	29	8.7	30.1	73.8	79.3	2604	794
TX	Mills	-0.43	1776	29.2	8.5	25.2	73.8	79.5	1462	446
WI	Juneau	-0.43	1777	29.9	7.9	22.8	74.1	80.1	949	289
WV	Putnam	-0.43	1778	29.4	10.4	27.7	75.5	79.3	792	241
TN	Sequatchie	-0.44	1779	35.8	9.6	30.7	72.7	79.1	1649	503
TN	Shelby	-0.44	1780	33.8	11.7	28.6	71.4	77.7	284	87
VA	Greene	-0.44	1781	30.5	8.7	23.2	74.7	80.1	1167	356
AR	Chicot	-0.45	1782	38.6	12.8	35.1	69.4	75.8	113	34
GA	Douglas	-0.45	1783	30.7	10.3	25.8	73.4	77.5	987	301
GA	Mitchell	-0.45	1784	34.1	11.6	30.2	69.8	76.7	217	66
KY	Anderson	-0.45	1785	35.3	11	34.5	75	79	776	237
MO	Webster	-0.45	1786	31.8	8.6	25.3	73.5	79.7	1411	430
MS	Pontotoc	-0.45	1787	33.8	10.7	34.3	72.1	79.4	409	125
PA	Perry	-0.45	1788	31.3	10	26.2	74.9	79.8	841	256
WI	Kenosha	-0.45	1789	28.3	7.9	23.3	75.3	80	739	225
GA	Jefferson	-0.46	1790	37.3	12.4	29.7	67.9	75.2	335	102
KY	Fulton	-0.46	1791	32.8	11	36	72.6	78.2	331	101
KY	Henry	-0.46	1792	35.1	11.4	32.4	73	78.9	775	236
MO	Henry	-0.46	1793	32.2	9	30	73.7	78.9	796	242
NC	Davie	-0.46	1794	28.5	8.9	27.7	74.7	80.2	749	228
OK	Harmon	-0.46	1795	32.5	9.8	34.4	72	77.9	1687	514
PA	Philadelphia	-0.46	1796	31.4	11.1	29.6	69.2	77.6	114	35
WI	Grant	-0.46	1797	29.1	7.6	19.5	76.2	80.8	931	284
AL	Dale	-0.47	1798	35.6	12.6	31	72.9	79	314	96
GA	Bacon	-0.47	1799	31	10	33.8	68.8	76.4	181	55
LA	Tensas	-0.47	1800	35.4	12.4	33.3	69.9	76.7	61	18
MO	Buchanan	-0.47	1801	37.4	10.3	30.1	73.8	79.6	923	281
VA	Scott	-0.47	1802	28.2	8.2	30	71.9	78.2	1822	555
AL	Sumter	-0.48	1803	42.4	16.8	32.3	67.9	76.6	173	53
KS	Lyon	-0.48	1804	30.5	8.1	24.7	75.5	79.5	1207	368
MO	St. Louis City	-0.48	1805	33.7	11.8	27.6	69.6	77.7	477	145
AL	Washington	-0.49	1806	36.3	11.4	32	72.9	78.5	148	45
GA	Coffee	-0.49	1807	29.5	11.3	32.2	70.2	78	254	77
GA	Randolph	-0.49	1808	36.1	13.4	31.9	67.6	74.7	386	118
IN	Ohio	-0.49	1809	29.4	9.5	28.2	74.7	79.5	712	217
NY	Rensselaer	-0.49	1810	28.7	8	23.3	75.8	80.3	823	251
AR	Union	-0.50	1811	31	10.1	27.3	71.2	77.6	170	52
GA	Franklin	-0.50	1812	28.1	9.5	24.7	72	78.9	760	232
LA	Avoyelles	-0.50	1813	36.9	11.2	36.1	69.4	76.3	47	14
AL	Geneva	-0.51	1814	35.9	12	34.2	71.6	78.4	212	65
IA	Appanoose	-0.51	1815	30	7.1	28.8	75	80.2	952	290
KY	Clark	-0.51	1816	28.8	10.5	29.5	74.1	78.8	900	274
NY	Wayne	-0.51	1817	29.4	8.7	23.3	75.6	80.7	434	132
TN	Montgomery	-0.51	1818	32.8	12.4	30.5	74.3	79.1	538	164
VA	Fluvanna	-0.51	1819	29.6	9.6	21.3	76	80.3	387	118
WI	Racine	-0.51	1820	31.2	7.8	24.6	75.7	80.6	759	231

HEALTHIEST PLACES TO LIVE

ST	COUNTY	USDA	AMEN	OBES	DIAB	INACT	M AGE	W AGE	ALT ft	ALT m
WV	Clay	-0.51	1821	37.3	13.4	33.2	71.9	78.3	1167	356
GA	Gordon	-0.52	1822	31.2	9.7	28.4	72	78.5	762	232
KY	Caldwell	-0.52	1823	35	10.4	31.7	73	79.3	507	155
ME	Penobscot	-0.52	1824	31	9.7	25.5	75	80.1	440	134
MI	Allegan	-0.52	1825	31.4	8.5	23.3	76	80.9	711	217
MO	Clark	-0.52	1826	32.5	8.6	30.6	74	80.2	644	196
NC	Harnett	-0.52	1827	31.6	9.5	27.6	72.6	78.2	247	75
NY	Niagara	-0.52	1828	28.4	8.1	28.1	74.9	80.1	459	140
TN	Morgan	-0.52	1829	32.3	9.9	29	71.5	77.7	1496	456
TX	Fort Bend	-0.52	1830	25.5	8.6	21.4	77.8	81.8	83	25
WI	Columbia	-0.52	1831	30.6	7.3	26.3	76.7	81.6	914	278
WV	Marion	-0.52	1832	35	10.9	32.1	73.9	79	1218	371
GA	Henry	-0.53	1833	27.8	10.6	23.5	74	78.7	784	239
NE	Madison	-0.53	1834	28.5	7.5	23.4	75.6	80.8	1703	519
PA	Montgomery	-0.53	1835	25	7.3	20.7	77.7	82	287	87
GA	Catoosa	-0.54	1836	32.8	10	29	73.3	79.2	857	261
GA	Macon	-0.54	1837	33.2	13.7	26.6	69.2	76.2	375	114
IN	Porter	-0.54	1838	29.6	9.1	25.8	76.2	80.5	693	211
GA	Webster	-0.55	1839	31.6	12.3	27.1	69.6	75.8	455	139
KY	Ballard	-0.55	1840	32.4	10.5	32.4	73.6	79.1	367	112
MI	Baraga	-0.55	1841	32.4	10.4	23.1	75.1	80.9	1336	407
MO	Macon	-0.55	1842	30.6	8.8	29.1	73.8	79.8	830	253
NE	Dodge	-0.55	1843	29.8	7.9	29	75.2	81.5	1301	397
OH	Licking	-0.55	1844	31.9	11.2	24.9	75.1	79.6	1030	314
SD	Ziebach	-0.55	1845	43.3	14.1	34.5	72.9	79.9	2278	694
TN	Bedford	-0.55	1846	34.1	11.8	30.5	71.9	79	842	257
WI	Crawford	-0.55	1847	28.2	7.7	22	75.1	80.2	937	286
WV	Berkeley	-0.55	1848	31.2	10.5	29.2	73.4	78.7	642	196
WV	Braxton	-0.55	1849	34.4	12.5	33.6	71.9	78.3	1186	361
AL	Macon	-0.56	1850	41.7	14.2	31.1	68.4	75.3	328	100
LA	Evangeline	-0.56	1851	33	10.5	30	69.8	75.5	69	21
LA	Iberville	-0.56	1852	36.8	12.2	32.6	69.4	76.3	8	3
SC	Florence	-0.56	1853	34.5	11.8	32.9	70.7	77.1	85	26
TN	Bledsoe	-0.56	1854	32.8	11.1	34.6	72.7	79.1	1601	488
VA	Tazewell	-0.56	1855	32.7	10.2	36.1	70.8	78.4	2697	822
WI	Bayfield	-0.56	1856	29.1	7.1	21.2	76.2	80.9	1117	340
GA	Lamar	-0.57	1857	29.8	10.8	26.8	72.1	77.9	746	227
IN	Jackson	-0.57	1858	30.6	8.9	32.4	74.7	79.4	626	191
MD	Montgomery	-0.57	1859	18.1	6.5	16.6	80.7	84.5	404	123
MO	Grundy	-0.57	1860	28.9	8	26.2	73.9	80	835	254
MS	Bolivar	-0.57	1861	39.2	13.3	31.4	67.9	75.2	136	42
NJ	Middlesex	-0.57	1862	23.5	8.1	27.1	78	82.4	85	26
PA	Cumberland	-0.57	1863	27.2	9.1	22.7	77	81.3	713	217
PA	Erie	-0.57	1864	29.4	8.6	28.8	75.3	80.3	1158	353
PA	Franklin	-0.57	1865	31.1	8.6	24.9	76.1	81.4	893	272
TX	Montague	-0.57	1866	29.2	8.7	28.7	73.2	79.6	971	296

ST	COUNTY	USDA	AMEN	OBES	DIAB	INACT	M AGE	W AGE	ALT ft	ALT m
VT	Orange	-0.57	1867	27.3	6.7	20	76.3	81.1	1269	387
KY	Calloway	-0.58	1868	29.4	10.8	24	74.7	79.7	493	150
KY	Washington	-0.58	1869	31.6	11.2	29.4	73.3	79.6	757	231
MI	Houghton	-0.58	1870	26.2	8.8	26.2	75.2	80.1	1026	313
MT	Carter	-0.58	1871	23.9	6	30.7	75	80.7	3426	1044
NY	Orleans	-0.58	1872	29.4	8	27.5	75.5	80.6	476	145
PA	York	-0.58	1873	31.6	8.9	22.6	76.1	81.6	595	182
AR	Lafayette	-0.59	1874	31	10.5	31.8	70.2	77.1	252	77
GA	Meriwether	-0.59	1875	31.4	11.9	26.5	69.4	76	827	252
KS	Hamilton	-0.59	1876	31.7	7.8	25.9	75.9	81.2	3446	1050
TX	Delta	-0.59	1877	29	9.2	28.2	73.8	80	453	138
GA	Jeff Davis	-0.60	1878	26.9	10.1	25.8	68.8	76.4	219	67
MS	Kemper	-0.60	1879	38.1	14.3	32.9	68.9	76.5	344	105
NE	Greeley	-0.60	1880	33.1	7.6	28.3	76.2	80.7	2052	625
NE	Platte	-0.60	1881	27.9	6.9	23.6	77.2	82.1	1620	494
VA	Craig	-0.60	1882	27	8.1	24.7	72.8	79	2175	663
KS	Haskell	-0.61	1883	30.4	9.3	27.2	75.3	80.2	2917	889
MD	Prince George's	-0.61	1884	33.8	11	24.9	73.5	79.2	147	45
MI	Van Buren	-0.61	1885	30.1	9.2	27.3	73.9	79.6	737	225
NE	Deuel	-0.61	1886	27.9	6.5	28.2	76.1	81.4	3731	1137
NE	Stanton	-0.61	1887	32.5	6.5	30.8	75.7	81.6	1609	490
NJ	Gloucester	-0.61	1888	26.7	9.4	25.1	74.6	80	78	24
SC	Abbeville	-0.61	1889	32.6	11.5	31.6	72	78.1	575	175
GA	Taylor	-0.62	1890	33.8	11.9	29.1	70.6	76.6	503	153
MO	Polk	-0.62	1891	33.2	10	27.2	73.7	79	1050	320
MS	Oktibbeha	-0.62	1892	31.6	11.4	26.9	73.9	79.3	301	92
GA	Pierce	-0.63	1893	28.8	10.6	27.6	70.3	77.5	103	32
GA	Pike	-0.63	1894	29.7	10.4	25.4	72.1	77.9	825	251
KY	Christian	-0.63	1895	31.3	11.1	33.2	72.7	78.6	568	173
KY	Nelson	-0.63	1896	30	10.3	28.5	73.9	80.4	639	195
MN	Washington	-0.63	1897	25.4	6.8	16.6	78.8	82	918	280
NY	Franklin	-0.63	1898	28.2	8.2	25.4	75	80.1	1397	426
OH	Cuyahoga	-0.63	1899	27.8	9.5	25	74	79.7	852	260
PA	Snyder	-0.63	1900	31.3	9.9	24	75.1	81.2	855	261
VA	Loudoun	-0.63	1901	22.8	7.9	21	79	82.2	461	140
VT	Washington	-0.63	1902	22.3	6.2	17	77.7	81.2	1338	408
WI	Ashland	-0.63	1903	29.5	7.8	20.4	74.4	80.9	1281	390
GA	Peach	-0.64	1904	30.2	12.4	28.5	70.6	76.3	435	133
KY	Owen	-0.64	1905	33.8	11.4	36.3	72.8	78.6	762	232
MA	Norfolk	-0.64	1906	20	6.4	19.4	78.2	82.6	191	58
NY	Washington	-0.64	1907	28.2	8.9	30	76.1	80.2	590	180
OH	Coshocton	-0.64	1908	31.1	9.5	29.5	74.5	79.6	946	288
OH	Vinton	-0.64	1909	30.9	9.9	29.3	71.9	78.5	834	254
SD	Gregory	-0.64	1910	30.6	7.8	29.5	75	80.8	1919	585
AR	Hempstead	-0.65	1911	36.4	12.4	31.6	71.5	77.2	343	105
MS	Coahoma	-0.65	1912	44.3	14.7	36.1	66.8	75	158	48

ST	COUNTY	USDA	AMEN	OBES	DIAB	INACT	M AGE	W AGE	ALT ft	ALT m
NC	Northampton	-0.65	1913	34.3	12.1	31.9	68.9	77	97	30
OK	Woodward	-0.65	1914	31.3	9.6	31.5	74.5	80.4	1941	591
SD	Harding	-0.65	1915	30.6	6.7	30.2	74.8	80.5	3077	938
TX	Hamilton	-0.65	1916	29.3	8.5	29	73.8	79.5	1200	366
TX	Sherman	-0.65	1917	29.2	8.6	27.7	73.7	78.9	3524	1074
AL	Coffee	-0.66	1918	32.2	12.5	28.2	73.4	79	328	100
MN	St. Louis	-0.66	1919	27.5	6.9	17.5	75.8	80.9	1378	420
PA	Lebanon	-0.66	1920	30.7	9	22.7	75.7	80.9	612	187
WI	Douglas	-0.66	1921	29.4	7.4	20.9	74.6	80.6	1061	323
WI	Vernon	-0.66	1922	27.9	7.2	22.9	75.2	80.4	1061	324
LA	Calcasieu	-0.67	1923	34.5	11.6	29.4	71.2	78.1	17	5
NE	Sioux	-0.67	1924	28.4	6.5	27.5	75.4	80.3	4450	1356
NY	Ontario	-0.67	1925	26.2	7.7	19.2	76.9	81.7	918	280
PA	Bedford	-0.67	1926	29.5	9.4	25.9	75.2	80.6	1458	444
AR	Phillips	-0.68	1927	39.7	13.2	37.8	66.8	75	174	53
KY	Warren	-0.68	1928	29.2	9.5	28.7	73.9	80	574	175
LA	Madison	-0.68	1929	36.7	12.6	34.5	69.3	75.3	72	22
NC	Lee	-0.68	1930	30.2	10.3	23.5	73.3	80	324	99
OH	Hocking	-0.68	1931	33.9	10.9	27.3	73.4	79	907	277
SC	Dillon	-0.68	1932	38.7	11.9	37.3	67.9	75.4	101	31
VA	Louisa	-0.68	1933	31.7	9.9	29.1	73.4	80.2	362	110
KY	Hardin	-0.69	1934	30.9	11.5	29.7	75.2	80.2	718	219
NC	Scotland	-0.69	1935	36	13.4	28.4	70.5	76.9	252	77
PA	Delaware	-0.69	1936	26.5	8.9	23.6	74.8	80	235	72
SC	Hampton	-0.69	1937	41.1	14.3	30	69.9	76.7	82	25
VA	Appomattox	-0.69	1938	31.8	10.8	26.4	73.1	79.7	658	201
WI	La Crosse	-0.69	1939	24.1	7.2	18.4	76.9	81.9	891	272
GA	Barrow	-0.70	1940	28.7	10.9	28	72.5	78.6	863	263
KS	Sedgwick	-0.70	1941	29.3	9.1	23.1	74.3	79.8	1361	415
MD	Wicomico	-0.70	1942	33.3	10.4	27.5	73	78.9	31	9
MS	Tate	-0.70	1943	35.5	12.4	32.2	72	77.2	302	92
NY	Erie	-0.70	1944	28.4	9	25.6	75.3	80.2	936	285
WI	Iron	-0.70	1945	27.8	7.5	21.4	75.3	80.7	1531	467
CO	Phillips	-0.71	1946	22.1	5.8	18.5	75.8	80.2	3819	1164
GA	Clarke	-0.71	1947	28.1	11	20.3	74.3	79.6	722	220
KY	Shelby	-0.71	1948	34.3	10.9	28	75.4	80.2	783	239
LA	St. Landry	-0.71	1949	38.1	12.6	32.5	70.7	77.2	34	10
MS	Jefferson	-0.71	1950	44.9	15.3	37.2	67.8	74.5	256	78
NC	Cumberland	-0.71	1951	33.1	12.4	29.8	72.6	78.4	147	45
PA	Warren	-0.71	1952	28.3	9.5	28.3	75.4	79.9	1623	495
SD	Corson	-0.71	1953	41.7	13	31.6	72.9	79.9	2088	636
TN	Obion	-0.71	1954	32.5	11.4	35.2	71.8	77.9	354	108
TN	Wayne	-0.71	1955	32.2	9.6	29.4	71.1	77.6	785	239
WI	Pepin	-0.71	1956	28.7	7.8	25.1	76.8	81.8	910	277
AL	Marengo	-0.72	1957	40.4	14.8	34.8	69.9	76.3	181	55
IL	Clinton	-0.72	1958	28.2	8	27.3	74.9	81.2	454	138

ST	COUNTY	USDA	AMEN	OBES	DIAB	INACT	M AGE	W AGE	ALT ft	ALT m
KY	Henderson	-0.72	1959	33.5	10.4	26.9	73.6	78.7	399	122
MI	Ontonagon	-0.72	1960	32.5	9.3	20.9	75	80.7	1110	338
MO	Ray	-0.72	1961	31.7	9.4	30.9	74.8	79.6	849	259
NE	Colfax	-0.72	1962	32.6	7.9	28.2	75.5	81.1	1498	457
LA	E Baton Rouge	-0.73	1963	31.5	11.1	25.9	72.3	78	59	18
PA	Berks	-0.73	1964	29	7.9	23.6	76	81.5	566	172
SD	Perkins	-0.73	1965	29.3	7.3	30.6	74.8	80.5	2611	796
KY	Letcher	-0.74	1966	38.9	15.2	36.1	69.4	76.8	1717	523
KY	Pendleton	-0.74	1967	35.9	10.1	31.6	72.3	78.5	729	222
MI	Huron	-0.74	1968	30.9	7.8	22.6	75.1	80	682	208
NE	Cherry	-0.74	1969	27.3	6.5	28.6	75.6	81.2	3201	976
IL	Calhoun	-0.75	1970	27.9	8.1	32.3	74.5	79.5	557	170
KY	Logan	-0.75	1971	34.1	10.3	33.5	72.5	78.1	597	182
NE	Banner	-0.75	1972	30.4	7.9	26.9	75.8	80.7	4655	1419
NY	Monroe	-0.75	1973	30.1	8.5	20.4	76.9	81.4	492	150
SC	Bamberg	-0.75	1974	41.5	12.6	33.1	68.7	76.2	159	48
SD	Jackson	-0.75	1975	34.1	10.9	30.8	71	78.3	2525	770
DC	Dist of Columbia	-0.76	1976	21.6	8.5	19.9	71.6	78.5	139	42
IN	Owen	-0.76	1977	35	9.7	29.5	73.6	79	672	205
KS	Atchison	-0.76	1978	33.4	7.8	29.5	75.2	79.9	1033	315
MI	Wexford	-0.76	1979	33.3	8.4	27.3	74.9	79.9	1181	360
MO	Atchison	-0.76	1980	29.7	8.5	27	76.2	80.7	998	304
MO	Oregon	-0.76	1981	32.7	9.6	32.7	71.9	78.7	767	234
ND	Billings	-0.76	1982	29.2	6.9	26.3	75.7	82.2	2591	790
NY	Steuben	-0.76	1983	30.9	9.7	25	75.4	80.8	1602	488
SD	Mellette	-0.76	1984	36.7	12.8	33.1	71	78.3	2219	676
TN	White	-0.76	1985	33.2	10.1	34.6	71.6	78.2	1207	368
VA	Madison	-0.76	1986	31.9	8.3	24.2	74.7	80.1	1015	309
GA	Burke	-0.77	1987	37	11.4	30.7	68.3	75	255	78
IN	Greene	-0.77	1988	30.7	10.9	27.8	74.2	79.4	591	180
KS	Kingman	-0.77	1989	31	8.5	29.7	75.3	80.1	1575	480
NE	Cuming	-0.77	1990	29.3	6.6	28.4	75.7	81.6	1438	438
NY	Otsego	-0.77	1991	28.1	7.6	23.9	75.7	81.3	1559	475
OH	Jefferson	-0.77	1992	36.2	12	31.5	72.6	78.3	1073	327
OK	Kingfisher	-0.77	1993	35.7	10.3	30.5	73.6	79.4	1121	342
VA	Shenandoah	-0.77	1994	30.3	8.8	27.1	74.8	80.4	1240	378
GA	Glascock	-0.78	1995	27.4	10.2	28	68.4	75.4	445	136
IN	Harrison	-0.78	1996	29.6	9.5	28.4	75.1	80.2	673	205
ND	Slope	-0.78	1997	28.8	6.8	30.3	75.7	81.6	2845	867
VA	Emporia	-0.78	1998	33.5	11.5	28.7	70.5	75.4	103	31
VA	Greensville	-0.78	1999	34.1	12	29.9	70.5	75.4	147	45
AL	Houston	-0.79	2000	33.3	11.2	32.5	73.3	79.5	219	67
AR	Lonoke	-0.79	2001	33.8	11	30.8	73.3	79	233	71
IA	Dubuque	-0.79	2002	26.8	7	20.1	76.9	81.5	957	292
MS	Prentiss	-0.79	2003	34.1	11.6	32.1	71.3	78.9	445	136
MS	Wayne	-0.79	2004	35.5	10.2	32	71.1	77.2	253	77

HEALTHIEST PLACES TO LIVE

ST	COUNTY	USDA	AMEN	OBES	DIAB	INACT	M AGE	W AGE	ALT ft	ALT m
OH	Pike	-0.79	2005	32.2	10.5	35.2	71.4	78.4	833	254
TX	Throckmorton	-0.79	2006	29.4	8.6	27.4	72.6	79	1363	416
KS	Clay	-0.80	2007	30.9	8.1	26.9	75.8	81.2	1291	394
MS	Simpson	-0.80	2008	34.9	11.7	32.2	70.3	76.4	384	117
NJ	Mercer	-0.80	2009	24.8	8.7	25.2	76.2	81.4	130	40
SC	Union	-0.80	2010	35.8	11.9	33.6	69.3	77.1	499	152
TN	Lewis	-0.80	2011	31.7	10.3	36	71.1	77.6	842	257
IA	Fremont	-0.81	2012	32.2	7.1	29.8	76.2	81.1	1028	313
KS	Marion	-0.81	2013	31.4	8	27.7	75.1	81.2	1426	435
KS	Montgomery	-0.81	2014	30.9	9.1	30.3	73	79.9	826	252
MS	George	-0.81	2015	37.9	10.1	33	70.4	77	134	41
MT	Wibaux	-0.81	2016	26.1	6.5	29.9	75.7	81	2715	828
NE	Blaine	-0.81	2017	29.7	7	28.4	75.6	81.2	2651	808
VT	Bennington	-0.81	2018	22.9	5.9	19.5	76.8	81.5	1710	521
KY	Jackson	-0.82	2019	33.4	11.3	36	70.3	76.9	1216	371
TN	Wilson	-0.82	2020	29.8	9.3	28.6	74.7	78.9	664	203
TX	Victoria	-0.82	2021	30.4	9.2	24.9	74.5	80.1	87	27
VT	Lamoille	-0.82	2022	25.4	6.6	17.4	77.8	81.4	1284	391
KS	Decatur	-0.83	2023	32	9.5	26.1	76	80.6	2648	807
TN	Dickson	-0.83	2024	30.1	10.4	31.5	72.4	78.8	706	215
AR	White	-0.84	2025	31.5	9.4	27.8	73.2	78.8	352	107
KS	Ford	-0.84	2026	32.8	9.2	28.6	75.4	80	2492	759
KY	Hickman	-0.84	2027	33.7	11.4	32.2	72.6	78.2	375	114
MO	Butler	-0.84	2028	32.6	8.6	31.7	70.7	77.8	372	113
NY	Broome	-0.84	2029	29.5	8.4	23.6	75.5	81.2	1317	401
VA	Chesterfield	-0.84	2030	26.5	9.1	21.8	75.3	79.7	200	61
VA	Colonial Hghts	-0.84	2031	28.2	9	22.3	75	80.5	75	23
VA	Rappahannock	-0.84	2032	26.3	8.5	24.5	73.9	80	1031	314
WV	Preston	-0.84	2033	33.9	9.6	32.1	73.4	79.8	2020	616
AL	Lamar	-0.85	2034	32.6	11.1	34.4	71.7	77.3	397	121
IA	Jackson	-0.85	2035	31.2	6.6	23.5	76	80.8	794	242
KY	Oldham	-0.85	2036	29.2	9.3	27.5	76.4	80.7	694	211
MS	Union	-0.85	2037	34.4	10.8	31.9	72.3	78.4	422	128
NC	Guilford	-0.85	2038	28	9.8	23	74.9	80.5	787	240
TN	Rutherford	-0.85	2039	29.1	10.6	27.4	75.2	79.5	678	207
VA	Bland	-0.85	2040	30.6	9.4	24.9	72.5	78.8	2705	825
AR	Prairie	-0.86	2041	32.5	9.5	30.2	70.9	77.3	200	61
GA	Marion	-0.86	2042	31.1	11	26.4	71.9	78.2	563	172
KY	Fleming	-0.86	2043	34.7	10.6	34.6	71	77.5	862	263
MS	Lee	-0.86	2044	33.6	11.7	30.5	70.9	77	335	102
PA	Blair	-0.86	2045	31.9	9.1	29.3	73.4	80	1538	469
PA	Venango	-0.86	2046	31.4	7.9	27.2	74.5	80.1	1376	419
AR	Arkansas	-0.87	2047	36.5	11.3	35.6	71.5	78.5	177	54
KY	Bullitt	-0.87	2048	33.8	10.9	33.8	75.4	80.2	577	176
KY	McCracken	-0.87	2049	30.1	9.6	28.4	73.6	79.1	375	114
MS	Walthall	-0.87	2050	39.6	12.4	34.9	69.9	76.9	355	108

ST	COUNTY	USDA	AMEN	OBES	DIAB	INACT	M AGE	W AGE	ALT ft	ALT m
OH	Lucas	-0.87	2051	31.3	10.3	27.5	73.4	78.8	629	192
OK	Okmulgee	-0.87	2052	35.3	9.9	33.2	70.8	78.1	722	220
TN	Williamson	-0.87	2053	23.8	8.2	18.8	77.9	82	778	237
WI	Jackson	-0.87	2054	30.4	8.4	24.1	74.8	79.6	983	300
AR	Ouachita	-0.88	2055	37.4	11.6	34.2	71.1	76.9	185	56
IN	Morgan	-0.88	2056	30.1	9.2	27.2	74.6	79.2	729	222
KS	Barton	-0.88	2057	34.5	9.4	26.4	75.6	81.9	1891	576
KS	Chase	-0.88	2058	31.8	8.1	22.5	74.7	80.4	1361	415
MO	Douglas	-0.88	2059	31.7	9.3	28.1	72.5	79.3	1142	348
SC	Williamsburg	-0.88	2060	41.9	13.4	31.4	67.8	75.6	53	16
IN	Jefferson	-0.89	2061	30.4	8.8	30	74.4	79.9	738	225
MI	Otsego	-0.89	2062	30.4	8.5	23.6	76	80.4	1219	371
MS	Issaquena	-0.89	2063	37.8	13.2	33.8	69.9	75.9	90	27
TN	Coffee	-0.89	2064	33.4	11.1	25.6	72.3	78.5	1093	333
TN	Lawrence	-0.89	2065	30.1	10.7	32.2	71.5	78.6	876	267
TN	Marshall	-0.89	2066	30.7	9.6	32.9	72.4	79.1	818	249
VA	Orange	-0.89	2067	31.8	9.7	24.5	75.1	80.1	420	128
KS	Lane	-0.90	2068	34.3	8.3	24.8	75.9	81.2	2757	840
MO	Putnam	-0.90	2069	29.4	7.7	28.5	74.8	80.2	964	294
NE	McPherson	-0.90	2070	29.8	7.9	28.1	76.1	80.2	3326	1014
NY	Allegany	-0.90	2071	28.8	8.5	25.7	75.6	79.9	1826	557
AL	Crenshaw	-0.91	2072	37.4	12.2	32.5	69.9	76.4	422	129
MI	Alger	-0.91	2073	30.6	8.7	24	74.7	80	858	262
MS	Pearl River	-0.91	2074	32.9	11.6	28.8	71.8	78	184	56
MS	Yazoo	-0.91	2075	35.5	12.8	35.2	69.9	75.9	210	64
NY	Livingston	-0.91	2076	27.4	8.3	24.3	76.5	81.2	1046	319
OH	Erie	-0.91	2077	28.6	9.8	27.6	75.3	80.1	665	203
WV	Wetzel	-0.91	2078	33.9	10.6	30.5	73.7	79.7	1125	343
WY	Weston	-0.91	2079	28.4	6.3	26.9	75.9	81.5	4452	1357
KY	Martin	-0.92	2080	38.6	12.6	38.1	69.7	77.4	943	288
MI	Montmorency	-0.92	2081	31.9	8.9	24.4	74.7	80.4	960	293
MS	Holmes	-0.92	2082	40.8	14.1	35.3	65.9	73.5	246	75
MS	Tallahatchie	-0.92	2083	37.6	12.8	33.5	68.6	76.3	187	57
OH	Ashtabula	-0.92	2084	30.6	9.1	30.7	73.7	79.1	891	272
AL	Pike	-0.93	2085	37	15	32.3	71.7	77.1	430	131
KY	Grant	-0.93	2086	37.6	10.4	36.7	72.6	78.7	809	247
PA	Jefferson	-0.93	2087	29.5	10.7	28.8	74.9	80.3	1569	478
VA	Henrico	-0.93	2088	28.5	8.7	25.6	75.6	80.3	142	43
VA	Richmond City	-0.93	2089	31.4	11.4	28	69.2	78.6	160	49
GA	Walton	-0.94	2090	28.2	10.3	30.5	74.4	79.6	809	247
KS	Hodgeman	-0.94	2091	32.9	9	27.1	75.2	80.6	2386	727
KS	Rooks	-0.94	2092	30.3	8.7	25.8	75.7	82	2013	614
KS	Smith	-0.94	2093	31.7	7.3	30.9	75.7	82	1830	558
MO	Monroe	-0.94	2094	31	9.6	27.1	74.4	80.1	722	220
NC	Granville	-0.94	2095	31.9	10.9	26.6	71.8	78.4	424	129
NY	Madison	-0.94	2096	26.3	7.1	22.4	76	80.5	1224	373

HEALTHIEST PLACES TO LIVE

ST	COUNTY	USDA	AMEN	OBES	DIAB	INACT	M AGE	W AGE	ALT ft	ALT m
VA	Franklin City	-0.94	2097	32.8	10.3	30.5	72.8	78.9	31	10
VA	Manassas	-0.94	2098	28.4	9.9	24.9	76.5	80.4	249	76
VA	Manassas Park	-0.94	2099	29.7	9.5	25.9	76.5	80.4	235	72
VA	Prince William	-0.94	2100	26.8	9.4	21.3	77.5	80.6	270	82
VA	Southampton	-0.94	2101	28.5	11.6	27.2	72	77.8	65	20
AR	Cross	-0.95	2102	34.5	10.6	35	70.7	77.2	234	71
KS	Coffey	-0.95	2103	34.9	9.2	23.4	75.2	80.6	1106	337
MI	Mackinac	-0.95	2104	33.8	9	25.3	75	80.3	733	223
OH	Holmes	-0.95	2105	30.6	8.9	26.7	73.5	78.5	1079	329
KS	Dickinson	-0.96	2106	31.3	8.3	25.9	75.1	81.2	1272	388
KS	Gray	-0.96	2107	29.5	8.7	25.8	75.3	80.2	2738	834
NC	Alamance	-0.96	2108	33.6	10.1	27.7	74.2	79.4	643	196
ND	Sioux	-0.96	2109	41.8	13.5	32.3	74.6	80.6	2029	618
KS	Grant	-0.97	2110	33.4	8.5	20.1	74.6	79.4	3056	931
NE	Hitchcock	-0.97	2111	32.9	7.5	31	76	81	2858	871
OH	Scioto	-0.97	2112	33.7	10.2	30.3	71.3	78.3	784	239
VA	Fredericksburg	-0.97	2113	29.7	9.7	25	73.5	80.6	103	31
VA	Spotsylvania	-0.97	2114	28	9.5	20	75.4	80.8	282	86
KS	Cherokee	-0.98	2115	35.7	9.1	25.5	73.2	78.9	867	264
KY	Todd	-0.98	2116	32.3	10.2	35.9	72.5	78.1	623	190
MS	Chickasaw	-0.98	2117	35.3	11.7	33.1	69.8	77.5	335	102
MT	Chouteau	-0.98	2118	29.7	7.9	27.7	74.4	80.2	3231	985
SD	Todd	-0.98	2119	41	14.4	31.5	71	78.3	2697	822
WI	Iowa	-0.98	2120	29.9	8.2	23.6	76.6	81.5	1006	307
WV	Lewis	-0.98	2121	30.4	11.1	31.9	72	78.5	1216	371
LA	Lincoln	-0.99	2122	34.4	10.8	30.8	74	78.9	229	70
MS	Lincoln	-0.99	2123	36.1	11.8	34.1	71.8	77.9	418	127
TX	Wharton	-0.99	2124	30.5	9.8	27.6	73.2	79.2	101	31
AL	Conecuh	-1.00	2125	33.5	14.1	34.9	69.6	77.2	323	98
IA	Adams	-1.00	2126	32.5	7	24.1	76.4	80.9	1214	370
IA	Mills	-1.00	2127	25.7	6.8	23.5	75.9	80.4	1089	332
KS	Crawford	-1.00	2128	34.8	9.4	27.7	73.9	79.6	938	286
KY	Wolfe	-1.00	2129	31.8	10.6	33	68.2	76.2	1063	324
MO	Saline	-1.00	2130	31.3	9.4	28.7	74	78.6	720	219
MS	Marshall	-1.00	2131	38.8	14.7	37.5	68.5	76	438	134
NC	Gates	-1.00	2132	34.7	11.2	29.4	72.9	78.2	28	9
SC	Lee	-1.00	2133	38.2	13.1	34.9	68.3	75.4	217	66
IA	Clayton	-1.01	2134	29.2	6.5	28.3	76.1	81.5	968	295
KS	Neosho	-1.01	2135	36.3	10	30	74	79.6	945	288
MO	Andrew	-1.01	2136	31.1	8.5	24.3	74.8	79.6	979	298
MS	Amite	-1.01	2137	37.8	11.9	32.3	69.3	76.1	351	107
MT	Dawson	-1.01	2138	27.8	6.7	29.7	75.3	80.5	2575	785
ND	Bowman	-1.01	2139	30	7.5	29.5	75.7	81.6	2974	906
OK	Grant	-1.01	2140	33.6	9.1	29	74.7	80.3	1122	342
TX	Jim Hogg	-1.01	2141	29.1	8.7	27	73.4	78.6	542	165
VT	Essex	-1.01	2142	26.1	6.6	23	75.4	80.3	1595	486

PEGGY FORNEY

ST	COUNTY	USDA	AMEN	OBES	DIAB	INACT	M AGE	W AGE	ALT ft	ALT m
WI	Sauk	-1.01	2143	29.7	8	23.5	76.2	81.9	981	299
MS	Carroll	-1.02	2144	34.7	10.9	31.6	70.7	77.9	312	95
MT	Powder River	-1.02	2145	24	6.4	29.1	75	80.7	3503	1068
OH	Gallia	-1.02	2146	32.2	10.4	38	72.1	79.3	732	223
IA	Monona	-1.03	2147	27.2	7	29.7	75.1	80.4	1153	352
IA	Pottawattamie	-1.03	2148	29.9	7.3	26.7	74.9	80	1188	362
KS	Saline	-1.03	2149	34.2	8	24.2	75.5	80.1	1332	406
KY	Carlisle	-1.03	2150	32.6	11.1	29.5	73.6	79.1	383	117
MS	Washington	-1.03	2151	38.2	11.6	36.1	68.1	75.3	109	33
WV	Logan	-1.03	2152	37.8	13.6	42.7	68.9	76.4	1355	413
AR	Desha	-1.04	2153	37.9	12.1	31.9	69.4	75.8	141	43
GA	Oconee	-1.04	2154	25.6	8.4	21.5	76.8	81.3	700	213
IL	Cook	-1.04	2155	26	8.8	23.6	75.1	80.7	659	201
IN	Floyd	-1.04	2156	30.9	8.7	24.1	74.9	79.3	709	216
LA	Jefferson Davis	-1.04	2157	33.2	12	31	72.6	78	22	7
MI	Arenac	-1.04	2158	35.2	8.6	24	74.1	79.6	683	208
MS	Benton	-1.04	2159	36.4	11.8	33.3	70.6	77.9	503	153
AR	Crittenden	-1.05	2160	37.2	13.1	33.1	69.6	75.9	207	63
GA	Madison	-1.05	2161	30.5	10.1	24	72.5	78.7	740	225
KS	Labette	-1.05	2162	32.2	9.3	31.4	73.8	79	867	264
MI	Schoolcraft	-1.05	2163	30	9.3	24.8	74.7	80	745	227
NY	Tioga	-1.05	2164	28.3	7.5	25	76	80.6	1248	380
TN	Hardeman	-1.05	2165	38.6	11.4	33.8	70.7	77.2	459	140
VA	Floyd	-1.05	2166	27.6	9.2	23.3	73.4	78.9	2581	787
WV	Lincoln	-1.05	2167	38.4	10.7	37.7	70.6	76.6	911	278
AR	Bradley	-1.06	2168	32.3	11.9	32	72	78.3	169	52
IA	Harrison	-1.06	2169	30.9	7.2	27.2	75	80.4	1171	357
KS	Jefferson	-1.06	2170	37.5	9.4	22.8	75.4	80	1026	313
MT	Custer	-1.06	2171	23.3	7.1	24	75	80.7	2845	867
NC	Forsyth	-1.06	2172	25.5	8.8	21	74.5	79.5	848	258
NE	Rock	-1.06	2173	30.9	7.8	29.5	75.6	80.9	2391	729
VA	Goochland	-1.06	2174	26.5	9.2	21.4	75.6	81.2	276	84
IA	Van Buren	-1.07	2175	32.3	7.4	24.3	76.9	80.9	705	215
KS	Osborne	-1.07	2176	32.9	9	25.3	75.7	82	1751	534
AL	Bullock	-1.08	2177	39.2	15.6	30.9	68.4	75.3	415	126
AR	Jefferson	-1.08	2178	38.2	12.9	34	70.4	77.2	216	66
GA	Chattooga	-1.08	2179	30.7	10.1	27.6	70.1	76.9	899	274
MS	Copiah	-1.08	2180	36	12.2	37.1	69.6	76.7	325	99
NC	Cabarrus	-1.08	2181	30.7	9.4	23.1	74.2	79	644	196
NE	Gosper	-1.08	2182	28.6	7.6	25.8	75.6	80.9	2452	747
NY	Seneca	-1.08	2183	30.9	8	31.1	75.4	80.4	608	185
OH	Lawrence	-1.08	2184	39.5	11.3	35.4	71.7	77.4	756	230
PA	Union	-1.08	2185	30.2	9	24.4	76	80.5	956	291
MI	Marquette	-1.09	2186	29.8	7.9	20.9	76.3	80.4	1246	380
OH	Warren	-1.09	2187	26.1	9.2	22.1	76.7	80.5	848	259
PA	Forest	-1.09	2188	31.7	10	24.4	74.9	80.7	1570	479

HEALTHIEST PLACES TO LIVE

ST	COUNTY	USDA	AMEN	OBES	DIAB	INACT	M AGE	W AGE	ALT ft	ALT m
MS	Jefferson Davis	-1.10	2189	35.2	11.5	31	69.9	76.9	390	119
NE	Brown	-1.10	2190	28.6	8	27.1	75.6	81.2	2601	793
OH	Ross	-1.10	2191	34.2	10.1	28.8	73.3	78.6	840	256
MI	Kalkaska	-1.11	2192	30.4	10	25	74.8	80	1121	342
MO	Adair	-1.11	2193	28.4	9.3	31.5	74.8	80.2	896	273
MS	Covington	-1.11	2194	40.7	12	30.8	69.2	77	323	98
MS	Jasper	-1.11	2195	39.5	14.4	35.5	70.5	77.2	404	123
PA	McKean	-1.11	2196	32.2	9.1	27.7	74.3	80	1917	584
SC	Dorchester	-1.11	2197	29.6	10.1	26.5	74.1	79.4	62	19
VA	Sussex	-1.11	2198	32.8	11.5	29.9	70.5	75.4	95	29
AR	Ashley	-1.12	2199	39.4	10.4	37.4	72.4	77.4	134	41
GA	Miller	-1.12	2200	32.8	12.5	32.1	70.1	77.2	167	51
KY	Montgomery	-1.12	2201	31.7	10.2	31.6	72.3	79.1	929	283
LA	St. James	-1.12	2202	35.7	11.5	32.6	71.3	78.3	6	2
MA	Middlesex	-1.12	2203	23	7.6	20.8	78.8	82.9	226	69
WV	Jefferson	-1.12	2204	34.5	10.6	27.5	74.6	79.1	512	156
WV	Mingo	-1.12	2205	31.4	11.7	40	68.7	75.9	1249	381
AR	Monroe	-1.13	2206	36.8	11	35.2	69.5	76.3	171	52
MN	Wabasha	-1.13	2207	24	6.3	22.3	77.1	81.8	985	300
MS	Stone	-1.13	2208	34	11.4	30.6	70.4	77	177	54
NY	Chemung	-1.13	2209	26.3	8.8	26.2	75.4	80	1303	397
IN	Lake	-1.14	2210	33.9	11	29.8	72.6	78.6	656	200
OK	Woods	-1.14	2211	29.4	8.4	30.4	74.4	79.7	1573	479
GA	Oglethorpe	-1.15	2212	30.5	10.1	23.7	71.7	78.1	598	182
KS	Miami	-1.15	2213	29.5	8.1	25.2	75.9	80.2	985	300
KS	Sumner	-1.15	2214	34	9.1	27.3	75	79.7	1225	373
MS	Scott	-1.15	2215	38	13.6	35	69.3	77.8	422	128
NJ	Camden	-1.15	2216	27.8	9.2	27.9	74	79.7	86	26
VA	Culpeper	-1.15	2217	32.2	9.8	23.9	74.7	79.6	380	116
AL	Butler	-1.16	2218	41.3	14.6	35.9	69.6	77.2	385	117
IN	Johnson	-1.16	2219	29	9.9	27.6	76	80.3	778	237
MO	Pemiscot	-1.16	2220	38.2	10	35.8	68.5	76.5	261	79
NC	Johnston	-1.16	2221	33.9	10.5	27.7	73.2	79.4	204	62
VT	Caledonia	-1.16	2222	25.5	7.1	20.7	76.1	81.4	1350	411
KS	Osage	-1.17	2223	35.3	9.2	27.3	75.3	80.4	1095	334
MS	Humphreys	-1.17	2224	41.4	13.6	33.4	66.5	74.1	101	31
MS	Tippah	-1.17	2225	35.2	11.7	39.4	70.6	77.9	517	158
WI	Buffalo	-1.17	2226	32.4	7.9	23.3	76.8	81.8	947	289
KS	Stevens	-1.18	2227	29.9	9.7	26.4	74.6	79.4	3101	945
TN	Fayette	-1.18	2228	35.3	11.9	30.4	72.3	78.3	397	121
IA	Guthrie	-1.19	2229	30.3	6.6	25.8	76.2	82	1206	368
IL	Franklin	-1.19	2230	29.6	8.8	28.9	72.2	78.6	435	133
MO	Harrison	-1.19	2231	32.5	9	30.3	74.9	80.2	974	297
GA	Jackson	-1.20	2232	25.6	10.2	25.5	72.2	78.6	827	252
IL	Perry	-1.20	2233	29.3	8.3	29.8	73.4	79.1	462	141
KY	Daviess	-1.20	2234	30.5	10.1	27.8	74.3	79.7	429	131

ST	COUNTY	USDA	AMEN	OBES	DIAB	INACT	M AGE	W AGE	ALT ft	ALT m
MI	Roscommon	-1.20	2235	36.1	9.7	30.3	73.8	79.9	1169	356
MO	Ralls	-1.20	2236	30.5	8.5	27.9	74.4	80.1	679	207
PA	Fulton	-1.20	2237	29.7	8.9	26	74.6	80.4	1118	341
TN	Lincoln	-1.20	2238	34.1	9.2	33.6	72.8	79	848	258
GA	Banks	-1.21	2239	27.3	9.8	24.2	72.9	79	862	263
KS	Sheridan	-1.21	2240	29.9	7.7	25.7	76.3	81.5	2727	831
MI	Luce	-1.21	2241	31.8	9.1	26.6	75	80.3	780	238
MS	Hinds	-1.21	2242	36	12.4	35.2	71.1	79	259	79
NE	Boone	-1.21	2243	28.6	6.9	28.1	75.6	80.5	1904	580
SD	Day	-1.21	2244	31.9	6.9	28.5	74.9	81.2	1739	530
WI	Pierce	-1.21	2245	25.8	7.2	21	77.3	82.1	1025	312
KY	Larue	-1.22	2246	33	11.6	30.9	72.4	78.2	781	238
LA	Ascension	-1.22	2247	31.8	9.7	28.5	73.3	78.9	9	3
MT	Hill	-1.22	2248	32.4	7.3	28.8	74.6	80.7	2969	905
VA	Caroline	-1.22	2249	30.8	10.5	23.5	71.7	78.9	162	49
KY	Garrard	-1.23	2250	33.3	11.1	35.2	74.5	78.8	918	280
MI	Sanilac	-1.23	2251	35.4	8.8	27.8	75.2	79.5	765	233
MS	Smith	-1.23	2252	34.3	11.3	35	69.6	77	384	117
NC	Wilson	-1.23	2253	32.2	11.2	30.9	71.1	77.6	128	39
SD	Charles Mix	-1.23	2254	35.6	9.6	29	75	80.9	1567	478
AR	Drew	-1.24	2255	35.9	11	32.8	71.8	77.4	190	58
AR	Lincoln	-1.24	2256	36.2	10.6	31.3	71.8	77.4	200	61
LA	East Carroll	-1.24	2257	36.2	13.4	32.8	70.1	76.2	87	26
MI	Macomb	-1.24	2258	30.8	9.4	24.6	75.6	80.5	680	207
MO	Mercer	-1.24	2259	31.9	8.7	33	74.8	80.2	965	294
AL	Madison	-1.25	2260	31.3	11.2	24.9	74.7	79.3	795	242
KS	Cowley	-1.25	2261	32.9	8.5	28.4	73.1	79.9	1249	381
KY	Lincoln	-1.25	2262	40.1	11.7	37.8	71.7	78.2	1060	323
MI	St. Clair	-1.25	2263	30.6	9.3	24	75.5	79.8	697	213
NC	Hertford	-1.25	2264	35.5	12	33.6	69.8	75.8	40	12
OK	Garfield	-1.25	2265	32.5	8.4	28.9	73.9	79.3	1167	356
KS	Comanche	-1.26	2266	29.3	7.7	28.8	75.4	80	1937	590
KS	Harper	-1.26	2267	28.5	8.8	31.5	75.3	80.1	1374	419
MO	Linn	-1.26	2268	37.5	8.8	32.9	74.2	80.2	815	248
NC	Hoke	-1.26	2269	33.2	12.7	29.4	71	76.9	278	85
NY	Jefferson	-1.27	2270	31.3	8.7	26.8	75.8	80.7	544	166
AR	St. Francis	-1.28	2271	37.8	12.1	39.8	69.4	75.3	215	65
KS	Barber	-1.28	2272	34.5	8.9	32.4	75.3	80.1	1639	500
KS	Graham	-1.28	2273	32.2	8.2	23.6	76.3	81.5	2345	715
KY	Powell	-1.28	2274	35.4	12.8	40.4	70.8	77.6	915	279
OH	Jackson	-1.28	2275	33.8	11.2	37.5	71.4	78.2	782	238
SD	Lyman	-1.28	2276	36.7	9.3	32.1	76.2	81.5	1765	538
IL	Henderson	-1.29	2277	30.5	8	26.2	75.9	80.9	630	192
MS	Franklin	-1.29	2278	39	12.6	37.9	70.8	77.6	322	98
WI	Richland	-1.29	2279	31.3	7.8	24	76.2	81.1	953	290
MI	Newaygo	-1.30	2280	34.5	11.5	25.2	75	79.8	885	270

HEALTHIEST PLACES TO LIVE

ST	COUNTY	USDA	AMEN	OBES	DIAB	INACT	M AGE	W AGE	ALT ft	ALT m
MS	Alcorn	-1.30	2281	32.8	10.7	33.8	71.9	77.9	490	149
NC	Halifax	-1.30	2282	38.7	12.6	33.3	69.5	76.9	153	47
ND	Morton	-1.30	2283	30.9	7.1	26	74.6	80.6	2049	624
NJ	Burlington	-1.30	2284	27.2	8.4	23.4	76.5	81.3	70	21
VA	Fairfax	-1.31	2285	23.2	8.1	18.7	81.1	83.8	266	81
VA	Fairfax City	-1.31	2286	28.1	9	26.6	76.6	82.1	390	119
VA	Falls Church	-1.31	2287	26.1	8.9	21.7	79.7	83.3	324	99
KY	Marion	-1.32	2288	33.8	10.6	34.7	73.3	79.6	790	241
NE	Knox	-1.32	2289	27.8	7.2	29.5	75.3	81.4	1595	486
TN	Van Buren	-1.32	2290	33	10.2	32.9	71.6	78.2	1547	471
KS	Lincoln	-1.33	2291	28.3	7.6	24.2	75.2	80.7	1515	462
MT	Fallon	-1.33	2292	25	6.3	30.8	75.7	81	3018	920
KS	Sherman	-1.34	2293	32.2	9.7	26.9	76	80.6	3657	1115
MD	Carroll	-1.34	2294	27.5	8	20.8	76.6	80.5	646	197
MS	Sharkey	-1.34	2295	40.2	13.3	35.2	66.5	74.1	92	28
VA	Dinwiddie	-1.34	2296	33.3	10.4	24.1	71.3	78.6	220	67
VA	Petersburg	-1.34	2297	37.8	13.5	32.5	66.9	76.2	95	29
WA	Adams	-1.34	2298	36.8	10.4	26.7	74.2	79.4	1590	485
AR	Calhoun	-1.35	2299	34.5	10.5	35.2	70.8	77.4	171	52
LA	Franklin	-1.35	2300	36.2	10.6	36	70	76.6	66	20
ND	Mountrail	-1.35	2301	35	8.3	33.3	75.7	81.4	2190	668
KY	Breathitt	-1.36	2302	39.6	14.7	33.7	68.2	76.1	1045	318
VA	Lee	-1.36	2303	34.2	10.6	33.2	70.4	77	1776	541
WI	Brown	-1.36	2304	29.5	7.9	20.1	77.4	82	746	227
WI	Monroe	-1.36	2305	28.7	8.2	24.6	74.4	80.1	1050	320
WV	Harrison	-1.36	2306	32.4	11.7	31.2	72.7	79.3	1190	363
MI	Oscoda	-1.37	2307	31.6	9.8	26.7	75.2	79.6	1136	346
SD	Hamlin	-1.37	2308	30.1	7.5	28.3	74.9	80.6	1738	530
WI	St. Croix	-1.37	2309	27.9	7	17	77.8	82.2	1065	324
WI	Winnebago	-1.37	2310	29.4	7.7	19.4	76.6	81.5	788	240
WV	Wyoming	-1.37	2311	35.8	14.3	40.9	69.5	76.6	1898	579
KS	Marshall	-1.38	2312	34.5	8.1	25.3	76.3	81.7	1305	398
MN	Goodhue	-1.38	2313	27.5	7.4	18.1	77.7	82	1048	319
OH	Logan	-1.38	2314	32.6	10.8	29.7	74.5	79.4	1114	340
SD	Potter	-1.38	2315	28.1	6.7	26.8	72.9	79.9	1928	588
WV	Monroe	-1.38	2316	29.6	11.7	30.1	72.6	79.2	2308	704
MO	Mississippi	-1.39	2317	31.4	9.7	37.3	69.9	76.9	305	93
NC	Nash	-1.39	2318	33.6	10.7	28.3	71.9	78.5	187	57
NC	Orange	-1.39	2319	22.6	6.5	16.5	77.4	81.5	604	184
OH	Hamilton	-1.39	2320	26.9	9.2	24.4	73.9	79.4	708	216
IA	Wapello	-1.40	2321	29.1	8.7	25.5	75.1	80.8	782	238
MI	Chippewa	-1.40	2322	31.4	10	22.9	75.9	80.7	722	220
ND	Kidder	-1.40	2323	30.7	7.3	29.6	75.2	81.3	1852	564
NE	Custer	-1.40	2324	29.5	6.8	29.3	75.6	81.2	2616	797
MS	Leflore	-1.41	2325	39	13.8	35.2	68.5	75.5	122	37
NC	Wayne	-1.41	2326	32.8	10.9	31.4	71.6	77.6	126	38

ST	COUNTY	USDA	AMEN	OBES	DIAB	INACT	M AGE	W AGE	ALT ft	ALT m
ND	McLean	-1.41	2327	30.9	7.3	29.4	75.8	80.8	1966	599
NE	Logan	-1.41	2328	27.6	6.9	26.6	76.1	80.2	2988	911
NY	Chenango	-1.41	2329	27	7.1	23.9	74.9	79.8	1448	441
OH	Ottawa	-1.41	2330	33.3	9.5	24	75.1	79.9	589	180
GA	Schley	-1.42	2331	30.4	11.3	27.3	70.9	77	483	147
KS	Pratt	-1.42	2332	32	7.5	29.2	75.4	80.6	1923	586
MD	Howard	-1.42	2333	24.4	7.3	17.6	79.8	82.6	442	135
NE	Garfield	-1.42	2334	27.2	6.8	23.8	76.2	80.7	2281	695
NE	Loup	-1.42	2335	29.2	7.5	27.1	75.6	81.2	2424	739
WI	Sawyer	-1.42	2336	26.6	7.7	21.9	75.5	80.4	1377	420
WI	Trempealeau	-1.42	2337	32.9	7.6	24.9	75.4	81.2	930	283
IL	Pulaski	-1.43	2338	31.4	9.8	29.3	69.9	77	367	112
KS	Allen	-1.43	2339	34.5	9	26.2	74.7	79.4	1018	310
KS	Logan	-1.43	2340	32.4	8.9	29.4	76.3	81.5	3090	942
KY	Nicholas	-1.43	2341	33.6	11.4	34.9	72.5	78	851	259
MI	Monroe	-1.43	2342	34.7	10.1	27	74.6	79.7	635	194
NC	Franklin	-1.43	2343	34.2	9.8	28.1	72.4	78.8	314	96
IA	Taylor	-1.44	2344	30.2	7.2	23.5	76.4	80.9	1204	367
MO	Scott	-1.44	2345	34.4	10	32.7	73	79	345	105
NJ	Somerset	-1.44	2346	21.3	6.2	21.2	78.7	82.5	196	60
NY	Cayuga	-1.44	2347	24.3	7.9	24.9	76	80.8	781	238
TN	Madison	-1.44	2348	34.3	10.9	28.8	72.7	78.9	434	132
VA	Brunswick	-1.44	2349	36.2	12.2	28.9	69.9	76.6	279	85
IA	Sac	-1.45	2350	29.1	7.1	24.9	76.3	81.2	1331	406
IN	Franklin	-1.45	2351	27.9	11	25.5	74.7	80.7	902	275
KS	Wallace	-1.45	2352	32	8	27.6	75.9	81.2	3620	1103
LA	Beauregard	-1.45	2353	32.6	10.8	30.2	72.2	77.7	114	35
SD	Campbell	-1.45	2354	29.4	6.7	33	74.1	80.3	1807	551
SD	Walworth	-1.45	2355	33.2	8.8	30.5	74.1	80.3	1916	584
TN	Warren	-1.45	2356	34.9	10.1	30.8	71.4	78	1111	339
KY	Clay	-1.46	2357	32.4	13.2	35.4	69.2	76.1	1178	359
LA	East Feliciana	-1.46	2358	34.9	11.9	27.6	69.9	76.7	197	60
TN	Giles	-1.46	2359	36.5	9.9	30	72.2	78.9	831	253
AR	Woodruff	-1.47	2360	34.2	10.6	33.9	70.9	77.3	198	60
KY	Barren	-1.47	2361	29.2	11.8	30.4	73.4	78.6	725	221
MO	Knox	-1.47	2362	31.9	8.6	29.4	73.8	79.8	774	236
MS	Sunflower	-1.47	2363	41.4	14.4	34.6	67.1	73.6	122	37
NE	Chase	-1.47	2364	26.1	6.8	26.4	76.1	81.4	3335	1017
MO	Marion	-1.48	2365	29	7.9	30.2	74	79.2	621	189
SD	Jones	-1.48	2366	31.9	6.9	30.6	76.6	81.5	2070	631
KS	Cloud	-1.49	2367	31.3	9.7	23	75.8	81.2	1444	440
KY	Knox	-1.49	2368	35.6	13.2	35.6	69.9	76.4	1238	377
MO	Clinton	-1.49	2369	31	9.9	29	74.2	80.1	981	299
MO	Jackson	-1.49	2370	32.5	8.9	25.4	73.2	79.2	894	272
OH	Highland	-1.49	2371	31.9	9.3	33.6	73.1	78.9	983	299
OK	Craig	-1.49	2372	34.7	10.9	32.7	73.2	79	803	245

HEALTHIEST PLACES TO LIVE

ST	COUNTY	USDA	AMEN	OBES	DIAB	INACT	M AGE	W AGE	ALT ft	ALT m
OK	Major	-1.49	2373	30.9	8.9	32.4	74.4	79.7	1421	433
VA	Charlotte	-1.49	2374	30.7	9.8	25.6	71.1	78.1	491	150
WI	Calumet	-1.49	2375	30.2	6.9	18.6	78.3	82.3	853	260
KS	Rawlins	-1.50	2376	33.3	7.8	26.3	76	80.6	3060	933
KS	Scott	-1.50	2377	29.1	7.2	23.1	75.9	81.2	2984	910
KY	Allen	-1.50	2378	33.5	10.6	28.6	71.5	77.9	689	210
VA	Cumberland	-1.50	2379	33.8	11	27.8	72.4	78.7	335	102
IA	Dickinson	-1.51	2380	26.6	6.8	20.9	78	82.1	1470	448
IA	Woodbury	-1.51	2381	30.5	8.4	29.1	75.4	80.5	1230	375
IN	Union	-1.51	2382	32.2	9.5	25.3	74.7	80.7	973	296
NC	Duplin	-1.51	2383	34.5	11.5	33.1	71.3	78.3	89	27
IL	Putnam	-1.52	2384	28.1	7.9	27	75.9	80.7	591	180
KS	Stafford	-1.52	2385	33.6	8.7	31.1	74.9	80.1	1901	579
KY	McLean	-1.52	2386	31.3	11.2	34.1	72.4	78.9	416	127
MN	Houston	-1.52	2387	26.5	7.1	19.1	76.9	81.8	974	297
MO	New Madrid	-1.52	2388	31.8	10	30.3	69.9	76.9	283	86
NC	Robeson	-1.52	2389	40.9	13.3	38.5	68.7	76.8	150	46
VA	Amelia	-1.52	2390	32.5	9.4	25	72.4	78.7	303	92
WV	Upshur	-1.52	2391	30.4	12.5	30.1	73.3	78.7	1807	551
IN	Posey	-1.53	2392	30.2	9.3	26.7	75.1	80.9	402	123
KS	Linn	-1.53	2393	34.8	8.8	28.8	74.7	79.4	931	284
MI	Bay	-1.53	2394	34.5	9.2	24.7	74.7	80.4	632	193
PA	Chester	-1.53	2395	20.8	7.5	18.5	77.9	82.2	442	135
VA	Fauquier	-1.53	2396	26.4	8.7	20.5	76.7	80.8	528	161
WI	Lafayette	-1.53	2397	31	7.2	21.5	75.8	81.2	954	291
KS	Ness	-1.54	2398	29.1	8.2	24.8	75.2	80.6	2379	725
SD	Brule	-1.54	2399	34.6	6.5	32.3	75	80.8	1663	507
WI	Dunn	-1.54	2400	29.1	6.5	23.9	76.3	81.6	983	300
ND	Golden Valley	-1.55	2401	30.2	6.6	30.2	75.7	82.2	2696	822
NY	Cortland	-1.55	2402	26.7	7.8	26.7	75.2	80.2	1479	451
VA	Smyth	-1.55	2403	32.7	8.2	23.3	71.7	78.1	2679	816
IN	Gibson	-1.56	2404	28	8.6	26.5	74.8	80	439	134
LA	Acadia	-1.56	2405	32.5	8.9	31.6	70	76.7	27	8
MO	Scotland	-1.56	2406	34.4	7.9	27.9	74	80.2	759	231
MO	Worth	-1.56	2407	30.4	8.6	28.3	74.9	80.2	1035	315
NE	Franklin	-1.56	2408	28.5	7.8	31.8	75.6	80.3	2038	621
LA	Washington	-1.57	2409	34.3	13.5	34.7	68.8	75.7	204	62
VA	Nottoway	-1.57	2410	32.7	10.3	27.2	71.6	77.6	372	114
KS	Thomas	-1.58	2411	31.4	8.1	20.8	76	80.6	3170	966
MO	Sullivan	-1.58	2412	28.7	9.3	29.1	73.9	80	927	282
WI	Green Lake	-1.58	2413	30.1	8	23.9	76.3	81	857	261
WI	Vilas	-1.58	2414	26.2	6.4	23.2	77	81.8	1672	510
AR	Cleveland	-1.59	2415	32.9	10.7	27.5	72	78.3	224	68
IA	Adair	-1.59	2416	30.7	8	28.7	76.1	82.6	1276	389
KS	Morton	-1.59	2417	33.1	8.1	29.8	74.6	79.4	3429	1045
KS	Stanton	-1.59	2418	31.2	8.5	25.5	75.9	81.2	3367	1026

ST	COUNTY	USDA	AMEN	OBES	DIAB	INACT	M AGE	W AGE	ALT ft	ALT m
NC	Jones	-1.59	2419	34.8	12.1	31.4	71.3	78.3	45	14
NY	Herkimer	-1.59	2420	31.9	8	26.1	75.4	79.8	1534	468
SD	Bon Homme	-1.59	2421	30.4	7.5	30.1	75	80.9	1432	437
SD	Buffalo	-1.59	2422	41.2	17.2	36.8	75.8	81.4	1650	503
AL	DeKalb	-1.60	2423	34	10.3	27	71.9	78.1	1216	371
MO	Vernon	-1.60	2424	34	9.4	30.5	73.2	78.6	824	251
ND	Mercer	-1.60	2425	31.5	8.1	27.1	75.8	80.8	2015	614
OH	Delaware	-1.60	2426	25.5	8.8	21.6	77.5	81.2	942	287
IN	Steuben	-1.61	2427	31.9	10.9	27.3	75.2	80.5	999	305
KS	Republic	-1.61	2428	32.7	8.3	26.5	76.3	81.7	1537	468
MI	Menominee	-1.61	2429	30.9	8.3	25.6	76.2	81	799	243
MN	Winona	-1.61	2430	30.5	7.2	19.5	77.3	82.2	1063	324
NE	Thomas	-1.61	2431	33.3	7.2	27.7	75.6	81.2	2979	908
VA	Buchanan	-1.61	2432	33.6	12.3	30.8	69	76.7	1876	572
WV	Randolph	-1.61	2433	33.6	11.3	32.7	73.3	79.2	2938	896
KS	Rice	-1.62	2434	37.4	9	23.8	74.9	80.1	1694	516
KY	Kenton	-1.62	2435	30.2	10.1	27.1	73.5	78.6	767	234
TN	Weakley	-1.62	2436	31.9	10.1	34.9	72.9	78.4	399	121
AR	Columbia	-1.63	2437	32.2	11.8	29	71.8	77.7	271	83
IL	Hancock	-1.63	2438	27.9	8	29	76	81.2	632	193
MI	Tuscola	-1.63	2439	30.6	9	26.4	74.7	79.7	709	216
NC	Sampson	-1.63	2440	35.8	10.9	28.4	70.9	77.6	124	38
NE	Furnas	-1.63	2441	33.2	8.2	25.7	75.6	80.3	2287	697
WI	Jefferson	-1.63	2442	32.1	7.9	21.8	76.8	82.5	848	259
NE	Hooker	-1.64	2443	33.4	7.3	26.7	76.1	80.2	3386	1032
MO	Bates	-1.65	2444	30.1	8.9	27.4	73.8	79.5	848	259
NY	Oneida	-1.65	2445	28.7	8.1	25.7	75.5	80.7	899	274
OH	Butler	-1.65	2446	31.2	11.3	26	74.9	79	788	240
SD	Marshall	-1.65	2447	28.6	8.1	29.2	74.9	81.2	1559	475
SD	Meade	-1.66	2448	25.9	7.5	27	74.8	80.5	2760	841
WV	Roane	-1.66	2449	34.2	12.9	32.2	72	78	939	286
IA	Montgomery	-1.67	2450	30.5	7.7	24.4	76.2	81.1	1161	354
KS	Ottawa	-1.67	2451	32	7.7	31.2	75.5	80.1	1345	410
KY	Magoffin	-1.67	2452	32.1	11.8	41.1	70.8	76.9	1076	328
KY	Owsley	-1.67	2453	32.7	11	33.6	68.2	76.1	1025	313
NE	Holt	-1.67	2454	28.7	7.4	30.8	75.6	80.9	2041	622
VA	Prince Edward	-1.67	2455	32	9.9	29	71.5	77	462	141
WV	Mercer	-1.67	2456	34.3	11	33.6	71	77.5	2462	750
IL	Jersey	-1.68	2457	27.1	7.4	27.2	75.3	79.8	575	175
IL	Wabash	-1.68	2458	28.4	7.9	28.8	75.2	80.1	430	131
MD	Caroline	-1.68	2459	32.1	11.1	29.2	73.2	78.7	40	12
MI	Lake	-1.68	2460	32.4	10	24.5	74.1	78.9	969	295
MO	Cass	-1.68	2461	33.1	9.8	27.1	75	79.4	921	281
NE	Cheyenne	-1.68	2462	29.1	6.8	24	75.8	80.7	4268	1301
SD	Deuel	-1.68	2463	33.1	6.5	26.7	76.2	82.2	1771	540
SD	Roberts	-1.68	2464	36.8	9.5	29.2	74.9	81.2	1320	402

HEALTHIEST PLACES TO LIVE

ST	COUNTY	USDA	AMEN	OBES	DIAB	INACT	M AGE	W AGE	ALT ft	ALT m
IL	Madison	-1.69	2465	29.7	9.6	27.3	74.5	79.5	512	156
IL	Massac	-1.69	2466	31.4	8.8	29.5	72.8	78.8	394	120
KS	Johnson	-1.69	2467	23.6	6.4	17.5	78.9	82.6	991	302
MI	Gogebic	-1.69	2468	30.9	8.4	24.7	75	80.7	1481	451
TN	McNairy	-1.69	2469	37.3	11	32.1	71.4	78.4	490	149
IA	Carroll	-1.70	2470	30.8	6.2	27.9	76.7	82	1311	400
IN	Daviess	-1.70	2471	32.3	9.7	26.3	74.2	79.8	494	150
MO	Lafayette	-1.70	2472	30.8	8.4	26.8	73.9	79.9	804	245
TN	Haywood	-1.70	2473	36.3	12.1	32.6	68.8	77	333	101
KS	Harvey	-1.71	2474	29.2	7.5	23.6	76	80.9	1445	440
NC	Lenoir	-1.71	2475	32.4	11.4	33.2	70.6	77.8	77	24
NE	Dixon	-1.71	2476	33.9	6.7	30.3	74.8	79.6	1406	429
KY	Harrison	-1.72	2477	30	11.6	33.5	72.5	78	808	246
OH	Mahoning	-1.72	2478	28.9	9.3	26.8	73.3	79.6	1087	331
MI	Wayne	-1.73	2479	34	11.6	27.6	71.9	78	642	196
NE	Burt	-1.73	2480	30.9	8.1	31.5	74.2	79.8	1226	374
SD	Codington	-1.73	2481	30	6.3	26.6	76.2	82.2	1813	553
IL	Jefferson	-1.74	2482	32.4	9	29.4	74.3	79.7	489	149
MN	Aitkin	-1.74	2483	27.9	7.6	20.2	76.2	81.6	1274	388
MN	Mille Lacs	-1.74	2484	26.5	7.1	22.6	75.1	80.6	1185	361
NC	Pitt	-1.74	2485	35.6	9.3	25.3	72.9	78	46	14
ND	Stark	-1.74	2486	29.2	7.8	27.1	75.7	81.6	2498	761
IN	Pike	-1.75	2487	30.5	9.2	28.1	74.8	80	479	146
KS	Wilson	-1.75	2488	34.9	9	25.3	74	79.6	919	280
LA	Richland	-1.75	2489	36.3	10.4	29.1	69.3	75.3	71	22
VA	Clarke	-1.75	2490	28.4	8.8	23.4	75.2	79.8	631	192
AR	Mississippi	-1.76	2491	38.8	12.1	42	68.7	76.2	234	71
KS	Shawnee	-1.76	2492	32.8	8.9	23.4	74.6	80.4	1007	307
MO	Gentry	-1.76	2493	31.2	9.5	28.2	74.9	80.2	951	290
NE	Dakota	-1.76	2494	34.5	9.3	30.9	74.8	79.6	1227	374
NE	Red Willow	-1.76	2495	30.8	7.6	24.2	76	81	2551	777
SD	Yankton	-1.76	2496	33.2	7.2	23.4	76.9	81.5	1333	406
AR	Grant	-1.77	2497	35.7	9.2	33.1	73.7	79.6	252	77
IL	Fulton	-1.77	2498	30.3	7.3	29.9	73.9	79.8	604	184
MI	Oakland	-1.78	2499	27	8.7	20.3	77.3	81.5	935	285
SD	Union	-1.78	2500	29.9	5.9	23.7	77.4	82.7	1253	382
IA	Cass	-1.79	2501	35.7	6.5	25.3	77	81.6	1270	387
KS	Gove	-1.79	2502	31.1	9	27.7	76.3	81.5	2676	816
ND	Grant	-1.79	2503	37.9	7	29.8	75.7	81.6	2239	682
ND	Stutsman	-1.79	2504	30	7.7	26.9	75.2	81.3	1674	510
KS	Greeley	-1.80	2505	34.1	8.5	28.6	75.9	81.2	3661	1116
KS	Wichita	-1.80	2506	31.9	8.8	28.7	75.9	81.2	3295	1004
IL	St. Clair	-1.81	2507	29.7	8.8	28.7	72.2	78.5	466	142
IN	Warrick	-1.81	2508	31.4	9.5	22.8	76.2	79.7	437	133
KS	McPherson	-1.81	2509	31.2	8.4	24	76.7	81.3	1501	458
ND	Emmons	-1.81	2510	32.1	7.5	28.6	74.6	80.6	1893	577

ST	COUNTY	USDA	AMEN	OBES	DIAB	INACT	M AGE	W AGE	ALT ft	ALT m
ND	Hettinger	-1.81	2511	27.2	7	29.1	75.7	81.6	2571	784
IA	Mahaska	-1.82	2512	28	7.4	29.4	76.3	81.6	808	246
IL	White	-1.82	2513	28.9	8.1	30.7	73.5	79.5	403	123
MI	Livingston	-1.82	2514	26.2	7.6	19	77.2	81.2	935	285
ND	Adams	-1.82	2515	30.6	7.5	26.2	75.7	81.6	2654	809
IA	Louisa	-1.83	2516	33.8	7	26.8	76.4	82	623	190
IA	Page	-1.83	2517	32.6	8.5	28.2	76.3	80.7	1107	337
IA	Union	-1.83	2518	30.2	7.2	27.6	76.5	81.5	1219	371
NE	Hall	-1.83	2519	31.6	8	26.1	75.1	80.8	1931	589
WI	Dodge	-1.83	2520	35.8	7.4	23.7	76.1	80.8	920	280
OH	Adams	-1.84	2521	30.7	9.1	33.6	72.2	77.8	850	259
AR	Dallas	-1.85	2522	34.2	10.7	32.8	70.8	77.4	276	84
AR	Jackson	-1.85	2523	32	11	35.8	70.6	76.9	255	78
KS	Bourbon	-1.85	2524	34.8	7.9	26.1	74.6	79.4	919	280
LA	Morehouse	-1.85	2525	37.8	11.6	35.7	69.5	75.6	90	28
NE	Nuckolls	-1.85	2526	30.3	6.8	27.6	76.8	81.8	1719	524
VA	Powhatan	-1.85	2527	27.1	8.8	26.9	75.9	80.1	275	84
IL	Mason	-1.86	2528	30.5	7.6	28.6	74.4	79.5	502	153
SD	Lake	-1.86	2529	32.3	6.9	26.6	76.8	82.3	1704	519
TN	Gibson	-1.86	2530	37.3	11	37.3	70.3	77.5	371	113
IL	Rock Island	-1.87	2531	27.2	7.6	26.4	75.7	81	654	199
IN	LaPorte	-1.87	2532	30.9	9.7	25.9	73.7	80.1	729	222
SD	Clay	-1.87	2533	32.5	6.4	23.6	77.4	82.7	1230	375
IL	Pike	-1.88	2534	28.2	7.6	26	75	80.5	601	183
NE	Nemaha	-1.88	2535	33.2	7.3	29	75.4	80.8	1049	320
NE	Webster	-1.88	2536	30.5	8.5	31.1	76.8	81.8	1880	573
OH	Mercer	-1.88	2537	27.4	9.4	26.1	75.7	80.7	872	266
WV	McDowell	-1.88	2538	32.6	14.2	42.1	66.3	74.7	1869	570
IA	Crawford	-1.89	2539	31.4	7	30.8	75.4	81.7	1361	415
IL	Marshall	-1.89	2540	26.1	7.7	28.5	74.9	80.3	656	200
KY	Scott	-1.89	2541	32.5	10.1	31.7	74.9	80.4	871	265
MI	Ogemaw	-1.89	2542	34	9	29.2	73.1	78.6	1033	315
ND	Sheridan	-1.89	2543	30.7	7.3	29.5	74.3	81.1	1865	568
IA	Ringgold	-1.90	2544	29.4	6.9	26.1	76.4	80.9	1174	358
IA	Wayne	-1.90	2545	33.5	6.7	25.1	74.7	80.9	1042	318
MI	Genesee	-1.90	2546	35.9	10.6	29.7	73.2	78.6	787	240
MO	Schuyler	-1.90	2547	32	9.1	28.4	74.8	80.2	892	272
WV	Boone	-1.90	2548	34.3	13.8	40.2	69.9	76.7	1340	408
KY	Robertson	-1.91	2549	32	10.8	33.9	72.3	78.5	782	238
NE	Richardson	-1.91	2550	33.1	8.3	31.5	75.4	80.8	1022	312
TN	Carroll	-1.91	2551	37.5	11.1	33	70.1	77.2	469	143
IN	Scott	-1.92	2552	28.9	10.8	31.5	72	77.9	626	191
NE	Douglas	-1.92	2553	27.1	8.1	23.6	75.6	80.7	1159	353
SD	Kingsbury	-1.92	2554	27.1	5.7	29	74.9	80.6	1667	508
TN	Robertson	-1.92	2555	32.2	11.5	33.1	72.8	78.5	664	202
WI	Fond du Lac	-1.92	2556	30.7	7.3	25	76.5	81.4	940	287

ST	COUNTY	USDA	AMEN	OBES	DIAB	INACT	M AGE	W AGE	ALT ft	ALT m
IN	Noble	-1.93	2557	30.6	9.4	27.2	74.4	79.9	929	283
MO	Barton	-1.93	2558	32.5	9.6	27.7	73.9	80	944	288
NE	Dundy	-1.93	2559	30.2	8.2	30.4	76.1	81.4	3287	1002
IA	Audubon	-1.94	2560	33.1	7.8	26.5	76.1	82.6	1380	421
IL	Cass	-1.94	2561	29.3	8.2	29.1	74.8	80	533	162
MI	Delta	-1.94	2562	30.1	8.7	24.3	76.5	80.9	733	224
MI	Mecosta	-1.94	2563	32.6	9.6	25.5	75.3	80.6	1002	306
IA	Lee	-1.95	2564	30.6	7.3	26.7	74.5	80.1	646	197
MI	Missaukee	-1.95	2565	33.4	9.7	25.1	75.1	79	1213	370
WI	Oconto	-1.95	2566	27.6	6.9	23.9	75.9	81.3	872	266
IA	Davis	-1.96	2567	30.7	7.2	27.9	74.7	80.9	841	256
IL	Moultrie	-1.96	2568	28.3	8.2	28.5	75.1	81	662	202
NE	Thurston	-1.96	2569	37.1	12.9	34.2	74.2	79.8	1345	410
IL	Fayette	-1.97	2570	30	7.7	30.9	73.6	79.2	550	168
KS	Franklin	-1.97	2571	33.5	9.2	27.1	75.7	79.6	986	300
KY	Casey	-1.97	2572	36.5	12.2	35.6	71.1	78.2	1008	307
MS	Quitman	-1.97	2573	40.1	15.1	34.8	66	74.1	156	48
OH	Greene	-1.97	2574	29.6	9.3	22.7	76.5	80.5	966	294
OH	Preble	-1.97	2575	30	9.9	28.5	74.7	79.8	1035	315
IN	Knox	-1.98	2576	31.9	8.9	32.9	73.5	79.9	462	141
SD	McPherson	-1.98	2577	29.2	6.4	25.8	74.1	80.3	1827	557
KY	Jessamine	-1.99	2578	30.4	11.4	30.6	74.3	79.5	886	270
PA	Crawford	-1.99	2579	28.6	10.1	24.9	74.8	80.1	1299	396
AR	Greene	-2.00	2580	34.4	10	27	72.7	78.5	302	92
MO	Johnson	-2.00	2581	33.5	10.1	29.5	74.6	80.1	830	253
IA	Shelby	-2.01	2582	32.1	7.6	24.1	77	81.6	1335	407
IL	Bond	-2.01	2583	29.1	8.6	30.8	74.1	79.5	537	164
ND	Burleigh	-2.01	2584	25	6.9	21.1	77.4	83	1900	579
ND	Ward	-2.01	2585	30.2	8.1	27.4	75.7	81.4	1934	589
ND	Williams	-2.01	2586	30.1	7.3	30.8	76.5	81.9	2205	672
NE	Cedar	-2.01	2587	27.9	6.9	28.6	76.5	82	1486	453
TN	Chester	-2.01	2588	36.4	11.1	28.3	72.9	78.2	492	150
LA	St. Helena	-2.02	2589	36.4	13	33.9	69.9	76.7	210	64
NE	Sarpy	-2.03	2590	28.9	7.7	20.8	77.6	80.9	1121	342
OH	Clark	-2.03	2591	31.8	10.4	29.1	73.5	78.5	1050	320
IA	Decatur	-2.04	2592	29.4	6.6	25.3	75.5	80.8	1054	321
IA	Des Moines	-2.04	2593	33.8	8.5	28.5	75.9	81.6	691	210
IN	Dearborn	-2.04	2594	32.7	9.5	28	75.3	80.6	796	243
KY	Woodford	-2.04	2595	31.5	9.6	27.3	75.5	80.1	811	247
MO	Livingston	-2.04	2596	28.4	9.3	32.5	74.2	80.2	770	235
NE	Wheeler	-2.04	2597	26.8	6.9	28.6	76.2	80.7	2104	641
IN	Wabash	-2.05	2598	35.7	9.3	25.2	74.9	80.5	779	237
MN	Jackson	-2.05	2599	30.3	6.6	22.2	77.5	82.9	1435	437
MO	Pettis	-2.05	2600	29.5	8.4	31.8	74.7	79.7	825	251
MO	Daviess	-2.06	2601	32.2	9.1	27.4	74.9	80.2	870	265
ND	Divide	-2.06	2602	29.8	6.5	30.5	76.5	81.9	2146	654

ST	COUNTY	USDA	AMEN	OBES	DIAB	INACT	M AGE	W AGE	ALT ft	ALT m
NY	Schenectady	-2.06	2603	27.9	8.7	24.3	76	81.2	713	217
SD	Brookings	-2.06	2604	27	6	22.6	77	81.8	1710	521
IN	Sullivan	-2.07	2605	31.2	8.8	32.1	73.1	79	507	154
KS	Doniphan	-2.07	2606	35.6	8.5	27.6	75.2	79.9	985	300
KS	Pawnee	-2.07	2607	34	8.8	28.7	75.2	80.6	2089	637
ND	Burke	-2.07	2608	28.8	7.8	30.1	76.5	81.9	2108	643
OH	Clinton	-2.07	2609	28.7	9.8	31.7	74.7	80	1017	310
IL	Schuyler	-2.08	2610	27	7.4	29.9	74.4	79.5	584	178
KS	Kiowa	-2.08	2611	31.2	7.8	24.4	75.4	80	2185	666
MN	Ramsey	-2.08	2612	24.1	7	15	77.4	82.5	918	280
VA	Hanover	-2.08	2613	26.4	8.4	19.9	76.5	80.8	181	55
IA	Emmet	-2.10	2614	31.4	7.4	27.2	75.7	81.2	1304	397
IL	Adams	-2.10	2615	30.7	8.7	32.8	74.4	80.7	648	197
MI	Kalamazoo	-2.10	2616	28.4	9.3	22.3	75.7	80.8	880	268
MO	Dunklin	-2.10	2617	34.9	10.6	40.7	69.8	76.6	267	81
IL	Grundy	-2.11	2618	31.3	7.5	34.8	75.8	80.5	584	178
NY	St. Lawrence	-2.11	2619	31.8	9.3	30.5	74.5	79.1	804	245
TN	Macon	-2.11	2620	35.2	11.5	28.8	71	77.4	858	262
WI	Waukesha	-2.11	2621	25.6	5.9	18.5	78.7	82.2	894	272
AR	Nevada	-2.12	2622	35.6	12	33.6	70.2	77.1	292	89
IN	Vigo	-2.12	2623	32.6	8.7	27.8	73.6	79.2	540	165
MI	Lapeer	-2.12	2624	33.3	8.3	25.8	76.1	80.1	862	263
MT	Sheridan	-2.12	2625	27.4	6	28.5	73.6	79.5	2233	681
NE	Cass	-2.12	2626	28.2	8.1	26	76.1	81.2	1165	355
OH	Trumbull	-2.12	2627	29.6	9.4	29.2	73.7	79.5	973	297
IA	Polk	-2.13	2628	27.5	7.7	23.9	76.4	81.2	904	276
IN	Washington	-2.13	2629	29.7	9.1	32.5	73.7	79	761	232
NC	Edgecombe	-2.13	2630	39.7	12.1	30.4	68.9	75.6	71	22
IA	Ida	-2.14	2631	27.3	6.5	24.2	75.1	80.4	1357	414
MI	Cass	-2.14	2632	30.6	8.5	27.4	74.6	79.6	846	258
MN	Crow Wing	-2.14	2633	24.8	6.4	17.3	77.3	81.8	1256	383
IA	Madison	-2.15	2634	28.5	7.4	20.6	76.5	81.5	1072	327
MI	Barry	-2.15	2635	35.2	8.3	25.7	75.4	80.7	878	268
MN	Carlton	-2.15	2636	27.9	8.1	19.1	74.9	81	1195	364
MN	Hennepin	-2.15	2637	21	6	16.3	78.1	82.4	924	282
IA	Warren	-2.16	2638	35	7.6	26.6	77.1	81.8	906	276
MN	Lincoln	-2.16	2639	27.5	6.6	21.6	75.1	81.8	1689	515
WI	Marinette	-2.16	2640	30.3	7.1	25.3	75.1	81.2	906	276
MN	Le Sueur	-2.17	2641	29	6.9	21	77.6	81.9	1016	310
OH	Portage	-2.17	2642	29.4	8.6	28.3	75.8	80.1	1098	335
VA	Lunenburg	-2.17	2643	34.3	11.3	31.4	71.1	78.1	431	131
IL	Marion	-2.18	2644	29.3	6.7	29.3	73.6	79.5	535	163
IL	Montgomery	-2.18	2645	24.5	8.3	27.4	74.1	79.8	640	195
ND	Oliver	-2.18	2646	29.1	7.4	24.7	77.4	83	2030	619
TN	Hickman	-2.18	2647	32.4	10.5	31.8	71.7	79	679	207
IL	Christian	-2.19	2648	29.1	8.3	25.9	73.6	80.2	617	188

HEALTHIEST PLACES TO LIVE

ST	COUNTY	USDA	AMEN	OBES	DIAB	INACT	M AGE	W AGE	ALT ft	ALT m
MI	Washtenaw	-2.19	2649	24.4	8.5	19.4	77.9	81.7	881	268
WI	Oneida	-2.19	2650	26.8	6.9	20.4	76	81.3	1603	489
IL	Richland	-2.20	2651	29.9	8.2	29.2	74.4	80	474	145
IN	Spencer	-2.20	2652	30.4	9.4	25.2	75.3	80.3	434	132
MN	Rice	-2.20	2653	24	7.3	17.2	77.3	82	1095	334
MN	Murray	-2.21	2654	30.6	7	18.9	75.8	82.1	1611	491
ND	McIntosh	-2.21	2655	32.9	6.7	31.4	75.2	81.3	2052	626
ND	Rolette	-2.21	2656	39.5	13.3	35.4	74.4	80.2	1799	548
NE	Phelps	-2.21	2657	30.9	6.8	25.2	75.6	80.9	2324	708
OH	Pickaway	-2.21	2658	33.3	10.6	29.9	74.1	79.2	768	234
TN	Crockett	-2.21	2659	34.4	11.9	32.2	70.7	77.4	339	103
IL	Washington	-2.23	2660	30.2	7.6	27.3	75.3	80.6	482	147
MI	Gladwin	-2.23	2661	34	8.8	26.7	74.2	79.6	792	242
MN	Chisago	-2.23	2662	26.7	7.9	18.8	76.7	81	907	276
MN	Douglas	-2.23	2663	27.8	6.8	19	78	82.8	1385	422
OH	Montgomery	-2.23	2664	30.9	10.9	24.6	73.9	79.6	902	275
AR	Craighead	-2.24	2665	33.1	10.9	32	72.3	78.5	257	78
IL	Greene	-2.24	2666	31.6	8.5	31	74.5	79.5	545	166
NE	Perkins	-2.24	2667	26.8	6.9	29	76.1	81.4	3393	1034
WI	Burnett	-2.24	2668	31.6	7.7	22.8	75.5	81.1	994	303
IL	Jasper	-2.25	2669	28.8	7.5	30.7	75.3	80.2	528	161
IL	Morgan	-2.25	2670	29.2	7.4	28.6	74.6	79.5	613	187
IN	Kosciusko	-2.25	2671	32.4	9.2	26.3	75.2	80.8	853	260
SD	Tripp	-2.25	2672	36.7	9.1	30.9	75	80.8	2096	639
VA	Alexandria	-2.25	2673	20.2	7.8	18.7	78.3	83.6	112	34
VA	Arlington	-2.25	2674	19.4	7.5	17.6	79.7	83.3	207	63
WI	Marquette	-2.25	2675	33.3	7.1	25.5	74.9	80.2	840	256
AR	Poinsett	-2.26	2676	36.9	10.4	37.3	69.3	76.6	231	71
IL	Woodford	-2.26	2677	28.7	7.4	23.5	76.6	81.4	706	215
MO	Jasper	-2.26	2678	33.1	8.2	26.5	73.1	78.9	991	302
NE	Gage	-2.26	2679	32.9	8.2	27	76.3	80.9	1366	416
NY	Onondaga	-2.26	2680	28.2	8.4	21.6	76.3	81.3	780	238
WI	Washburn	-2.26	2681	30.6	8.5	21	75.6	81.2	1178	359
ND	Wells	-2.27	2682	28.6	6.4	27.4	74.3	81.1	1681	512
SD	Clark	-2.27	2683	32.7	6.9	28.7	74.9	80.6	1705	520
IA	Marion	-2.28	2684	31.5	7.2	23.7	75.7	81.1	832	254
MI	Kent	-2.28	2685	30.1	8.9	21.3	76.5	81	796	243
IA	Palo Alto	-2.29	2686	28.5	7.4	24.9	75.7	81.2	1285	392
MO	Shelby	-2.29	2687	32.9	10	28.4	73.8	79.8	764	233
NE	Merrick	-2.29	2688	34.9	7.8	26.8	75.6	80.5	1712	522
AR	Clay	-2.30	2689	33.2	10.6	32.6	70.3	78.1	300	91
IN	Parke	-2.30	2690	28.3	9.8	32.5	74.5	80.1	637	194
IN	Vermillion	-2.30	2691	30.4	10.9	26.8	73.8	79.2	599	182
KY	Webster	-2.30	2692	36.9	11.6	33.8	72.4	78.9	436	133
KS	Ellis	-2.31	2693	31.1	7.5	24.3	76.6	81.6	2039	621
MI	Lenawee	-2.31	2694	33.4	8.5	23.8	76.2	79.8	828	252

ST	COUNTY	USDA	AMEN	OBES	DIAB	INACT	M AGE	W AGE	ALT ft	ALT m
IL	Whiteside	-2.32	2695	27.4	7.8	29.2	75.2	80.2	657	200
SD	Faulk	-2.32	2696	28.8	6.9	29.2	76.3	82.4	1627	496
WI	Green	-2.32	2697	25.5	6.7	18.1	76.5	81.2	924	282
WI	Rusk	-2.32	2698	28.7	7.4	25.4	74.8	80.2	1250	381
IL	DuPage	-2.33	2699	24.2	6.8	18.9	79	82.4	733	223
MO	DeKalb	-2.33	2700	31.9	8.4	29.8	74.8	79.6	967	295
NC	Greene	-2.33	2701	33.3	11.3	29.2	70.4	76.7	79	24
OH	Miami	-2.33	2702	30	10.2	28.4	75.5	80.3	953	290
IL	Lawrence	-2.34	2703	29.2	7.8	28.8	73.7	79.3	454	138
IL	Shelby	-2.34	2704	27.4	7.6	30.6	75.9	80.5	635	194
IN	Huntington	-2.34	2705	34.8	10.3	29.8	75.7	81	804	245
MN	Becker	-2.34	2706	28.5	7.5	21.1	75.7	81.2	1454	443
IA	Clinton	-2.35	2707	29.8	7.3	28.7	75.5	80.7	726	221
IL	Clark	-2.35	2708	30.3	8.1	30.3	74.5	80.5	590	180
MI	Osceola	-2.35	2709	33.2	9.1	26.6	74.1	78.9	1194	364
MN	Cottonwood	-2.35	2710	27.4	7.7	25.2	76.3	81.8	1364	416
NE	Washington	-2.35	2711	29.4	7.3	21.7	77	81.2	1200	366
OH	Champaign	-2.35	2712	33.4	9.2	25.7	74.2	79.1	1117	341
WV	Webster	-2.35	2713	34.8	11.5	35.6	72	78.5	2404	733
IA	Monroe	-2.36	2714	32.5	7.2	34.4	74.7	80.9	887	270
IL	Macoupin	-2.36	2715	28.7	8.2	25.4	74.6	80.2	630	192
IN	LaGrange	-2.36	2716	29.5	8.8	24.3	74.1	79.7	907	276
MI	Clare	-2.36	2717	30.3	8.9	30.4	72.7	79	1069	326
MN	Itasca	-2.36	2718	26	7	18	76	81.1	1363	416
MN	Waseca	-2.36	2719	30.3	7.7	23	77.5	81.3	1124	343
NE	Adams	-2.36	2720	29.7	7.3	23.5	76.8	81.8	1949	594
NE	Otoe	-2.36	2721	32.2	7.7	27.2	76.6	80.9	1149	350
WI	Chippewa	-2.36	2722	31.5	8.3	17.4	76.7	81	1064	324
IA	Greene	-2.37	2723	29.1	6.8	26.3	76.2	82	1106	337
IA	Muscatine	-2.37	2724	31.6	6.7	23.8	75.7	80.7	670	204
MI	Crawford	-2.37	2725	30.1	8.3	23.4	74.1	79.2	1218	371
OH	Allen	-2.37	2726	36.6	9.7	26.2	74.9	79.7	842	257
WV	Calhoun	-2.37	2727	34.9	10.5	30.8	72.1	78.7	966	295
IN	Bartholomew	-2.38	2728	30.5	9.8	25.9	75.3	80.4	677	206
LA	Allen	-2.38	2729	38.4	12.2	33.8	73.1	78.7	77	24
MN	Cass	-2.38	2730	27.5	6.8	21	75.3	81.1	1345	410
MN	Freeborn	-2.38	2731	28.7	7	21.5	76.6	81.7	1257	383
IA	Scott	-2.39	2732	27.2	7.6	20.8	76	80.9	707	216
IL	Brown	-2.39	2733	29.7	8.5	28.2	74.4	79.5	625	191
KY	Fayette	-2.39	2734	30.7	9.7	24.7	75.4	80.3	944	288
SD	Hyde	-2.39	2735	37.2	8	30	76.3	82.4	1849	564
IL	McHenry	-2.40	2736	23.8	6.4	23.5	77.7	81.6	873	266
IN	Ripley	-2.40	2737	30.6	8	29.5	74.9	79.8	933	284
MI	Hillsdale	-2.40	2738	28	9.1	25.8	75.2	80.5	1057	322
MI	St. Joseph	-2.40	2739	32	9.5	25.5	73.5	79.8	848	258
OH	Summit	-2.40	2740	28.5	9.4	23.6	74.8	80	1023	312

HEALTHIEST PLACES TO LIVE

ST	COUNTY	USDA	AMEN	OBES	DIAB	INACT	M AGE	W AGE	ALT ft	ALT m
IL	Peoria	-2.41	2741	28.6	9.6	25.6	74.5	79.9	651	198
IL	Will	-2.41	2742	30.3	8.6	25	77	80.9	661	202
IN	Marshall	-2.41	2743	28.7	8.4	28.6	75	81.1	803	245
MN	Anoka	-2.41	2744	30	7.7	20.8	78.3	82.4	909	277
MN	Otter Tail	-2.41	2745	30.2	6.7	22.7	76.5	82.4	1355	413
IA	Clarke	-2.42	2746	29.5	6.7	28	75.5	80.8	1095	334
KS	Anderson	-2.42	2747	32.1	7.4	25.8	75.2	80.6	1049	320
NE	Jefferson	-2.42	2748	30.7	8.1	30.6	75.9	80.7	1434	437
PA	Potter	-2.42	2749	30.5	9.1	26.9	75.2	80	1996	608
WV	Ritchie	-2.42	2750	33.8	11.3	33.8	73.3	79	939	286
IL	Knox	-2.43	2751	32.9	8	31	74.2	79.3	714	218
MO	Audrain	-2.43	2752	31.1	8.4	31.1	73.6	79.3	790	241
MO	Stoddard	-2.43	2753	29	8.7	39.4	71.8	78.2	343	105
OH	Franklin	-2.43	2754	30.7	10.5	25.5	73.7	79	833	254
WI	Adams	-2.43	2755	32.7	7.9	24.9	74.7	80	984	300
IA	Buena Vista	-2.44	2756	28.5	7.1	26.4	76.7	81.2	1376	419
IL	Crawford	-2.44	2757	30.4	7.9	31.1	74.9	79.6	503	153
OH	Shelby	-2.44	2758	29.8	9.6	29.2	75.4	80.3	994	303
WI	Wood	-2.44	2759	26.3	7.5	18.5	77	82.7	1081	330
MI	Branch	-2.45	2760	32.9	9.2	28.9	74.7	79.6	949	289
MI	Jackson	-2.45	2761	36.4	9.4	27	74.4	79.3	983	300
MN	Pope	-2.45	2762	28	7.1	23.4	77.8	81.9	1281	391
MT	Roosevelt	-2.45	2763	34.8	12.1	32.4	73.6	79.5	2288	697
OH	Geauga	-2.45	2764	23.6	8	19.9	78.1	82.5	1166	355
MO	Lawrence	-2.46	2765	29.8	8.4	28.5	73.3	79.4	1239	378
WI	Walworth	-2.46	2766	25.3	6.8	21.3	77.2	80.8	927	283
IL	Mercer	-2.47	2767	30.4	7.5	25	75.9	80.9	677	206
IL	Sangamon	-2.47	2768	28.8	8.6	25.6	74.8	80	597	182
IL	Scott	-2.47	2769	28.5	7.9	28.9	75	80.5	530	162
LA	Lafayette	-2.47	2770	29.1	7.8	25.1	73.3	78.7	29	9
ND	Eddy	-2.47	2771	26.9	7.4	29.9	75.2	81.1	1517	462
IN	Jennings	-2.48	2772	29.2	9	28.1	73.2	79.2	699	213
IN	Vanderburgh	-2.48	2773	28.8	9.3	27.1	73.8	79.4	424	129
KY	Graves	-2.48	2774	33.8	10.5	31	72.6	78.2	465	142
MI	Montcalm	-2.48	2775	33.6	9	22.6	74.4	79	883	269
MN	Blue Earth	-2.48	2776	27.4	7.2	25	77.4	81.6	997	304
MN	Martin	-2.48	2777	26.9	6.6	20.4	76.5	82.8	1205	367
MN	Nobles	-2.48	2778	26.8	8.2	22.1	77.5	82.9	1607	490
WI	Waupaca	-2.48	2779	32.4	7.4	21.6	74.3	80.2	873	266
IN	Clark	-2.49	2780	30.7	8.7	31.3	73.3	78.8	606	185
NE	Antelope	-2.49	2781	28.9	8	27.3	75.3	81.4	1872	570
SD	Grant	-2.49	2782	32.2	8.7	28.9	76.2	82.2	1441	439
IL	Winnebago	-2.50	2783	28.6	9.1	26.2	75.1	80.8	803	245
MN	Wright	-2.50	2784	24.4	6.2	17.9	77.8	82.1	1005	306
NE	Pawnee	-2.50	2785	31.2	8	31.5	75.4	80.8	1276	389
OH	Stark	-2.50	2786	31.7	9.8	25.8	75.6	80.4	1108	338

ST	COUNTY	USDA	AMEN	OBES	DIAB	INACT	M AGE	W AGE	ALT ft	ALT m
IN	Marion	-2.51	2787	30.1	10.5	26.1	72.6	78.7	794	242
IN	St. Joseph	-2.51	2788	29.2	8.9	26.7	74.4	80.8	770	235
IA	Clay	-2.52	2789	30.5	6.8	26.5	77	81.6	1391	424
IL	De Witt	-2.52	2790	28.5	7.5	27.9	73.9	79.6	723	220
WV	Doddridge	-2.52	2791	32.3	11.1	36.3	73	78.9	1051	320
IN	Hamilton	-2.53	2792	21.9	8.1	19.4	78.6	82.7	851	259
ND	Foster	-2.53	2793	28.4	7	27.5	75.2	81.1	1531	467
IN	Wayne	-2.54	2794	27.8	7.6	27.6	73.4	79.6	1048	319
OH	Sandusky	-2.54	2795	31.8	10.6	26.3	74.6	79.7	650	198
WI	Portage	-2.54	2796	27.7	6.9	23	77.3	81.8	1111	339
IL	Tazewell	-2.55	2797	26.7	6.6	26.6	75.4	80.3	614	187
NE	Hayes	-2.55	2798	28.3	6.5	28.2	76.1	81.4	3023	922
NE	Lancaster	-2.55	2799	27.4	7.4	20.3	77.8	82.3	1296	395
IA	Dallas	-2.56	2800	30	8.1	23.9	77	81.9	992	302
IN	Clay	-2.56	2801	35.7	9.2	28.6	73.7	78.7	610	186
IN	Whitley	-2.56	2802	32.3	7.7	20.1	75.2	80.6	871	265
WI	Forest	-2.56	2803	31	8.7	24.2	75.8	80.6	1594	486
KS	Rush	-2.57	2804	29	7.6	25.7	75.2	80.6	2082	635
MN	Nicollet	-2.58	2805	27.8	7.5	17	78	82.1	987	301
NE	Pierce	-2.58	2806	31.7	7.2	32.6	75.3	81.4	1718	524
SD	Minnehaha	-2.58	2807	29.1	6.9	23.6	77.1	82.3	1544	471
ND	Logan	-2.59	2808	33	7.7	32	75.2	81.3	2002	610
IN	Delaware	-2.60	2809	32.7	9.4	29.3	73.6	78.9	938	286
MN	Kandiyohi	-2.60	2810	28.7	6.5	22.8	77.2	82.5	1176	358
NE	Johnson	-2.60	2811	33.2	7.8	28.9	75.4	80.8	1243	379
NE	Saunders	-2.60	2812	29.3	7.1	24.8	76.6	81.5	1290	393
OH	Defiance	-2.60	2813	28.8	9.9	27.5	75.6	80.7	727	222
IA	Lucas	-2.61	2814	31.3	6.7	28.3	75	80.2	979	298
IL	Wayne	-2.61	2815	29.1	7.3	26	74.6	80.3	435	132
IN	Henry	-2.61	2816	30.8	9.1	30.1	73.2	79.3	1051	320
WI	Florence	-2.61	2817	28.2	6.9	22.4	75.8	80.6	1391	424
WI	Waushara	-2.61	2818	32.9	8.1	23.2	75.2	80.6	945	288
WI	Rock	-2.62	2819	31	8	23.7	75.8	80.5	887	270
NY	Montgomery	-2.63	2820	30	7.4	27.9	74.3	80.7	712	217
OH	Hancock	-2.63	2821	29.7	8.4	24.5	76.5	81.3	805	245
WI	Washington	-2.63	2822	28.1	6.6	21.8	77.6	82.5	982	299
IA	Johnson	-2.64	2823	23.6	6.5	19.3	79.3	82.5	745	227
KS	Brown	-2.64	2824	36.7	9.2	28.9	75.1	80.9	1091	333
NE	Boyd	-2.64	2825	28.2	6.2	28.7	75.6	80.9	1726	526
WV	Gilmer	-2.64	2826	36.6	11.5	34.2	72.1	78.7	1004	306
MN	Meeker	-2.65	2827	25.7	8.2	23.6	76.4	80.8	1139	347
IA	Cherokee	-2.66	2828	26	6.8	21.3	75.9	81.8	1365	416
MN	Isanti	-2.66	2829	28.6	7.6	18.7	76.7	81.7	956	291
WI	Price	-2.66	2830	31.9	7.8	24.3	75.3	80.7	1534	468
OH	Morrow	-2.67	2831	29.8	9	31.6	74.5	79.1	1167	356
OH	Paulding	-2.67	2832	29.9	8.9	29.3	74.4	80.2	714	218

HEALTHIEST PLACES TO LIVE

ST	COUNTY	USDA	AMEN	OBES	DIAB	INACT	M AGE	W AGE	ALT ft	ALT m
IN	Fountain	-2.68	2833	28.9	9.5	28.7	74.3	79.5	649	198
OH	Henry	-2.68	2834	33	9.5	28.6	75.6	81	689	210
SD	Edmunds	-2.68	2835	39.2	6.5	27.1	74.1	80.3	1696	517
IA	Plymouth	-2.69	2836	30.3	7.3	28.7	76.4	81.8	1329	405
MN	Grant	-2.69	2837	26.9	6.8	20.8	76.5	82.4	1143	348
NY	Wyoming	-2.69	2838	28.7	7.8	22.7	74.9	80.5	1479	451
MN	Carver	-2.70	2839	25.9	6.6	16.9	78.6	83	971	296
MN	Lyon	-2.70	2840	29.3	7.1	22.5	76.9	81.6	1306	398
ND	Renville	-2.70	2841	26.6	6.8	25.1	74.4	80.2	1713	522
IN	Putnam	-2.71	2842	31.1	10.1	29.8	75.8	79.7	795	242
IN	Elkhart	-2.72	2843	28.3	9	25.7	75.6	80.3	817	249
ND	Pierce	-2.72	2844	31.9	7.4	31.6	74.3	81.1	1576	480
SD	Brown	-2.72	2845	31.9	6.8	29.5	76.3	82.4	1337	408
IA	Calhoun	-2.73	2846	30.7	7.9	27.7	76.3	81.2	1198	365
IN	White	-2.73	2847	33.3	8.6	27.6	74.5	80.7	693	211
MI	Calhoun	-2.73	2848	35.5	10.3	27.3	73.1	79.1	938	286
WI	Polk	-2.73	2849	28.4	6.9	19	76.1	81.7	1121	342
IL	La Salle	-2.75	2850	29.6	8.1	25.7	74.4	80.1	658	201
TN	Cannon	-2.75	2851	31.7	9.6	31.8	71.5	78.4	980	299
IL	Kane	-2.77	2852	27.5	8.1	23.6	77.4	81	816	249
MN	Big Stone	-2.77	2853	27.7	6.7	20.2	76.5	82.2	1096	334
MN	Pine	-2.77	2854	27.1	7	19.7	75.3	80.1	1079	329
PA	Mercer	-2.78	2855	29.8	10.1	23.9	74.7	80.2	1211	369
IL	Macon	-2.79	2856	32.3	7.9	27	74	80.1	665	203
IN	Tippecanoe	-2.79	2857	28.1	9.4	24.2	75.6	80.7	676	206
LA	West Carroll	-2.79	2858	31.5	11.2	32.1	70.1	76.2	95	29
NY	Lewis	-2.79	2859	28.3	8.4	26.1	75.4	81	1300	396
IL	Cumberland	-2.80	2860	27.8	8.2	29.9	75.3	80.2	602	184
OH	Wood	-2.80	2861	29.7	8.4	25	76.4	81.3	677	206
IL	Effingham	-2.81	2862	27.7	7.6	28.3	75.3	80.7	575	175
IN	DeKalb	-2.81	2863	31	8.8	26.3	75.4	80.4	884	269
IL	Ogle	-2.82	2864	27.6	7.4	28	75.8	80.5	812	247
IA	Linn	-2.83	2865	28.1	7.8	23.4	77.6	81.5	851	259
IN	Carroll	-2.83	2866	31.7	9.2	26	75.3	80.8	680	207
IN	Miami	-2.83	2867	31.8	10.3	30.2	74.2	79.9	775	236
MO	Caldwell	-2.83	2868	34.7	9.2	30.2	74.5	80.4	895	273
ND	Barnes	-2.83	2869	26.7	5.6	25.6	75.9	81.3	1394	425
NE	Hamilton	-2.83	2870	31.1	6.9	27.8	77.1	81.3	1798	548
SD	Aurora	-2.83	2871	29.6	6.5	34.1	74.9	81.2	1573	479
MN	Todd	-2.84	2872	30	7.4	25.8	75.7	81.1	1335	407
OH	Ashland	-2.84	2873	30.1	10.1	28.6	75.7	80.5	1122	342
IL	Kendall	-2.85	2874	25.3	6.6	24.8	77.4	81.9	654	199
IN	Starke	-2.85	2875	32.1	9.9	33.8	72.1	77.8	700	213
KS	Jackson	-2.85	2876	31.5	8.2	26.3	75.8	80.8	1115	340
MN	Watonwan	-2.85	2877	27.8	7.2	21.7	76.3	81.8	1106	337
MO	Nodaway	-2.85	2878	30.7	8.2	30.5	76.2	80.7	1049	320

ST	COUNTY	USDA	AMEN	OBES	DIAB	INACT	M AGE	W AGE	ALT ft	ALT m
WI	Barron	-2.86	2879	31.1	6.9	23.7	75.8	81.2	1199	365
MN	Stearns	-2.87	2880	28.4	7.6	19	78.8	83.9	1197	365
MI	Iron	-2.88	2881	30.2	9.2	23	75.1	80.9	1538	469
MN	Sherburne	-2.88	2882	30.4	7.9	22.4	77.3	80.8	979	298
OH	Richland	-2.88	2883	29.4	9.3	27	74.8	79.4	1195	364
MN	Beltrami	-2.89	2884	30.2	7.4	21.3	74.6	81	1261	384
OH	Knox	-2.89	2885	27.9	10.1	25.9	74.8	79.8	1114	340
IL	Edwards	-2.90	2886	26.6	7.5	26.5	75.2	80.1	440	134
MN	Faribault	-2.91	2887	28.5	7.2	22.8	76	81.8	1114	340
SD	Jerauld	-2.91	2888	28.9	5.5	29.8	75.8	81.4	1641	500
IL	Lee	-2.93	2889	26.4	8.5	27.2	74.8	79.9	789	240
MN	Fillmore	-2.93	2890	28.4	6.7	21.7	76.4	82	1194	364
MN	McLeod	-2.93	2891	28.6	6.9	18.6	77.3	82.4	1057	322
NC	Martin	-2.93	2892	35.8	12	27.8	69.5	76.4	45	14
NY	Genesee	-2.94	2893	27.8	8.7	23.7	76.3	81.2	834	254
IA	Henry	-2.95	2894	30.1	8	24.2	76	81.4	690	210
IA	Pocahontas	-2.95	2895	29.6	8	24.5	75.9	81.1	1243	379
KS	Washington	-2.95	2896	33.3	8.2	22.5	76.3	81.7	1393	425
MN	Scott	-2.95	2897	24.6	6.2	17.4	78.3	82.4	928	283
IA	Cerro Gordo	-2.96	2898	26.5	8	23.5	75.7	81.5	1183	361
MN	Clearwater	-2.96	2899	30.4	7.5	21	74.9	81	1427	435
ND	Dickey	-2.96	2900	29.5	7.5	28.4	75.8	82	1534	468
SD	Moody	-2.96	2901	32.5	7.3	27	76.8	82.3	1629	497
IL	Hamilton	-2.97	2902	29.7	7.8	30.4	73	79.5	441	134
IN	Allen	-2.97	2903	32.8	9.9	25.3	75.4	80.6	793	242
OH	Williams	-2.97	2904	30.3	9.2	23.7	75.8	80.7	832	254
WI	Lincoln	-2.98	2905	28.7	8	23	76	81	1476	450
IL	Coles	-2.99	2906	29.2	7.3	24.8	74.7	80.1	677	206
IL	Clay	-3.01	2907	28.3	7.6	29.9	74.4	80	487	148
KS	Edwards	-3.01	2908	34.6	8.5	26.7	74.9	80.1	2173	662
IL	Menard	-3.04	2909	25.9	7.5	29	74.8	80	570	174
IN	Cass	-3.04	2910	34	9.3	27.9	74.5	79.4	731	223
MN	Kanabec	-3.04	2911	28.2	7.4	21.3	76.2	80.7	1087	331
NE	Saline	-3.04	2912	32.9	7.4	27.2	76.9	81.8	1466	447
IL	Bureau	-3.05	2913	27.8	7.5	28.1	75.9	80.7	708	216
MN	Dakota	-3.05	2914	26	6.3	16.9	78.7	81.7	922	281
MN	Steele	-3.05	2915	29.5	6.6	21.2	77.7	82.5	1215	370
SD	McCook	-3.05	2916	26.6	7	27.7	76.2	81.6	1513	461
IA	Black Hawk	-3.07	2917	28.8	8.5	23	76.8	80.8	921	281
MI	Ionia	-3.07	2918	33.2	9.8	23.4	75.1	80	799	244
MN	Brown	-3.07	2919	30.6	7.4	22.1	77.4	82	1019	310
OH	Madison	-3.07	2920	31.1	11.3	32.6	74.9	79.5	985	300
ND	Benson	-3.08	2921	33.3	9.7	33	74.3	81.1	1549	472
IN	Decatur	-3.09	2922	30.4	9.4	24.5	74.3	80.2	885	270
MI	Midland	-3.09	2923	31	8.1	21.6	77.1	81.2	669	204
MN	Lk of the Woods	-3.09	2924	27.8	7.1	21.6	75.3	81.1	1134	345

172

HEALTHIEST PLACES TO LIVE

ST	COUNTY	USDA	AMEN	OBES	DIAB	INACT	M AGE	W AGE	ALT ft	ALT m
MN	Mahnomen	-3.09	2925	31.6	9.1	27	74.9	81	1365	416
MN	Morrison	-3.09	2926	28.3	6.8	20.6	75	81.1	1221	372
OH	Huron	-3.09	2927	31.8	10.1	31.7	74.6	79.4	883	269
MI	Isabella	-3.10	2928	32.8	8.5	24.2	75.5	80.4	859	262
MN	Sibley	-3.10	2929	29.8	6.9	23.1	76.6	81.5	1012	308
ND	Ramsey	-3.10	2930	31.9	6.8	24.9	75	81.2	1493	455
NE	Thayer	-3.12	2931	29.5	7.6	27.5	75.9	80.7	1563	476
IN	Fulton	-3.13	2932	31.2	9	25.9	73.3	79.3	791	241
NE	Polk	-3.13	2933	33.7	8.3	28.4	77.1	81.3	1633	498
WI	Langlade	-3.13	2934	30.1	7.6	22.3	75.1	80.9	1535	468
MI	Eaton	-3.14	2935	31.1	8.5	22.4	76	80.4	892	272
IA	Bremer	-3.16	2936	27.4	7.1	22.7	77.6	82.2	1022	312
KY	Metcalfe	-3.16	2937	35.3	10.9	33.7	71.9	77.9	850	259
OH	Medina	-3.16	2938	27.2	8.5	23	77.4	81.3	1019	311
WI	Eau Claire	-3.16	2939	28.2	6.5	23.2	77.3	81.9	987	301
IL	Warren	-3.17	2940	29.1	8.1	26.8	75.1	79.6	715	218
KY	Bourbon	-3.18	2941	35	11.8	35.3	74	79.2	891	271
ND	Griggs	-3.18	2942	28.1	6.5	24.3	75.2	81.1	1449	442
IA	Jasper	-3.19	2943	35.1	8.3	23.5	76.9	80.9	902	275
IA	Osceola	-3.19	2944	30.9	6.5	23.9	75.8	81.2	1542	470
IL	McDonough	-3.19	2945	29.5	7.4	27.4	76.1	80.5	667	203
OH	Wyandot	-3.19	2946	32.5	10.6	30.5	75.3	80.2	847	258
IA	Webster	-3.20	2947	30	8.6	30.4	75.1	80.2	1131	345
OH	Fayette	-3.20	2948	29.8	9.9	30.4	73.2	78.6	970	296
SD	Hand	-3.20	2949	31.3	6.8	31.9	75.8	81.4	1652	504
IL	Vermilion	-3.21	2950	28.5	9	30.1	73.1	78.7	683	208
NE	Seward	-3.21	2951	29.1	8	23	76.7	81.5	1499	457
OH	Wayne	-3.22	2952	31.7	8.9	23.5	75.4	80.4	1071	326
OH	Meigs	-3.23	2953	31.2	9.6	31.2	71.9	78.5	759	231
IA	Buchanan	-3.24	2954	29.3	7.8	25.7	76.2	81.3	987	301
MN	Hubbard	-3.24	2955	24.9	6.9	18.7	76	81.5	1453	443
IN	Warren	-3.25	2956	29.4	10.2	29.9	74.8	80.6	701	214
OH	Auglaize	-3.25	2957	34.4	9.1	25.4	75.8	80.9	918	280
SD	Beadle	-3.25	2958	32.9	6	29.3	75.8	81.4	1331	406
IN	Blackford	-3.27	2959	33	10	28.7	74.2	79.5	868	265
IA	Cedar	-3.28	2960	32.9	7.1	24	76.9	82.2	798	243
IA	Washington	-3.28	2961	30.6	7	22.9	76.4	82	727	222
OH	Fulton	-3.29	2962	30.1	11.1	26.1	75.8	81.1	734	224
SD	Davison	-3.29	2963	28	6.7	27.2	76.2	81.6	1382	421
IL	Kankakee	-3.30	2964	30.9	8.2	27.9	73.3	79	646	197
ND	McHenry	-3.30	2965	32.7	7.8	36.1	74.4	80.2	1541	470
WI	Marathon	-3.30	2966	30.7	7.9	26	77.8	82.6	1307	398
MN	Stevens	-3.31	2967	27.4	7.1	21.3	77.8	81.9	1133	345
OH	Darke	-3.31	2968	31.6	9.4	30.6	75	81.2	1037	316
IL	Boone	-3.32	2969	29	7.3	26	76.5	80.6	864	263
MI	Saginaw	-3.33	2970	39.9	9.8	30.2	73.5	79.1	624	190

ST	COUNTY	USDA	AMEN	OBES	DIAB	INACT	M AGE	W AGE	ALT ft	ALT m
SD	Hutchinson	-3.33	2971	31.8	6.4	27.5	74.9	81.2	1391	424
IA	Tama	-3.34	2972	25.7	7.8	28.5	77.1	81.4	951	290
NE	Kearney	-3.34	2973	26.9	6	24.7	75.6	80.3	2141	653
IA	Boone	-3.35	2974	33.7	6.8	26.4	76.4	81.5	1058	322
IA	Jefferson	-3.35	2975	29	7.9	22.1	76.9	80.9	741	226
IN	Fayette	-3.35	2976	34	9.2	30.4	72.9	79.2	974	297
IN	Montgomery	-3.35	2977	31	9.4	30.1	74.9	80.3	803	245
ND	LaMoure	-3.35	2978	26.8	6.5	25.8	75.8	82	1543	470
WI	Outagamie	-3.35	2979	28.7	8.8	21.6	77.8	82.4	774	236
NE	Clay	-3.36	2980	34.7	8.4	30.3	75.9	80.7	1772	540
NE	Butler	-3.37	2981	27.9	6.3	27.7	75.5	81.1	1543	470
OH	Seneca	-3.37	2982	29.8	9	28.5	74.8	79.9	811	247
MI	Ingham	-3.38	2983	30.9	8.3	22.4	76.1	80.4	914	279
WI	Menominee	-3.38	2984	35.5	12.4	30.8	75.1	80.9	1051	320
WI	Taylor	-3.39	2985	27.2	7.7	24.2	76	81.1	1398	426
WI	Shawano	-3.40	2986	30.2	8.1	25.4	76.3	81	979	298
IA	Poweshiek	-3.42	2987	30.5	7.5	24.8	77.4	80.8	920	280
IN	Newton	-3.42	2988	30.3	9.8	28.6	74	79.3	671	205
MN	Chippewa	-3.42	2989	31.6	7.3	20.7	76.8	81.7	1036	316
SD	Hanson	-3.42	2990	29.1	6.2	25.8	76.2	81.6	1338	408
IL	Henry	-3.43	2991	27.1	7.8	29.4	75.9	81	704	215
MN	Benton	-3.43	2992	27.3	8.4	21.6	75.4	80.2	1123	342
MN	Lac qui Parle	-3.43	2993	29.4	7.7	19.8	76.5	82.2	1068	326
ND	Bottineau	-3.44	2994	31.8	8.1	26.1	74.4	80.2	1584	483
IA	Delaware	-3.45	2995	32.4	6.9	27.4	77.4	81.7	1016	310
IA	Jones	-3.45	2996	30	7.4	24.7	76.1	81.4	879	268
SD	Miner	-3.45	2997	30.8	6.3	33.9	76.2	81.6	1489	454
IN	Madison	-3.47	2998	36.6	11	32.8	74.1	79.1	864	263
SD	Sanborn	-3.47	2999	35.4	6.9	33.2	75.8	81.4	1295	395
IN	Pulaski	-3.48	3000	33.7	9.7	26.9	73.3	79.3	698	213
MI	Shiawassee	-3.48	3001	31.7	9.5	25.6	75.2	80.5	787	240
SD	Turner	-3.48	3002	31.3	6.5	30.7	76.9	81.5	1384	422
MI	Clinton	-3.49	3003	31.2	9	24.9	77	81.5	768	234
IL	Douglas	-3.50	3004	29.6	7.1	27.8	74.6	80.3	659	201
OH	Union	-3.50	3005	33.9	8.9	26.4	75.3	79.8	982	299
IA	Worth	-3.51	3006	28.7	7.5	24.2	76.5	81.8	1232	375
ND	Cavalier	-3.52	3007	31.3	7	27	75	81.2	1549	472
IA	Story	-3.54	3008	26	6.5	21.1	78.5	83.1	1006	307
IN	Grant	-3.54	3009	29.6	10.2	31.4	73	79.2	842	257
IN	Adams	-3.55	3010	33.3	7.9	24.6	75.9	80.8	810	247
IA	Wright	-3.56	3011	30	7	28	76	81.9	1179	359
ND	Steele	-3.56	3012	32.9	6.9	26.3	75.2	81.1	1266	386
IL	McLean	-3.57	3013	30.2	7.6	24.7	76.6	80.9	767	234
IN	Jasper	-3.57	3014	32.1	9.9	29.1	74.9	80.6	681	208
MN	Traverse	-3.57	3015	28.2	7.2	21.8	76.5	82.2	1041	317
OH	Hardin	-3.57	3016	31	10.5	26.4	73.7	79.8	968	295

HEALTHIEST PLACES TO LIVE

ST	COUNTY	USDA	AMEN	OBES	DIAB	INACT	M AGE	W AGE	ALT ft	ALT m
IL	DeKalb	-3.58	3017	29.7	7.9	25.4	77	81	832	254
IN	Hancock	-3.58	3018	27.1	8.7	23.6	76.2	80.4	868	264
MI	Dickinson	-3.58	3019	27.4	8.4	22.4	76.5	81.9	1186	362
SD	Douglas	-3.59	3020	31.8	6.7	31.6	74.9	81.2	1564	477
OH	Van Wert	-3.60	3021	34.5	9.9	23.5	75.2	80.5	766	233
IN	Hendricks	-3.61	3022	33.1	8.9	23.4	76.9	80.8	888	271
IN	Howard	-3.61	3023	34.1	9.7	31	73.8	79.3	814	248
ND	Sargent	-3.61	3024	30.2	8	29.1	75.8	82	1239	378
KS	Nemaha	-3.62	3025	28.2	8.7	25.4	75.1	80.9	1257	383
SD	Spink	-3.62	3026	35.9	7	30.7	74.9	81.2	1314	400
IA	Hardin	-3.63	3027	33.4	7	29.6	76	81.1	1113	339
IA	Chickasaw	-3.65	3028	31.1	7.1	26.4	76.3	81	1137	346
IL	Edgar	-3.65	3029	30.3	8.1	28.4	73.8	79.7	666	203
IA	Benton	-3.66	3030	30.3	7	25	77.7	82	893	272
MN	Redwood	-3.67	3031	29.2	6.9	21	76	81.1	1073	327
IN	Boone	-3.68	3032	29.8	8.5	29.8	76.6	80.9	918	280
NE	Keya Paha	-3.69	3033	28.7	7.1	32.7	75.6	80.9	2271	692
IA	Marshall	-3.70	3034	31.6	7.3	24.2	74.4	81.7	985	300
IA	Sioux	-3.70	3035	26.3	5.7	23.3	77.5	82.8	1367	417
OH	Putnam	-3.70	3036	30.8	8.8	26.8	76.3	81.6	732	223
OH	Crawford	-3.71	3037	33.9	9.6	27.1	73.8	79.6	1001	305
IN	Randolph	-3.72	3038	34.5	10.2	36.5	74.2	79.5	1083	330
KY	Green	-3.72	3039	32	11.4	36.2	71.9	77.9	711	217
ND	Nelson	-3.72	3040	30.2	7.2	28.1	75.2	81.1	1487	453
IN	Wells	-3.73	3041	31.5	8.7	25.9	75.7	81.4	820	250
IA	Hamilton	-3.74	3042	31.6	7.2	23.6	76.7	82.4	1127	344
MN	Swift	-3.74	3043	28.7	8.2	26.5	76.8	81.7	1076	328
MN	Wadena	-3.74	3044	30.7	7.8	21.7	76	81.5	1358	414
IL	Stephenson	-3.75	3045	29.9	8	27.9	75.5	80.8	871	265
IN	Shelby	-3.76	3046	35.1	10	32.4	74.4	79.6	771	235
MN	Polk	-3.76	3047	30.5	7.7	26	75.3	81.4	1012	308
IA	Winnebago	-3.81	3048	26.1	7.4	22.7	76.5	81.8	1264	385
ND	Richland	-3.81	3049	32.3	6.4	27.8	76.8	82.2	1022	311
MT	Daniels	-3.82	3050	22.9	6.5	23.6	73.6	79.5	2635	803
IA	Iowa	-3.84	3051	28.7	6.9	29.1	76.6	81.8	811	247
IL	Stark	-3.87	3052	29.4	7.6	28.1	74.9	80.3	721	220
IL	Logan	-3.89	3053	34.6	8.3	28.9	74	79.8	599	183
MN	Renville	-3.90	3054	32	7.4	23	76.2	80.9	1066	325
SD	Lincoln	-3.91	3055	26.3	5.8	22.8	77.3	81.4	1380	421
MI	Gratiot	-3.92	3056	37.7	9.1	27.9	75.2	79.6	735	224
OH	Marion	-3.93	3057	31.6	10.4	30.4	74	78.8	928	283
IA	Butler	-3.94	3058	25.4	6.1	25.9	76.3	81	998	304
IA	Keokuk	-3.95	3059	33.5	6.6	24.3	76.6	81.8	784	239
IL	Livingston	-3.95	3060	29	8.3	30.9	74	79.3	683	208
ND	Walsh	-3.95	3061	32.5	6.6	27.3	75.8	81.4	1124	343
MN	Olmsted	-3.96	3062	28	7	17.4	78.3	83.7	1172	357

ST	COUNTY	USDA	AMEN	OBES	DIAB	INACT	M AGE	W AGE	ALT ft	ALT m
IN	Rush	-3.97	3063	32	9.9	30.2	74.5	80.1	951	290
IN	Jay	-3.98	3064	34.3	9.6	31.2	74.2	79.5	905	276
KY	Simpson	-3.98	3065	32.3	11.5	35.4	73.1	79.3	668	204
MN	Yellow Medicine	-3.98	3066	25	7	19.5	76	81.1	1127	343
ND	Towner	-3.99	3067	29.7	7.1	24.6	75	81.2	1562	476
IL	Iroquois	-4.00	3068	31.3	7.8	30.4	74.6	79.5	665	203
NE	Fillmore	-4.00	3069	29.1	6.9	26.7	75.9	80.7	1636	499
IL	Ford	-4.02	3070	31.8	7.9	29.4	74.6	79.5	748	228
NE	Wayne	-4.02	3071	29	6.8	25.8	76.5	82	1611	491
IA	Floyd	-4.03	3072	29.5	7.3	24.6	76.5	81.1	1072	327
IA	Humboldt	-4.05	3073	30.6	7.4	24.7	75.9	81.1	1140	347
MN	Marshall	-4.05	3074	26.1	6.9	20.7	75.3	82.4	1025	312
NE	York	-4.05	3075	35	7.4	28.1	76.9	81.8	1642	500
IA	Hancock	-4.06	3076	28.6	7.1	23.8	76.6	81.4	1233	376
IA	Fayette	-4.09	3077	33.5	6.4	24.1	76.1	80.8	1100	335
IA	Mitchell	-4.10	3078	26	6.4	26.9	76.6	81.4	1196	365
MN	Pipestone	-4.13	3079	27.8	7.4	19.2	75.1	81.8	1714	522
IA	Howard	-4.16	3080	28.3	6.8	22	76.6	81.4	1271	387
MN	Clay	-4.17	3081	29.9	7.9	22.3	77.3	82.6	1022	312
IA	Franklin	-4.18	3082	32.6	7.8	26.5	76.6	81.4	1174	358
MN	Koochiching	-4.20	3083	29.4	8.1	19.8	75.3	81.1	1215	370
IL	Piatt	-4.21	3084	28.4	7.9	30.2	75.1	81	695	212
ND	Ransom	-4.21	3085	31.6	7.5	28.2	75.9	81.3	1199	365
IA	O'Brien	-4.23	3086	30.1	7.5	24.2	75.9	81.8	1455	443
MN	Rock	-4.25	3087	24.3	6.7	22.2	75.8	82.1	1547	471
MN	Roseau	-4.30	3088	31.6	6.7	22.2	75.9	81.3	1092	333
WI	Clark	-4.34	3089	31.1	6.8	24.1	75.7	81.2	1166	355
IN	Clinton	-4.37	3090	28.4	11.9	26.3	74.6	79.9	844	257
IA	Winneshiek	-4.44	3091	24.5	7.2	21.6	77.6	82.9	1142	348
IA	Kossuth	-4.47	3092	28.9	6.7	32.2	77.1	82.7	1182	360
IA	Lyon	-4.49	3093	26.5	6.5	26.6	75.8	81.2	1417	432
IL	Champaign	-4.55	3094	26.6	7.7	25.6	76.6	80.8	714	218
IN	Benton	-4.71	3095	32.3	9.8	33	74.8	80.6	757	231
ND	Cass	-4.84	3096	28.2	7	22.3	77.2	82.9	1008	307
IA	Grundy	-4.86	3097	31.2	7.4	23.4	77.1	81.4	1036	316
MN	Kittson	-4.90	3098	28.8	7.6	22.3	75.3	82.4	904	276
MN	Pennington	-4.97	3099	28.1	8.6	23.1	74.9	81	1121	342
ND	Grand Forks	-5.01	3100	30.9	7.4	23	76.5	81.4	1015	309
MN	Dodge	-5.08	3101	31.3	7.2	19.6	77.5	82.3	1259	384
ND	Traill	-5.12	3102	32.6	6.3	29.8	76.5	81.4	943	287
MN	Mower	-5.18	3103	28.5	7.2	21.8	77.6	82.6	1309	399
ND	Pembina	-5.18	3104	32.7	8	29.7	75.8	81.4	888	271
MN	Norman	-5.37	3105	30.4	8.1	21.2	75.7	81.2	984	300
IN	Tipton	-5.40	3106	30.4	9.3	28.2	75.7	80.7	872	266
MN	Wilkin	-6.10	3107	28.6	7.2	25	76.5	82.4	993	303
MN	Red Lake	-6.40	3108	31.8	7.2	19.8	75.3	81.4	1089	332

CHAPTER 7

Obesity Ratings for 3,108 Lower Forty-Eight Counties

There is no data on weight loss when you go to a health club, either.
—Thomas Wadden, University of Pennsylvania weight loss expert.[1]

This section ranks the 3,108 lower forty-eight counties by CDC obesity rate. The obesity rates range from 13.5%-47.9%. CDC data from 2009 was used in the book. While minor shuffling between counties occurs from year to year, the 2009-2012 county obesity rates do not fluctuate significantly. As a general rule, diabetes and leisure-time physical inactivity rates correlate significantly with obesity rates; the higher the obesity rate the higher the diabetes and leisure-time physical inactivity rate. Longevity rates are inversely correlated; the higher the obesity rate the lower the longevity rate.

There are 53 counties that fall into the 13.5%-19.9% obesity rate category, 180 counties that are in the 20.0%-24.1% category, and 370 counties that are in the 24.2%-27.2% category. That's 603 counties or almost 20% of the 3,108 counties. If 80% equals a "B" grade, this may be a good place to start your search for the healthiest places to live.

The lowest obesity rates (13.5%-19.9%) are correlated with either high or low elevation. Santa Barbara, California, has an obesity rate of 19.9% and a mean altitude of 1,823'. Denver, Colorado, has an obesity rate of 18.2% and a mean altitude of 5,332'. There are no counties with an obesity rate of 13.5%-19.9% that are in the 3,509' elevation gap between Santa Barbara and Denver.

It is important to realize that the CDC obesity, diabetes, and leisure-time physical inactivity rates are "raw" numbers. This means they don't account for demographic factors such as race, income, education, etc. While there are some exceptions, the majority of the counties with the lowest obesity rates don't reflect demographics that are representative of their state as a whole. This can skew certain important characteristics of a county.

Let's take housing costs as an example. According to the US Census Bureau, of the 25 counties with the lowest obesity rates, only Lake County and Conejos County in Colorado have owner-occupied housing units, 2009-2013, with a median value of less than the state average. The other 23 counties with the lowest obesity rates have a higher-than-state-average median value of owner-occupied housing units; in some cases, much higher. So if you are seeking a healthy, but relatively low-cost, county in which to spend your retirement years, you will need to factor this type of information into your decision-making criteria. You can find a wealth of county-level facts and data on the US Census Bureau website at www.quickfacts.census.gov.

With the exception of a few very urban counties, low obesity rates are generally correlated with higher natural amenities. But, here's something interesting. The ten counties rated lowest for natural amenities don't have the highest obesity and diabetes rates. The longevity rates for these counties are also relatively high. Nine of the ten counties rated lowest for natural amenities are located in Minnesota and North Dakota where there are cold winters! So perhaps cold winter temperatures might actually be good for our health. There's some new research out there that indicates this may be true.

Researchers at the University of California, Berkeley have found that exposure to cold temperatures increases levels of a newly discovered protein that is critical for the formation of brown fat. Unlike white fat, brown fat is active, using up calories to keep the body warm. The study authors noted that there's an active area of research in the relationship between brown fat and diabetes. Higher levels of brown fat are associated with greater sensitivity to insulin. Resistance to insulin leads to Type 2 diabetes. Here is what principal investigator Hei Sook Sul, UC Berkeley professor of nutritional science and toxicology has to say.

> Knowing which proteins regulate brown fat is significant because brown fat is not only important for thermogenesis, but there is evidence that brown fat may also affect metabolism and insulin resistance. If you can somehow increase levels of this protein through drugs, you

could have more brown fat, and could possibly lose more weight even if eating the same amount of food.[2]

But, until our scientific community develops this or another "magic obesity pill," the best solution we have is to leverage Mother Nature. Natural amenities, altitude, and perhaps even cold winter temperatures can help tip the scales. Today, Mother Nature offers the very best weight loss program in the world.

The blue book dataset headers are as follows:

ABBREVIATION	DESCRIPTION
ST	State
COUNTY	County
USDA	USDA numerical rating with +11.17 denoting the highest number of natural amenities and -6.40 denoting the lowest number of natural amenities
AMEN	Numerical amenity ranking of the USDA natural amenities data with +11.17 being #1 and -6.40 being #3,108. #1 denotes highest ranking and #3,108 denotes lowest ranking
OBES	% obesity among adults ≥ 20
DIAB	% diabetes among adults ≥ 20
INACT	% leisure-time physical inactivity among adults ≥ 20
M AGE	Longevity for men in years
W AGE	Longevity for women in years
ALT ft.	Mean county altitude in feet
ALT m.	Mean county altitude in meters

Obesity Ratings for 3,108 Lower Forty-Eight Counties

ST	COUNTY	USDA	AMEN	OBES	DIAB	INACT	M AGE	W AGE	ALT ft	ALT m
CO	Routt	5.29	90	13.5	3.8	11.1	78.6	83.3	8197	2499
WY	Teton	5.39	87	13.8	4.4	10.6	79.9	84.7	8044	2452
CO	Eagle	4.57	156	13.9	4.2	11.8	79.1	83.1	9074	2766
NM	Santa Fe	3.02	306	14.1	3.9	12	78.1	82.9	6924	2110
CO	Pitkin	6.14	54	14.2	4.7	12.7	80	84.2	10010	3051
CO	Boulder	5.82	71	14.5	4.6	11.3	77.6	81.4	7381	2250
CA	Marin	8.14	18	15	5.4	12.1	80.8	84.5	426	130
CO	Summit	8.08	19	15.1	4.7	12.3	79.3	83	10481	3195
NY	New York	-0.31	1682	15.2	7.2	16.4	78.7	83.7	48	15
CO	Douglas	5.15	104	15.7	4.6	11.1	80.3	83.5	6876	2096
UT	Summit	4.96	131	15.7	4.5	13	78.7	82.8	8472	2582
CO	Gunnison	4.94	132	15.7	4.8	15.3	80	84.2	9548	2910

ST	COUNTY	USDA	AMEN	OBES	DIAB	INACT	M AGE	W AGE	ALT ft	ALT m
CO	Chaffee	6.46	47	15.9	4.6	15.6	77.1	81.1	9959	3035
CO	La Plata	5.83	69	15.9	4.6	15.5	77.9	82.2	7988	2435
CO	San Miguel	5.14	108	16.4	5.4	13.7	75.6	80.9	7943	2421
CO	Archuleta	5.58	80	16.5	5	16.7	76.8	81.4	8265	2519
CO	Ouray	6.08	57	17	5.4	15	75.7	81.2	8980	2737
NY	Westchester	0.80	913	17	6.7	18.6	79.2	83.3	340	104
CA	San Francisco	10.52	6	17.2	7.3	17	77.6	83.8	236	72
CO	Conejos	4.98	123	17.2	4.7	18.9	76.8	81.4	8951	2728
ID	Blaine	2.94	317	17.2	5.3	13.3	79.3	83.6	6103	1860
CO	Garfield	3.81	214	17.3	5.4	15.5	76.7	81.5	7893	2406
MT	Gallatin	3.86	210	17.4	4.4	17.3	78.3	82.4	6274	1912
CO	Lake	8.52	11	17.7	5.1	18.9	77.1	81.6	10931	3332
CO	Park	7.11	33	17.7	5	19.2	77.1	81.6	9672	2948
CO	Clear Creek	6.96	37	17.7	5.1	17.3	78.2	82	10296	3138
CO	Teller	6.29	52	17.8	6	18.7	77.9	81.8	9181	2798
CT	Fairfield	2.25	421	18	5.8	19.2	78.9	83.3	378	115
MA	Barnstable	1.52	592	18.1	6.1	16.6	78.1	82.9	55	17
MD	Montgomery	-0.57	1859	18.1	6.5	16.6	80.7	84.5	404	123
MA	Dukes	2.89	321	18.2	7.8	18.1	78.2	82.9	58	18
CO	Denver	2.88	323	18.2	6.1	16.3	74.4	80.9	5335	1626
CO	Grand	7.47	25	18.3	5.2	16.9	78.2	82	9259	2822
CO	Larimer	5.62	77	18.5	5	14.2	79.2	82.7	7725	2355
CO	Montrose	2.94	315	18.6	4.9	18.9	75.3	81	6943	2116
CO	Mineral	5.79	72	18.7	5.2	17.2	75.7	81.2	10492	3198
CO	Jefferson	5.61	79	18.7	5.2	15.7	77.6	81.4	7056	2151
CO	San Juan	7.16	31	18.8	5.3	18.4	75.6	80.9	11344	3458
NM	Taos	4.16	189	18.8	5.9	15.7	75.4	81.8	8533	2601
NM	Los Alamos	3.04	303	18.8	5.3	14.4	80.1	83	7655	2333
CO	Hinsdale	6.90	38	18.9	5.3	18.3	75.7	81.2	10935	3333
CO	Montezuma	4.41	167	18.9	5.7	19.8	75.6	80.9	6813	2077
CO	Gilpin	6.97	36	19.2	5.4	18.7	77.1	81.8	9303	2836
WA	San Juan	4.35	172	19.2	4.9	13.1	77.3	81.1	180	55
FL	Monroe	6.05	59	19.4	6.1	18.1	76	81.8	3	1
CO	Arapahoe	2.35	398	19.4	5.8	17.2	78.4	82.3	5468	1667
VA	Arlington	-2.25	2674	19.4	7.5	17.6	79.7	83.3	207	63
CA	Santa Cruz	8.49	12	19.5	6.1	12.4	78.1	82.6	939	286
CT	Litchfield	1.04	796	19.7	6.1	18.5	77.3	82.5	914	279
CA	San Mateo	8.19	17	19.8	6.5	16.1	79.8	84.5	669	204
CA	Santa Barbara	10.97	3	19.9	6.6	15.8	78.3	83.1	1823	556
NM	Bernalillo	3.77	216	19.9	6	15.9	74.8	81.1	5967	1819
UT	Grand	2.08	455	19.9	5.8	18.2	75.7	80	5752	1753
OR	Deschutes	6.10	56	20	6.6	15.3	78.4	81.7	4577	1395
CO	Rio Blanco	3.59	240	20	5.4	18.9	74.8	80.3	7231	2204
MA	Norfolk	-0.64	1906	20	6.4	19.4	78.2	82.6	191	58
CA	Nevada	7.26	28	20.1	5.5	12.9	78	81.8	4139	1262
CO	Huerfano	5.20	100	20.1	5.5	23.1	74.5	80.1	7507	2288
CA	Alameda	5.13	110	20.1	7.3	16.6	77.7	82.3	864	263

ST	COUNTY	USDA	AMEN	OBES	DIAB	INACT	M AGE	W AGE	ALT ft	ALT m
VT	Chittenden	0.09	1374	20.1	5.2	15	77.5	82.1	685	209
CO	Custer	5.61	78	20.2	5.4	20.5	74.9	79.9	9062	2762
VA	Alexandria	-2.25	2673	20.2	7.8	18.7	78.3	83.6	112	34
CA	Mono	8.21	16	20.3	6.5	13.6	77	80.7	7760	2365
CA	Placer	6.00	62	20.3	6.5	13.8	79	82.8	3812	1162
CO	Dolores	4.38	170	20.3	5.2	20.8	75.6	80.9	8330	2539
CO	Delta	3.64	232	20.3	5.6	22.7	75.9	81.5	6982	2128
CA	El Dorado	6.10	55	20.4	6.5	14.1	77.2	81.5	4256	1297
CO	Costilla	4.96	130	20.4	5.7	18.8	74.5	80.1	8861	2701
CO	Alamosa	1.59	571	20.4	6.2	19.9	74.5	80.1	7744	2360
CA	Orange	8.74	10	20.5	7.1	16.4	79.3	83.6	725	221
CO	Jackson	6.45	49	20.5	5.4	17.9	78.6	83.3	8919	2719
MT	Missoula	1.74	539	20.5	5.3	16.7	76.7	81	4954	1510
RI	Bristol	1.36	649	20.5	5.2	19	77	82.6	32	10
NJ	Hunterdon	0.83	898	20.5	6.2	18.4	79.4	82.7	400	122
CO	Saguache	4.91	137	20.7	4.8	18.2	74.9	79.9	9206	2806
NM	Lincoln	4.26	178	20.8	5.5	20	76.3	81.8	5852	1784
MT	Sweet Grass	3.19	282	20.8	6.2	27.9	75.8	80.9	5623	1714
MT	Ravalli	1.59	572	20.8	5.3	20	77.1	81.3	5918	1804
NY	Nassau	0.76	930	20.8	7.3	22.3	79.4	83.3	94	29
PA	Chester	-1.53	2395	20.8	7.5	18.5	77.9	82.2	442	135
RI	Washington	2.64	349	20.9	5.8	18.7	78.1	82	156	48
MT	Jefferson	2.27	419	20.9	6.6	19.9	75.9	80.9	5869	1789
CO	Cheyenne	-0.04	1470	20.9	5.4	19.6	74.4	80.6	4350	1326
CO	El Paso	5.15	105	21	6	18.2	76.6	81.1	6423	1958
MN	Hennepin	-2.15	2637	21	6	16.3	78.1	82.4	924	282
CA	Santa Clara	5.95	64	21.1	7.4	16.6	80.6	83.9	1226	374
CO	Rio Grande	5.26	92	21.1	6	22.5	75.7	81.2	9029	2752
NM	Colfax	3.70	226	21.1	6.2	23.7	75.4	80.3	7214	2199
CO	Washington	0.58	1027	21.1	5.6	24.3	75	80.7	4604	1403
MT	Park	3.61	237	21.2	5.2	21.4	78.3	82.4	6960	2122
CO	Elbert	0.90	859	21.2	4.5	18.9	77.9	81.9	5965	1818
FL	Sarasota	4.78	144	21.3	7.3	18.1	77.8	83.8	21	6
NJ	Monmouth	0.64	990	21.3	7.5	21.2	77.3	81.6	111	34
NJ	Somerset	-1.44	2346	21.3	6.2	21.2	78.7	82.5	196	60
CA	Los Angeles	10.33	7	21.4	7.7	18.9	77.4	82.5	2265	691
WY	Lincoln	5.12	111	21.4	7.8	20.7	76.8	81.4	7381	2250
RI	Newport	2.14	445	21.4	6.1	18.6	77.9	81.7	102	31
SC	Beaufort	1.66	555	21.4	7	17.2	78	83.3	10	3
NJ	Morris	1.30	677	21.4	6.6	20.5	79.5	82.2	636	194
CA	San Luis Obispo	7.87	21	21.5	5.9	14.2	77.9	82.2	1552	473
NM	Mora	5.22	96	21.5	6.7	21.8	75.4	81.8	7166	2184
FL	St. Johns	2.98	310	21.5	7.4	17.7	77.6	82.8	22	7
MT	Musselshell	1.22	724	21.5	6.6	26.7	75.8	80.9	3510	1070
NJ	Bergen	1.20	733	21.6	6.8	23.3	79.3	83.5	192	59
CO	Lincoln	1.05	789	21.6	6.4	23.1	74.4	80.6	5122	1561
ME	Cumberland	1.05	793	21.6	6.8	16.3	77.1	81.7	282	86

HEALTHIEST PLACES TO LIVE

ST	COUNTY	USDA	AMEN	OBES	DIAB	INACT	M AGE	W AGE	ALT ft	ALT m
DC	Dist of Columbia	-0.76	1976	21.6	8.5	19.9	71.6	78.5	139	42
NV	Douglas	7.61	22	21.7	6.3	16.4	79.1	82.7	6047	1843
FL	Martin	5.34	88	21.7	6.2	18.9	77.7	83.4	21	6
WY	Park	3.96	202	21.7	6	21.2	76.1	81.5	7529	2295
AZ	Santa Cruz	5.95	63	21.8	6.1	16.7	74.3	81	4548	1386
MT	Flathead	2.80	332	21.8	5.6	19.2	75.5	80.5	4908	1496
CO	Las Animas	3.60	238	21.9	6.2	23.3	75	80.5	5947	1813
IN	Hamilton	-2.53	2792	21.9	8.1	19.4	78.6	82.7	851	259
AZ	Yavapai	5.21	97	22	6.6	19.1	75.8	81.6	4508	1374
WY	Albany	4.91	138	22	5.7	19.4	77.2	81.1	7464	2275
NJ	Union	0.14	1341	22	8.2	25.2	77.2	81.1	127	39
CA	Napa	7.53	23	22.1	6.2	15.1	77.2	81.9	935	285
FL	Collier	5.00	120	22.1	7.2	16.2	80.2	86	11	3
MA	Suffolk	0.83	896	22.1	8.6	22.1	75.8	81.9	57	17
MA	Hampshire	-0.01	1445	22.1	6.6	16.9	77.5	81.6	739	225
CO	Phillips	-0.71	1946	22.1	5.8	18.5	75.8	80.2	3819	1164
FL	Palm Beach	5.14	109	22.2	8	21.6	77.1	83.5	15	5
CO	Fremont	4.82	143	22.2	6.8	19.6	74.9	79.9	7525	2294
FL	Indian River	4.72	147	22.2	8.4	22.6	77	82.6	25	8
ID	Bonner	4.57	157	22.2	6.6	19	76.1	80.7	3168	966
CO	Mesa	2.26	420	22.2	5.4	17.8	75.9	81.2	6846	2087
CT	Tolland	1.48	602	22.2	6.9	19.1	78.3	82.5	581	177
NY	Queens	0.01	1430	22.2	9	28	79	83.7	54	17
CA	Monterey	9.24	9	22.3	7.3	16	78	82.6	1464	446
OR	Hood River	4.54	158	22.3	7.4	16.8	76.3	81.5	3018	920
WA	King	4.53	160	22.3	6.6	16.7	78.6	82.8	1842	561
UT	Morgan	3.72	221	22.3	6.8	18.2	78.8	81.8	6736	2053
CO	Prowers	1.13	757	22.3	6.1	26.9	74.2	79.3	3801	1159
VT	Washington	-0.63	1902	22.3	6.2	17	77.7	81.2	1338	408
OR	Benton	3.10	296	22.4	6.8	14.8	78.7	81.9	787	240
CO	Crowley	2.60	359	22.5	6.4	22.9	74.1	80	4539	1383
CA	Mendocino	10.93	4	22.6	6.3	17	75.6	80.8	1827	557
NV	Washoe	6.77	40	22.6	6.4	17.2	75.2	80.3	5359	1633
MA	Nantucket	2.89	322	22.6	7.6	19.8	78.1	82.9	26	8
NC	Orange	-1.39	2319	22.6	6.5	16.5	77.4	81.5	604	184
CA	Sonoma	7.93	20	22.7	6.1	14.2	77.8	82.1	729	222
NV	Storey	5.11	113	22.7	7.4	22.4	74.5	79.9	5565	1696
NM	San Miguel	3.73	218	22.7	6.4	19	72.7	79.8	5930	1807
WY	Crook	2.57	365	22.7	6.1	22.2	75.9	81.5	4270	1301
MT	Granite	2.27	418	22.7	5.8	24.3	75.5	80.5	6118	1865
CO	Baca	0.48	1084	22.7	5.7	22.3	74.2	79.3	4292	1308
CA	San Diego	9.78	8	22.8	7.3	17.4	77.6	82.4	1975	602
OR	Jackson	4.50	164	22.8	6.6	13.9	76.2	81.5	3182	970
NC	Polk	1.84	512	22.8	7	23	74.9	80.8	1220	372
SD	Lawrence	1.76	531	22.8	5.7	23.6	77	81.3	4968	1514
MA	Plymouth	1.09	779	22.8	7.4	20.5	76.3	81.3	80	24
VT	Addison	-0.28	1659	22.8	5.6	18.5	77.1	82.3	849	259

183

ST	COUNTY	USDA	AMEN	OBES	DIAB	INACT	M AGE	W AGE	ALT ft	ALT m
VA	Loudoun	-0.63	1901	22.8	7.9	21	79	82.2	461	140
CA	Ventura	11.17	1	22.9	6.8	16.8	78.1	82.6	2690	820
CT	Middlesex	2.32	407	22.9	6.3	20.2	77.8	82.5	286	87
VT	Bennington	-0.81	2018	22.9	5.9	19.5	76.8	81.5	1710	521
MT	Daniels	-3.82	3050	22.9	6.5	23.6	73.6	79.5	2635	803
MT	Beaverhead	3.50	246	23	7.1	20	76.6	79.8	7078	2157
NM	De Baca	3.43	254	23	6.7	26.4	72.9	79.6	4435	1352
GA	Forsyth	0.99	817	23	9.2	20.2	77.2	81.8	1156	352
ID	Lemhi	0.43	1121	23	7.3	16.4	76.2	80.4	6928	2112
MA	Middlesex	-1.12	2203	23	7.6	20.8	78.8	82.9	226	69
NV	Carson City	7.29	27	23.1	7.1	19.8	74	79.6	5780	1762
CA	Tuolumne	7.10	34	23.1	6	18.1	77	80.7	5653	1723
CA	Inyo	7.08	35	23.1	6.9	16.7	75.5	81.1	4163	1269
MT	Sanders	2.33	406	23.1	7.1	25.5	74.7	79.8	4102	1250
CO	Logan	1.29	682	23.1	5.5	22.1	75.8	80.2	4193	1278
VT	Windham	0.04	1413	23.1	5.6	15.8	76.7	81.9	1353	412
NY	Tompkins	-0.28	1655	23.1	7	21.7	77.7	81.4	1200	366
CO	Moffat	4.14	190	23.2	6	26.1	74.8	80.3	6733	2052
MT	Lewis & Clark	3.16	286	23.2	6.2	19	76.7	80.5	5337	1627
ID	Boundary	2.61	357	23.2	7.1	25.9	76.1	80.7	4068	1240
ID	Ada	1.87	504	23.2	7	15.1	77.8	81.9	3074	937
MA	Essex	1.43	625	23.2	8.3	21.7	77.4	81.7	86	26
VA	Fairfax	-1.31	2285	23.2	8.1	18.7	81.1	83.8	266	81
WY	Johnson	2.78	335	23.3	7.2	21.9	76.6	81.5	5557	1694
CT	New London	2.43	384	23.3	7.4	22.1	76.4	81.5	248	76
NC	Ashe	2.28	417	23.3	7.4	24.7	73.7	79.2	3198	975
GA	Cobb	-0.17	1570	23.3	9.1	21.3	77.6	81.3	981	299
MT	Custer	-1.06	2171	23.3	7.1	24	75	80.7	2845	867
CA	Sierra	5.90	66	23.4	6.9	17.7	76.3	81.5	5746	1751
ID	Fremont	2.95	314	23.4	7.9	22.3	76.2	80.4	6163	1879
UT	Wasatch	4.92	136	23.5	6.3	15.5	77.5	80.5	8034	2449
MA	Berkshire	0.81	908	23.5	7.5	21.1	76.9	81.1	1404	428
NJ	Middlesex	-0.57	1862	23.5	8.1	27.1	78	82.4	85	26
AZ	Maricopa	4.87	139	23.6	7.6	19.3	76.8	81.6	1677	511
CA	Trinity	4.07	194	23.6	7.3	20.6	74.6	80.7	3805	1160
CO	Pueblo	2.11	450	23.6	6.9	19.3	74.1	80	5212	1589
GA	Fayette	-0.24	1628	23.6	9.8	20.3	77.8	82	865	264
KS	Johnson	-1.69	2467	23.6	6.4	17.5	78.9	82.6	991	302
OH	Geauga	-2.45	2764	23.6	8	19.9	78.1	82.5	1166	355
IA	Johnson	-2.64	2823	23.6	6.5	19.3	79.3	82.5	745	227
TX	El Paso	4.46	165	23.7	8.3	21.7	76.3	82	4069	1240
MT	Fergus	2.63	350	23.7	6	22.7	75.3	80.8	3779	1152
MT	Petroleum	1.86	509	23.7	6.6	24.5	76.1	81	2958	901
NH	Grafton	0.32	1206	23.7	7.1	19	78.8	82	1492	455
CO	Yuma	0.30	1213	23.7	5.3	21.1	75.2	79.9	3934	1199
WY	Niobrara	-0.01	1451	23.7	6.3	28.5	76.3	80.9	4532	1381
AZ	Cochise	7.13	32	23.8	7.2	22.3	75.8	81.1	4635	1413

HEALTHIEST PLACES TO LIVE

ST	COUNTY	USDA	AMEN	OBES	DIAB	INACT	M AGE	W AGE	ALT ft	ALT m
NM	Grant	6.45	50	23.8	6	19.2	74.7	80.6	5823	1775
TX	Kendall	4.72	148	23.8	7.8	23.9	76.5	81.2	1558	475
UT	Cache	2.63	353	23.8	6.5	17.9	78.8	81.8	6306	1922
ME	Lincoln	1.55	584	23.8	6.7	19.4	77.3	81	158	48
CT	Hartford	1.05	790	23.8	7.3	22.5	76.6	81.7	316	96
GA	Fulton	-0.24	1629	23.8	9.2	19.8	75	80.2	940	287
TN	Williamson	-0.87	2053	23.8	8.2	18.8	77.9	82	778	237
IL	McHenry	-2.40	2736	23.8	6.4	23.5	77.7	81.6	873	266
CA	Plumas	6.55	44	23.9	6.6	18.4	76.3	81.5	5309	1618
FL	Miami-Dade	5.48	84	23.9	8.6	23.6	76.6	82.8	5	1
CA	San Benito	5.20	99	23.9	7	16.1	77.7	82	1939	591
ID	Caribou	3.08	297	23.9	7	26.2	76.2	80.9	6494	1979
OR	Washington	2.65	347	23.9	6.1	16.5	78.9	82.5	743	227
CO	Kiowa	2.31	409	23.9	5.5	19.8	74.4	80.6	4157	1267
NJ	Hudson	0.49	1081	23.9	8.3	28.6	75.8	81.3	37	11
PA	Bucks	0.01	1433	23.9	8	22.1	77.1	81.4	337	103
WI	Dane	-0.17	1580	23.9	6.1	17.7	78.7	82.5	957	292
MT	Carter	-0.58	1871	23.9	6	30.7	75	80.7	3426	1044
FL	Pinellas	5.05	117	24	8.2	19.5	74.7	81.4	21	6
UT	Washington	2.57	364	24	6.5	17.1	78.8	83.5	5072	1546
NC	Buncombe	2.18	437	24	7.9	19.6	74.6	80.5	2684	818
WY	Washakie	1.10	777	24	7.2	23.8	75	80.6	5211	1588
IL	Lake	-0.30	1666	24	7.1	18.9	78.5	81.7	740	226
MT	Powder River	-1.02	2145	24	6.4	29.1	75	80.7	3503	1068
MN	Wabasha	-1.13	2207	24	6.3	22.3	77.1	81.8	985	300
MN	Rice	-2.20	2653	24	7.3	17.2	77.3	82	1095	334
CA	Mariposa	8.25	15	24.1	7.2	19.4	76.3	81.1	3637	1108
OR	Multnomah	4.33	174	24.1	7.5	16.4	75.3	80.2	1025	313
NM	Hidalgo	3.37	262	24.1	6.1	23.5	73.2	79.8	4735	1443
UT	Carbon	3.13	293	24.1	7.8	25.1	74.6	80.2	7129	2173
UT	Kane	2.97	312	24.1	7.5	21.6	74.9	80.2	5736	1748
WI	La Crosse	-0.69	1939	24.1	7.2	18.4	76.9	81.9	891	272
MN	Ramsey	-2.08	2612	24.1	7	15	77.4	82.5	918	280
CA	Contra Costa	8.36	13	24.2	6.9	17.3	78.3	82.4	486	148
WA	Whatcom	5.26	93	24.2	6.8	15.5	77.7	82.2	3024	922
MT	Madison	3.22	280	24.2	6	26.3	74.6	79.8	6657	2029
WA	Chelan	1.56	581	24.2	7.3	19.1	77.8	81.9	3944	1202
NJ	Passaic	1.30	678	24.2	8.2	27.4	76.3	81.1	587	179
WY	Hot Springs	1.08	782	24.2	7.3	22.9	76.1	81.5	6124	1867
OR	Grant	0.44	1116	24.2	7.6	18.4	75.9	80.4	4696	1431
NY	Albany	0.30	1216	24.2	7.1	22.4	76.1	80.8	770	235
VT	Windsor	0.14	1346	24.2	6.4	19.1	77.2	81.7	1273	388
MA	Franklin	0.00	1440	24.2	6.7	18.7	77.1	81.3	853	260
IL	DuPage	-2.33	2699	24.2	6.8	18.9	79	82.4	733	223
UT	Piute	3.87	209	24.3	6.9	24.4	75.2	79.9	7786	2373
NM	Sandoval	3.66	228	24.3	6.4	19.1	76.4	81.1	6720	2048
NC	Henderson	1.99	475	24.3	7.9	22.1	75.6	80.8	2413	736

ST	COUNTY	USDA	AMEN	OBES	DIAB	INACT	M AGE	W AGE	ALT ft	ALT m
TX	Collin	1.01	811	24.3	7.6	22.1	79.7	82.5	613	187
NM	Union	0.99	820	24.3	5.9	24.6	75.4	80.3	5423	1653
CO	Sedgwick	0.92	851	24.3	5.2	19.4	75.8	80.2	3761	1146
NY	Cayuga	-1.44	2347	24.3	7.9	24.9	76	80.8	781	238
MN	Rock	-4.25	3087	24.3	6.7	22.2	75.8	82.1	1547	471
CA	Colusa	4.34	173	24.4	7.4	17.2	74.2	80.3	767	234
UT	Salt Lake	4.21	187	24.4	7.5	18.4	77.1	81.3	5577	1700
MT	Powell	1.79	524	24.4	7	25.5	75.5	80.5	5676	1730
NY	Yates	-0.03	1467	24.4	7.5	26.1	76	81.5	1035	315
MD	Howard	-1.42	2333	24.4	7.3	17.6	79.8	82.6	442	135
MI	Washtenaw	-2.19	2649	24.4	8.5	19.4	77.9	81.7	881	268
MN	Wright	-2.50	2784	24.4	6.2	17.9	77.8	82.1	1005	306
NM	Rio Arriba	5.23	95	24.5	6.3	22.4	71	79.5	7657	2334
CO	Bent	2.45	379	24.5	6	22.6	74.2	79.3	4130	1259
NC	Transylvania	2.40	388	24.5	7.4	22.8	75.5	82.1	2824	861
WY	Sheridan	2.17	441	24.5	7.5	19.1	76.6	81.5	5151	1570
NY	Kings	-0.17	1575	24.5	9.5	27.6	76.8	82.3	40	12
IL	Montgomery	-2.18	2645	24.5	8.3	27.4	74.1	79.8	640	195
IA	Winneshiek	-4.44	3091	24.5	7.2	21.6	77.6	82.9	1142	348
CA	Imperial	6.45	48	24.6	7.3	22.6	75.1	81.7	415	126
NM	Catron	6.24	53	24.6	6.3	19.3	73.3	79.8	7377	2248
WY	Platte	4.10	193	24.6	8.6	26.8	75.9	81.2	5155	1571
WY	Fremont	3.71	225	24.6	7.3	24.6	73.3	79.7	7037	2145
CO	Adams	2.48	373	24.6	6.9	21.3	77.6	81.4	5088	1551
UT	Wayne	0.92	853	24.6	6.8	20.3	75.5	79.8	6110	1862
MT	Treasure	-0.02	1455	24.6	6.2	26.8	76.1	81	3032	924
MN	Scott	-2.95	2897	24.6	6.2	17.4	78.3	82.4	928	283
UT	Davis	5.54	82	24.7	6.8	16.5	78.2	81.1	4589	1399
CA	Modoc	4.99	121	24.7	6.7	18.9	75.5	79.8	4979	1517
TX	Travis	3.24	279	24.7	8	19.2	77.6	81.4	726	221
ID	Teton	1.90	497	24.7	7.7	17.4	76.7	80.4	6512	1985
MT	Judith Basin	1.89	499	24.7	5.8	28	75.6	81.2	5039	1536
NM	Quay	1.66	554	24.7	6.1	27.3	72.9	79.6	4323	1318
NH	Carroll	0.93	849	24.7	7.3	20	77.1	82.4	1033	315
NY	Hamilton	0.24	1266	24.7	8.6	21.4	75.6	80.7	1985	605
ID	Lincoln	-0.41	1762	24.7	7.4	23.2	74.3	80	4370	1332
CA	Amador	7.23	29	24.8	8	16.6	76.3	81.1	2655	809
WA	Jefferson	5.31	89	24.8	6.4	15.7	77.8	83.2	2186	666
CA	Butte	5.11	112	24.8	8	16.3	74	80	1558	475
UT	Garfield	4.00	200	24.8	7	23.2	75.2	79.9	6778	2066
MT	Teton	3.88	206	24.8	6.2	25.1	74.4	80.2	4502	1372
TX	Presidio	3.06	299	24.8	8.2	25.5	75	80.8	4287	1307
NC	Chatham	0.41	1134	24.8	8	21.7	75.4	80.5	424	129
NJ	Mercer	-0.80	2009	24.8	8.7	25.2	76.2	81.4	130	40
MN	Crow Wing	-2.14	2633	24.8	6.4	17.3	77.3	81.8	1256	383
CA	Alpine	7.41	26	24.9	7.9	19.4	77	80.7	7732	2357
AZ	Coconino	4.93	134	24.9	7.5	17	75.8	80.8	5914	1803

HEALTHIEST PLACES TO LIVE

ST	COUNTY	USDA	AMEN	OBES	DIAB	INACT	M AGE	W AGE	ALT ft	ALT m
NC	Watauga	1.82	519	24.9	8.8	20.8	76.7	80.8	3298	1005
NJ	Cape May	0.07	1392	24.9	8.4	22.3	74.2	80.2	13	4
MN	Hubbard	-3.24	2955	24.9	6.9	18.7	76	81.5	1453	443
OR	Josephine	4.26	179	25	8.1	20.7	73.9	80.3	2418	737
ID	Bear Lake	3.62	235	25	7.5	28.9	76.2	80.9	6769	2063
CA	Siskiyou	3.36	264	25	7	18.7	74.6	80.7	4254	1297
FL	Seminole	3.14	289	25	10.1	20.2	77.1	81.5	37	11
MT	Meagher	2.83	328	25	6.5	27.3	75.9	80.9	5861	1786
NM	Guadalupe	2.66	346	25	6.3	22.9	72.9	79.6	5179	1578
CO	Weld	1.70	543	25	6.2	18.5	77.6	81.4	4964	1513
PA	Montgomery	-0.53	1835	25	7.3	20.7	77.7	82	287	87
MT	Fallon	-1.33	2292	25	6.3	30.8	75.7	81	3018	920
ND	Burleigh	-2.01	2584	25	6.9	21.1	77.4	83	1900	579
MN	Yellow Medicine	-3.98	3066	25	7	19.5	76	81.1	1127	343
WY	Laramie	3.05	301	25.1	7.9	23.4	74.9	79.8	5987	1825
FL	Alachua	2.44	383	25.1	8.3	22.6	75.1	79.8	103	31
ME	Hancock	1.87	505	25.1	7.2	19.6	76	81.3	293	89
NM	Torrance	4.02	197	25.2	6.5	23.8	74.3	79.4	6455	1967
CA	Tehama	3.24	278	25.2	8.3	16.7	74.1	79.1	2144	653
UT	Iron	2.37	394	25.2	7.1	19.5	76.2	80.3	6376	1943
MT	Silver Bow	2.15	443	25.2	7.1	24.6	74.6	79.8	6456	1968
NY	Rockland	0.77	925	25.2	8.7	24.3	78.7	82.8	422	129
MA	Worcester	0.24	1264	25.2	8	22.6	76.4	81.2	709	216
MI	Ottawa	-0.04	1475	25.2	8.2	21.3	78.8	82.4	655	200
GA	Gwinnett	-0.35	1709	25.2	8.7	20.7	77.2	80.9	997	304
FL	Broward	4.98	124	25.3	8.3	22.5	76.5	82	11	3
OR	Sherman	1.61	566	25.3	7.6	17.8	75.9	80.8	1846	563
NY	Suffolk	1.52	593	25.3	7.1	22.2	77.6	81.7	76	23
ID	Jefferson	1.40	631	25.3	8.4	23.8	75.4	80.4	4879	1487
VA	Bedford	1.39	638	25.3	7.7	28.3	75.8	80.9	1050	320
GA	Bartow	1.17	741	25.3	9.3	24.8	71.9	78.2	856	261
NH	Rockingham	0.34	1193	25.3	6.8	20.1	77.8	81.7	266	81
NH	Merrimack	0.02	1423	25.3	6.9	20	77.1	81.4	729	222
NY	Columbia	-0.33	1691	25.3	6.7	21.1	75.9	80.6	620	189
WI	Walworth	-2.46	2766	25.3	6.8	21.3	77.2	80.8	927	283
IL	Kendall	-2.85	2874	25.3	6.6	24.8	77.4	81.9	654	199
ID	Kootenai	3.50	245	25.4	7.5	19.6	77.5	81.8	2940	896
MT	Wheatland	3.07	298	25.4	6.6	29.9	75.8	80.9	4859	1481
OR	Wallowa	2.68	343	25.4	6.9	19.3	75.7	80.2	4447	1355
MT	Lincoln	2.33	405	25.4	7.2	23.2	74.7	79.8	4259	1298
WA	Ferry	2.31	411	25.4	6.4	23.5	75.7	80.4	3275	998
GA	Columbia	0.79	915	25.4	9.3	22.2	75.4	80.2	357	109
NE	Grant	-0.08	1512	25.4	6.9	29.8	76.1	80.2	3773	1150
MN	Washington	-0.63	1897	25.4	6.8	16.6	78.8	82	918	280
VT	Lamoille	-0.82	2022	25.4	6.6	17.4	77.8	81.4	1284	391
IA	Butler	-3.94	3058	25.4	6.1	25.9	76.3	81	998	304
UT	Utah	4.93	135	25.5	7.3	16.4	78.5	81.7	6264	1909

ST	COUNTY	USDA	AMEN	OBES	DIAB	INACT	M AGE	W AGE	ALT ft	ALT m
OR	Lake	4.19	188	25.5	7.7	19.8	74.4	78.7	5132	1564
CO	Otero	2.24	425	25.5	6.4	22.1	74.4	80.6	4448	1356
MT	Cascade	2.20	431	25.5	7.6	23.4	75.6	81.2	4273	1302
NC	Alleghany	1.47	606	25.5	8.6	28.2	73.7	79.2	2868	874
NC	New Hanover	1.25	710	25.5	10.2	20.6	75.5	80.8	22	7
TX	Fort Bend	-0.52	1830	25.5	8.6	21.4	77.8	81.8	83	25
NC	Forsyth	-1.06	2172	25.5	8.8	21	74.5	79.5	848	258
VT	Caledonia	-1.16	2222	25.5	7.1	20.7	76.1	81.4	1350	411
OH	Delaware	-1.60	2426	25.5	8.8	21.6	77.5	81.2	942	287
WI	Green	-2.32	2697	25.5	6.7	18.1	76.5	81.2	924	282
CA	Calaveras	8.27	14	25.6	6.7	19.3	76.6	81.6	2430	741
NM	Dona Ana	4.77	146	25.6	6.9	17.5	76.3	80.9	4463	1360
TX	Henderson	2.72	338	25.6	9.2	28.4	73	79.2	410	125
NC	Mecklenburg	0.82	903	25.6	8.5	20.4	75.6	80.7	687	209
PA	Lackawanna	0.16	1333	25.6	8.1	28.3	74	80.3	1456	444
GA	Oconee	-1.04	2154	25.6	8.4	21.5	76.8	81.3	700	213
GA	Jackson	-1.20	2232	25.6	10.2	25.5	72.2	78.6	827	252
WI	Waukesha	-2.11	2621	25.6	5.9	18.5	78.7	82.2	894	272
WY	Sublette	5.29	91	25.7	5.8	23.2	76.8	81.4	8045	2452
OR	Clatsop	4.97	129	25.7	7.6	18.7	76.6	80.5	862	263
TX	Comal	3.25	276	25.7	8.3	25	76.8	81.8	1026	313
AL	Baldwin	1.82	516	25.7	9.9	24.2	74.4	80.3	121	37
ME	Sagadahoc	1.05	794	25.7	7.6	19.8	76.5	80.5	139	42
ME	York	0.86	880	25.7	7.2	20.4	77	81.5	309	94
NC	Wake	0.23	1278	25.7	7.8	18.5	77.6	82	324	99
WI	Ozaukee	-0.39	1750	25.7	6.9	17.5	78.6	82.7	777	237
IA	Mills	-1.00	2127	25.7	6.8	23.5	75.9	80.4	1089	332
MN	Meeker	-2.65	2827	25.7	8.2	23.6	76.4	80.8	1139	347
IA	Tama	-3.34	2972	25.7	7.8	28.5	77.1	81.4	951	290
MT	Broadwater	3.93	205	25.8	6.2	23.2	75.9	80.9	5015	1529
NC	Clay	3.05	300	25.8	8.1	22.3	73.4	79.7	2683	818
OR	Wheeler	2.79	333	25.8	7.7	18.8	75.6	80.5	3742	1141
TX	Randall	2.36	396	25.8	8.9	21.4	75.6	80.2	3623	1104
ME	Knox	2.06	457	25.8	7.6	20.7	76.7	81.4	235	72
MT	Garfield	0.65	985	25.8	6.2	26.8	75.7	81	2810	856
TX	Lamar	0.36	1180	25.8	9.4	31	72.5	78.2	492	150
IN	Monroe	0.29	1221	25.8	9.6	22.3	76.6	81.6	733	224
NY	Saratoga	0.11	1360	25.8	7.1	23.4	78	82.3	730	222
NJ	Essex	-0.02	1457	25.8	9.2	27.5	73.8	79.8	234	71
WI	Pierce	-1.21	2245	25.8	7.2	21	77.3	82.1	1025	312
CA	Humboldt	11.15	2	25.9	8.1	18.9	73.9	79.1	1754	535
FL	Manatee	4.66	152	25.9	8.9	24	75.9	82.8	55	17
AZ	Pima	4.04	196	25.9	7.1	19.3	75.8	81.7	2647	807
NM	Otero	4.00	198	25.9	7.8	22	75.6	79.7	5301	1616
FL	Volusia	3.45	250	25.9	9.6	24.6	74.3	80.6	28	9
ID	Camas	2.70	340	25.9	7.6	20.9	74.3	80	6320	1926
CO	Morgan	1.43	624	25.9	6.6	23	75	80.7	4492	1369

HEALTHIEST PLACES TO LIVE

ST	COUNTY	USDA	AMEN	OBES	DIAB	INACT	M AGE	W AGE	ALT ft	ALT m
SD	Custer	0.97	828	25.9	6.6	24	71.1	78.5	4234	1290
NY	Orange	0.09	1371	25.9	8.1	25.9	76.3	80.9	634	193
SD	Meade	-1.66	2448	25.9	7.5	27	74.8	80.5	2760	841
MN	Carver	-2.70	2839	25.9	6.6	16.9	78.6	83	971	296
IL	Menard	-3.04	2909	25.9	7.5	29	74.8	80	570	174
NV	Clark	4.86	140	26	8.8	25.6	74.1	79.7	3305	1008
FL	Hillsborough	4.32	175	26	9.6	24.1	74.7	80.4	63	19
UT	Sevier	3.66	229	26	8	21.9	75.5	79.8	7550	2301
OR	Morrow	3.34	265	26	8.3	24.1	75.6	80.5	2355	718
VA	Alleghany	1.77	527	26	8.4	23.8	72.8	79	2000	610
MT	McCone	0.52	1053	26	6	26.2	75.7	81	2483	757
GA	Paulding	0.44	1113	26	10.9	25.7	74.1	78.4	1026	313
IL	Cook	-1.04	2155	26	8.8	23.6	75.1	80.7	659	201
MN	Itasca	-2.36	2718	26	7	18	76	81.1	1363	416
IA	Cherokee	-2.66	2828	26	6.8	21.3	75.9	81.8	1365	416
MN	Dakota	-3.05	2914	26	6.3	16.9	78.7	81.7	922	281
IA	Story	-3.54	3008	26	6.5	21.1	78.5	83.1	1006	307
IA	Mitchell	-4.10	3078	26	6.4	26.9	76.6	81.4	1196	365
CA	Yolo	5.10	114	26.1	7.8	16.5	76.9	81.5	340	104
OR	Clackamas	3.64	234	26.1	7.9	16.9	77.8	81.4	2160	658
ID	Twin Falls	0.96	831	26.1	8.2	23.1	75.4	79.9	4795	1461
PA	Adams	-0.13	1549	26.1	8.9	27.1	76.1	80.5	758	231
GA	DeKalb	-0.30	1665	26.1	9.9	21.2	75.9	81.4	915	279
MT	Wibaux	-0.81	2016	26.1	6.5	29.9	75.7	81	2715	828
VT	Essex	-1.01	2142	26.1	6.6	23	75.4	80.3	1595	486
OH	Warren	-1.09	2187	26.1	9.2	22.1	76.7	80.5	848	259
VA	Falls Church	-1.31	2287	26.1	8.9	21.7	79.7	83.3	324	99
NE	Chase	-1.47	2364	26.1	6.8	26.4	76.1	81.4	3335	1017
IL	Marshall	-1.89	2540	26.1	7.7	28.5	74.9	80.3	656	200
IA	Winnebago	-3.81	3048	26.1	7.4	22.7	76.5	81.8	1264	385
MN	Marshall	-4.05	3074	26.1	6.9	20.7	75.3	82.4	1025	312
OR	Harney	3.45	252	26.2	7.7	19.5	75.9	80.4	4848	1478
SD	Pennington	1.27	693	26.2	7.3	22.1	76.6	81.5	3562	1086
MT	Liberty	0.45	1104	26.2	5.9	32.5	74.6	80.7	3372	1028
NC	Gaston	0.42	1128	26.2	9	28.4	71.9	78.1	763	233
NY	Sullivan	0.14	1342	26.2	8.6	23.8	74.6	79.9	1428	435
MD	Frederick	0.10	1367	26.2	8.2	21.8	76.8	81.2	599	183
VT	Grand Isle	-0.16	1568	26.2	5.5	18.1	76.4	81.1	106	32
MI	Houghton	-0.58	1870	26.2	8.8	26.2	75.2	80.1	1026	313
NY	Ontario	-0.67	1925	26.2	7.7	19.2	76.9	81.7	918	280
WI	Vilas	-1.58	2414	26.2	6.4	23.2	77	81.8	1672	510
MI	Livingston	-1.82	2514	26.2	7.6	19	77.2	81.2	935	285
NV	Lincoln	3.86	211	26.3	8.7	22.9	74.1	79.7	5266	1605
WA	Island	3.41	255	26.3	7.8	15.5	79.8	83.1	157	48
NC	Macon	3.33	266	26.3	8.1	23	74.5	80.8	3085	940
OR	Baker	2.42	386	26.3	7.9	18.8	75.7	80.2	4359	1329
TX	Montgomery	1.58	574	26.3	8.6	22.3	75.6	80.2	208	63

ST	COUNTY	USDA	AMEN	OBES	DIAB	INACT	M AGE	W AGE	ALT ft	ALT m
ID	Latah	1.13	760	26.3	7.8	17.7	77.6	81.6	2944	897
MD	Talbot	0.10	1368	26.3	7.5	20.9	76.4	81.7	26	8
VA	Rappahannock	-0.84	2032	26.3	8.5	24.5	73.9	80	1031	314
NY	Madison	-0.94	2096	26.3	7.1	22.4	76	80.5	1224	373
NY	Chemung	-1.13	2209	26.3	8.8	26.2	75.4	80	1303	397
WI	Wood	-2.44	2759	26.3	7.5	18.5	77	82.7	1081	330
IA	Sioux	-3.70	3035	26.3	5.7	23.3	77.5	82.8	1367	417
SD	Lincoln	-3.91	3055	26.3	5.8	22.8	77.3	81.4	1380	421
CA	Lassen	6.35	51	26.4	7.6	18.9	75.5	79.8	5361	1634
FL	Lee	5.23	94	26.4	8.6	22.3	76.4	83.1	15	5
WA	Kittitas	3.33	268	26.4	7.1	18.5	77.2	81.3	3169	966
FL	Walton	2.18	435	26.4	9.4	25.7	73.7	79.7	165	50
CA	Sutter	1.72	541	26.4	7.8	21.9	75	80.4	77	23
OR	Malheur	1.68	548	26.4	7.7	21	74.2	80	4291	1308
GA	Pickens	1.56	579	26.4	10	22.5	74.5	79.7	1417	432
NC	Catawba	1.32	667	26.4	8.2	26.1	74	79.1	981	299
NJ	Sussex	1.30	679	26.4	7.4	21.8	77.2	80.6	806	246
NH	Belknap	0.80	912	26.4	8	21.7	76	82	755	230
VA	Nelson	0.36	1182	26.4	9.1	22.7	73.1	79.7	1150	350
MT	Phillips	0.29	1225	26.4	6.2	30.4	75.3	80.8	2666	813
VA	Fauquier	-1.53	2396	26.4	8.7	20.5	76.7	80.8	528	161
VA	Hanover	-2.08	2613	26.4	8.4	19.9	76.5	80.8	181	55
IL	Lee	-2.93	2889	26.4	8.5	27.2	74.8	79.9	789	240
AZ	Gila	7.50	24	26.5	8.7	23.1	72.9	79.6	4662	1421
NM	Sierra	6.72	41	26.5	6.1	24.3	73.3	79.8	5445	1660
CA	Lake	6.55	43	26.5	7.8	16.6	73.2	78.4	2327	709
TX	Jeff Davis	5.93	65	26.5	8.8	22.6	76.3	82	4906	1495
OR	Tillamook	5.54	81	26.5	7.4	18.9	75.8	80.8	1113	339
OR	Klamath	5.15	107	26.5	7.3	20.4	74.4	78.7	4982	1518
UT	Beaver	2.39	392	26.5	7.5	22.3	75.2	79.9	6359	1938
TX	Midland	1.42	628	26.5	7.7	29.5	75.9	81.1	2765	843
TX	Rockwall	1.39	637	26.5	8.4	27.3	76.9	80.8	523	159
VA	Virginia Beach	1.18	740	26.5	8.7	24.6	76.8	81	9	3
TX	Grayson	0.78	922	26.5	8.6	25.6	73.6	79.1	707	216
NY	Ulster	0.70	961	26.5	7.5	22.9	76.6	80.9	1134	346
KS	Douglas	0.36	1175	26.5	7	19.6	78.1	81.9	966	295
KS	Riley	-0.11	1534	26.5	8	19.6	78.1	81.9	1244	379
VA	Augusta	-0.12	1541	26.5	8.7	25.1	75.1	80.6	1870	570
PA	Butler	-0.25	1638	26.5	8.6	22.5	75.9	80.8	1241	378
PA	Delaware	-0.69	1936	26.5	8.9	23.6	74.8	80	235	72
VA	Chesterfield	-0.84	2030	26.5	9.1	21.8	75.3	79.7	200	61
VA	Goochland	-1.06	2174	26.5	9.2	21.4	75.6	81.2	276	84
MN	Houston	-1.52	2387	26.5	7.1	19.1	76.9	81.8	974	297
MN	Mille Lacs	-1.74	2484	26.5	7.1	22.6	75.1	80.6	1185	361
IA	Cerro Gordo	-2.96	2898	26.5	8	23.5	75.7	81.5	1183	361
IA	Lyon	-4.49	3093	26.5	6.5	26.6	75.8	81.2	1417	432
UT	Rich	5.03	119	26.6	7.2	19.9	78.8	81.8	6822	2079

HEALTHIEST PLACES TO LIVE

ST	COUNTY	USDA	AMEN	OBES	DIAB	INACT	M AGE	W AGE	ALT ft	ALT m
FL	Orange	2.96	313	26.6	9.6	24.1	75.5	80.9	77	23
MT	Stillwater	2.63	351	26.6	6.3	22.3	75.8	80.9	5036	1535
GA	Dawson	2.48	374	26.6	9.2	22.9	74.6	80.2	1469	448
ID	Bonneville	2.00	471	26.6	8.3	20.4	76.4	80	6090	1856
ID	Payette	1.79	523	26.6	8.1	24.6	75	79.6	2596	791
AR	Carroll	1.75	535	26.6	9.1	26.8	74.3	79.4	1330	405
VA	Rockingham	1.25	714	26.6	8	20.1	75.8	81	1706	520
NC	Stanly	0.68	964	26.6	9.6	30.8	73.2	79.4	515	157
WI	Sawyer	-1.42	2336	26.6	7.7	21.9	75.5	80.4	1377	420
IA	Dickinson	-1.51	2380	26.6	6.8	20.9	78	82.1	1470	448
ND	Renville	-2.70	2841	26.6	6.8	25.1	74.4	80.2	1713	522
IL	Edwards	-2.90	2886	26.6	7.5	26.5	75.2	80.1	440	134
SD	McCook	-3.05	2916	26.6	7	27.7	76.2	81.6	1513	461
IL	Champaign	-4.55	3094	26.6	7.7	25.6	76.6	80.8	714	218
CA	Solano	5.88	67	26.7	9.7	21.2	76.1	81	167	51
UT	Sanpete	4.44	166	26.7	7.3	23.3	75.4	80.2	7311	2228
TX	Terrell	3.17	285	26.7	8.6	29.5	75	80.8	2398	731
CT	New Haven	2.52	369	26.7	8.2	26	76.3	81.3	319	97
RI	Kent	1.30	680	26.7	7.8	24.5	75.9	81	286	87
GA	Habersham	1.22	721	26.7	9	25.5	74.6	80	1527	465
NJ	Ocean	0.66	979	26.7	8.6	24	76	81.8	85	26
NH	Hillsborough	0.07	1391	26.7	7.9	21.8	77.3	81.4	652	199
IL	Carroll	-0.08	1507	26.7	8.6	30.3	75.6	81.1	765	233
NJ	Gloucester	-0.61	1888	26.7	9.4	25.1	74.6	80	78	24
NY	Cortland	-1.55	2402	26.7	7.8	26.7	75.2	80.2	1479	451
MN	Chisago	-2.23	2662	26.7	7.9	18.8	76.7	81	907	276
IL	Tazewell	-2.55	2797	26.7	6.6	26.6	75.4	80.3	614	187
ND	Barnes	-2.83	2869	26.7	5.6	25.6	75.9	81.3	1394	425
UT	Box Elder	3.29	273	26.8	7.6	22	76.8	81	4839	1475
FL	Bay	2.15	442	26.8	8.9	23.5	73.7	79.2	55	17
WY	Goshen	2.00	474	26.8	6.7	29.2	76.3	80.9	4650	1417
NV	Eureka	1.92	491	26.8	7.2	25.6	74.9	80.3	6211	1893
TX	Williamson	0.91	857	26.8	7.3	19.7	79.3	82.7	751	229
PA	Susquehanna	0.25	1255	26.8	9.9	25.5	74.7	80.1	1424	434
DE	New Castle	0.01	1427	26.8	7.2	21.9	75.2	80.1	90	27
MD	Queen Anne's	-0.08	1509	26.8	7.8	23.4	76.1	81.8	42	13
PA	Centre	-0.40	1758	26.8	8.4	20.4	77.8	81.3	1472	449
IA	Dubuque	-0.79	2002	26.8	7	20.1	76.9	81.5	957	292
VA	Prince William	-0.94	2100	26.8	9.4	21.3	77.5	80.6	270	82
NE	Wheeler	-2.04	2597	26.8	6.9	28.6	76.2	80.7	2104	641
WI	Oneida	-2.19	2650	26.8	6.9	20.4	76	81.3	1603	489
NE	Perkins	-2.24	2667	26.8	6.9	29	76.1	81.4	3393	1034
MN	Nobles	-2.48	2778	26.8	8.2	22.1	77.5	82.9	1607	490
ND	LaMoure	-3.35	2978	26.8	6.5	25.8	75.8	82	1543	470
FL	St. Lucie	5.03	118	26.9	10.9	24.3	75.1	81.5	23	7
CA	Glenn	4.38	169	26.9	7.3	18.5	73.6	79.2	1263	385
NV	Lander	3.67	227	26.9	7.6	24.3	74.9	80.3	6000	1829

ST	COUNTY	USDA	AMEN	OBES	DIAB	INACT	M AGE	W AGE	ALT ft	ALT m
NM	Socorro	3.13	292	26.9	7.3	21.8	74.3	79.4	5989	1825
MN	Cook	2.99	309	26.9	7.3	18.3	76.3	81.7	1617	493
TX	Brazoria	1.31	673	26.9	9.9	25.9	75.3	78.8	26	8
VA	Pulaski	1.29	686	26.9	9.8	23.5	72.9	78.8	2178	664
VA	Charlottesville	-0.02	1460	26.9	9.2	26.8	75.6	81.5	453	138
NE	Harlan	-0.41	1765	26.9	6.7	27.9	75.6	80.3	2133	650
GA	Jeff Davis	-0.60	1878	26.9	10.1	25.8	68.8	76.4	219	67
OH	Hamilton	-1.39	2320	26.9	9.2	24.4	73.9	79.4	708	216
ND	Eddy	-2.47	2771	26.9	7.4	29.9	75.2	81.1	1517	462
MN	Martin	-2.48	2777	26.9	6.6	20.4	76.5	82.8	1205	367
MN	Grant	-2.69	2837	26.9	6.8	20.8	76.5	82.4	1143	348
NE	Kearney	-3.34	2973	26.9	6	24.7	75.6	80.3	2141	653
OR	Lincoln	6.06	58	27	7.4	19	75.5	80.3	704	215
ID	Valley	4.59	154	27	6.8	23.3	76.7	81	6466	1971
OR	Lane	4.29	177	27	7.1	16.6	76.1	81.1	2146	654
MT	Carbon	4.22	186	27	6.1	24.8	74.6	80.3	5572	1698
GA	Glynn	2.06	456	27	9.3	24.6	73	79	13	4
NE	Sheridan	2.00	472	27	7.8	29.7	74.4	80.9	3829	1167
MT	Deer Lodge	1.51	596	27	6.7	22.9	76.6	79.8	6664	2031
VA	James City	1.15	753	27	8	20.1	78.1	82.5	65	20
RI	Providence	0.97	827	27	8.3	27.1	75.7	81.4	362	110
GA	Harris	0.18	1318	27	10.5	20	74.9	80.1	696	212
VA	Roanoke	0.01	1437	27	9.2	22.8	76	80.5	1680	512
CO	Kit Carson	-0.01	1442	27	5.5	26.4	75.2	79.9	4418	1347
VA	Craig	-0.60	1882	27	8.1	24.7	72.8	79	2175	663
NY	Chenango	-1.41	2329	27	7.1	23.9	74.9	79.8	1448	441
MI	Oakland	-1.78	2499	27	8.7	20.3	77.3	81.5	935	285
SD	Brookings	-2.06	2604	27	6	22.6	77	81.8	1710	521
IL	Schuyler	-2.08	2610	27	7.4	29.9	74.4	79.5	584	178
UT	Weber	3.71	224	27.1	8	19.3	76.3	80.5	5649	1722
FL	Lake	3.40	256	27.1	9.1	22.2	76.8	82.9	83	25
GA	Rabun	3.11	294	27.1	9.4	23.1	75.1	81	2289	698
WA	Stevens	2.58	363	27.1	7.7	22.3	74.5	80	2738	835
MO	Camden	1.68	547	27.1	8.3	30.7	75	81	864	263
TX	Kimble	1.02	806	27.1	8.3	25.4	75.5	81	2031	619
NJ	Warren	0.95	838	27.1	7.5	25.4	76.7	80.7	604	184
NM	Curry	0.94	842	27.1	8.6	27.4	74.2	79.1	4437	1352
MO	Christian	0.08	1380	27.1	7.7	26.2	75.1	80.1	1246	380
VA	Albemarle	-0.02	1459	27.1	8.7	19.1	77.8	81.7	741	226
IL	Jersey	-1.68	2457	27.1	7.4	27.2	75.3	79.8	575	175
VA	Powhatan	-1.85	2527	27.1	8.8	26.9	75.9	80.1	275	84
NE	Douglas	-1.92	2553	27.1	8.1	23.6	75.6	80.7	1159	353
SD	Kingsbury	-1.92	2554	27.1	5.7	29	74.9	80.6	1667	508
MN	Pine	-2.77	2854	27.1	7	19.7	75.3	80.1	1079	329
IL	Henry	-3.43	2991	27.1	7.8	29.4	75.9	81	704	215
IN	Hancock	-3.58	3018	27.1	8.7	23.6	76.2	80.4	868	264
CA	Del Norte	10.75	5	27.2	7.6	18.1	72.8	79.8	2189	667

HEALTHIEST PLACES TO LIVE

ST	COUNTY	USDA	AMEN	OBES	DIAB	INACT	M AGE	W AGE	ALT ft	ALT m
FL	Charlotte	5.10	115	27.2	8.7	19.4	76.2	83.1	27	8
TX	Brewster	4.58	155	27.2	8	25.1	75	80.8	3614	1102
OR	Yamhill	3.25	275	27.2	6.9	18.7	76.6	80.6	678	207
WY	Natrona	2.49	372	27.2	7.1	23.6	74.9	81.1	6069	1850
TX	Cameron	2.46	377	27.2	8.5	22.8	76.9	83	26	8
GA	Cherokee	1.93	488	27.2	7.8	22.3	76	79.7	1072	327
NC	Lincoln	1.49	600	27.2	10	22.9	73.3	78.9	879	268
NM	Roosevelt	1.44	620	27.2	5.9	28	73.6	79.3	4240	1292
ID	Custer	0.86	879	27.2	7.3	22.7	75.8	80.4	7615	2321
LA	St. Tammany	0.76	928	27.2	8.9	23.9	74.1	79.6	48	14
TX	Franklin	0.76	931	27.2	8.8	30.1	73.8	80	404	123
VA	Chesapeake	0.48	1089	27.2	9.1	22	74.6	79.6	13	4
OR	Gilliam	0.45	1108	27.2	7.5	17.8	75.9	80.8	1934	590
VA	Highland	0.30	1219	27.2	8.4	21.8	75.1	80.6	2850	869
NC	Moore	0.12	1356	27.2	7.8	22.5	75.3	80.9	426	130
MT	Golden Valley	0.06	1398	27.2	6.5	24.2	75.8	80.9	4220	1286
MT	Valley	-0.03	1465	27.2	7.8	28.7	75.7	81	2581	787
MD	Baltimore City	-0.37	1730	27.2	8.6	27.1	75.1	80.3	202	62
PA	Cumberland	-0.57	1863	27.2	9.1	22.7	77	81.3	713	217
IA	Monona	-1.03	2147	27.2	7	29.7	75.1	80.4	1153	352
NJ	Burlington	-1.30	2284	27.2	8.4	23.4	76.5	81.3	70	21
NE	Garfield	-1.42	2334	27.2	6.8	23.8	76.2	80.7	2281	695
ND	Hettinger	-1.81	2511	27.2	7	29.1	75.7	81.6	2571	784
IL	Rock Island	-1.87	2531	27.2	7.6	26.4	75.7	81	654	199
IA	Scott	-2.39	2732	27.2	7.6	20.8	76	80.9	707	216
OH	Medina	-3.16	2938	27.2	8.5	23	77.4	81.3	1019	311
WI	Taylor	-3.39	2985	27.2	7.7	24.2	76	81.1	1398	426
ID	Adams	3.83	212	27.3	7.6	22	76.7	81	4804	1464
NY	Bronx	1.04	799	27.3	9.6	30.1	73.9	80.5	77	24
NY	Richmond	0.23	1279	27.3	8.7	28.8	76.6	81.4	87	27
NY	Schuyler	-0.03	1466	27.3	7.1	28.8	76.2	80.5	1312	400
NY	Dutchess	-0.07	1502	27.3	9	22.5	77.4	81.6	537	164
VT	Orange	-0.57	1867	27.3	6.7	20	76.3	81.1	1269	387
NE	Cherry	-0.74	1969	27.3	6.5	28.6	75.6	81.2	3201	976
GA	Banks	-1.21	2239	27.3	9.8	24.2	72.9	79	862	263
IA	Ida	-2.14	2631	27.3	6.5	24.2	75.1	80.4	1357	414
MN	Benton	-3.43	2992	27.3	8.4	21.6	75.4	80.2	1123	342
WA	Skagit	4.94	133	27.4	6.8	17.3	76.9	81.1	2403	732
TX	Llano	3.75	217	27.4	9.1	26.9	76.6	81.3	1230	375
GA	Towns	3.18	283	27.4	9.4	26.2	75.1	81	2551	778
NC	Cherokee	3.00	308	27.4	9.7	25.5	73.4	79.7	2133	650
AR	Cleburne	2.19	433	27.4	10.4	30.4	74.4	79.5	714	218
WA	Klickitat	1.97	480	27.4	7.3	21.4	76.3	81	2020	616
ME	Oxford	1.28	689	27.4	8.3	24.1	74.5	80	1175	358
TX	Lubbock	1.14	756	27.4	8.3	26.2	74	79.2	3232	985
ID	Madison	0.92	852	27.4	8	22.9	76.7	80.4	5579	1700
MO	Cape Girardeau	0.91	854	27.4	9	27.2	75	80.2	462	141

ST	COUNTY	USDA	AMEN	OBES	DIAB	INACT	M AGE	W AGE	ALT ft	ALT m
TX	Bosque	0.84	893	27.4	8.2	24.8	73.8	79.5	830	253
MD	Anne Arundel	0.71	952	27.4	8.5	20.1	75.7	80.2	88	27
PA	Wayne	0.44	1117	27.4	8.9	23.9	74.3	80	1463	446
NY	Delaware	0.35	1188	27.4	7.6	26.3	75	80	1824	556
TX	Dallam	0.22	1288	27.4	8.9	28.8	73.7	78.9	4150	1265
MO	Boone	-0.02	1454	27.4	7.5	21.6	76.5	80.5	765	233
NE	Arthur	-0.25	1635	27.4	7.3	26.8	76.1	80.2	3671	1119
NY	Essex	-0.26	1645	27.4	7.9	22.4	75.6	80.7	1541	470
GA	Glascock	-0.78	1995	27.4	10.2	28	68.4	75.4	445	136
NY	Livingston	-0.91	2076	27.4	8.3	24.3	76.5	81.2	1046	319
OH	Mercer	-1.88	2537	27.4	9.4	26.1	75.7	80.7	872	266
MT	Sheridan	-2.12	2625	27.4	6	28.5	73.6	79.5	2233	681
IL	Whiteside	-2.32	2695	27.4	7.8	29.2	75.2	80.2	657	200
IL	Shelby	-2.34	2704	27.4	7.6	30.6	75.9	80.5	635	194
MN	Cottonwood	-2.35	2710	27.4	7.7	25.2	76.3	81.8	1364	416
MN	Blue Earth	-2.48	2776	27.4	7.2	25	77.4	81.6	997	304
NE	Lancaster	-2.55	2799	27.4	7.4	20.3	77.8	82.3	1296	395
IA	Bremer	-3.16	2936	27.4	7.1	22.7	77.6	82.2	1022	312
MN	Stevens	-3.31	2967	27.4	7.1	21.3	77.8	81.9	1133	345
MI	Dickinson	-3.58	3019	27.4	8.4	22.4	76.5	81.9	1186	362
CA	Riverside	6.64	42	27.5	8.9	21.5	75.8	81.3	1857	566
CA	Kings	3.48	247	27.5	7.6	22.4	74.6	79.6	343	105
NM	Valencia	3.04	304	27.5	7	24.1	73.4	79.6	5424	1653
FL	Franklin	2.66	345	27.5	9.1	28.9	72.4	78.5	13	4
SC	Charleston	1.45	613	27.5	9.7	23.6	73.8	80	13	4
OR	Union	1.38	641	27.5	7.4	18.1	76.3	80.5	4331	1320
WA	Okanogan	1.36	651	27.5	7.9	22	75.4	81.1	3741	1140
GA	Lumpkin	1.28	688	27.5	8.6	20.3	73.6	79	1658	505
TX	Hemphill	1.27	695	27.5	8.5	28.4	73.8	79.3	2523	769
MI	Manistee	0.89	864	27.5	8.5	27.2	75.3	80.8	790	241
IL	Jackson	0.71	950	27.5	8.3	27.7	75.3	80.1	449	137
IN	Switzerland	-0.20	1595	27.5	9.7	27.1	74.7	79.5	749	228
NY	Schoharie	-0.30	1669	27.5	7.9	26.8	75.7	81.2	1503	458
MT	Prairie	-0.39	1745	27.5	6.6	27.8	75.7	81	2724	830
MN	St. Louis	-0.66	1919	27.5	6.9	17.5	75.8	80.9	1378	420
MD	Carroll	-1.34	2294	27.5	8	20.8	76.6	80.5	646	197
MN	Goodhue	-1.38	2313	27.5	7.4	18.1	77.7	82	1048	319
IA	Polk	-2.13	2628	27.5	7.7	23.9	76.4	81.2	904	276
MN	Lincoln	-2.16	2639	27.5	6.6	21.6	75.1	81.8	1689	515
MN	Cass	-2.38	2730	27.5	6.8	21	75.3	81.1	1345	410
IL	Kane	-2.77	2852	27.5	8.1	23.6	77.4	81	816	249
OR	Crook	5.06	116	27.6	7.9	18.9	75.6	80.1	4355	1328
UT	Duchesne	3.73	220	27.6	8.6	24.5	75	79.8	7792	2375
NM	Luna	2.87	324	27.6	7.1	21.4	73.2	79.8	4514	1376
WY	Big Horn	2.49	371	27.6	7	25.7	75	80.6	5422	1653
TX	Mason	1.54	588	27.6	8.4	27	76.4	81.6	1631	497
AL	Shelby	1.12	763	27.6	8.3	23.5	75.6	80	578	176

HEALTHIEST PLACES TO LIVE

ST	COUNTY	USDA	AMEN	OBES	DIAB	INACT	M AGE	W AGE	ALT ft	ALT m
MT	Yellowstone	1.08	781	27.6	7.3	23.5	76.1	81	3482	1061
TX	Tarrant	1.02	807	27.6	8.7	22.8	75.3	79.9	656	200
GA	Lee	0.22	1284	27.6	9.7	24.3	74.9	80	271	83
MO	Clay	0.15	1336	27.6	8.5	26.5	76.1	80.3	883	269
VA	Washington	-0.23	1625	27.6	9.8	28.4	73.3	78.9	2170	662
VA	Floyd	-1.05	2166	27.6	9.2	23.3	73.4	78.9	2581	787
NE	Logan	-1.41	2328	27.6	6.9	26.6	76.1	80.2	2988	911
WI	Oconto	-1.95	2566	27.6	6.9	23.9	75.9	81.3	872	266
IL	Ogle	-2.82	2864	27.6	7.4	28	75.8	80.5	812	247
UT	Daggett	4.30	176	27.7	7	19.4	75	79.8	7536	2297
VA	Bath	2.19	434	27.7	9	25.3	75.1	80.6	2213	674
ID	Washington	2.17	440	27.7	8.7	24.9	76.7	81	3698	1127
TX	Coleman	2.14	446	27.7	8.3	31.8	73.1	79.5	1705	520
TX	Baylor	1.70	545	27.7	8.8	26.6	72.6	79	1254	382
MO	Ozark	1.60	569	27.7	8.2	29	72.5	79.3	904	276
WA	Douglas	0.42	1133	27.7	7.8	20	76.3	81.1	2237	682
WI	Portage	-2.54	2796	27.7	6.9	23	77.3	81.8	1111	339
MN	Big Stone	-2.77	2853	27.7	6.7	20.2	76.5	82.2	1096	334
IL	Effingham	-2.81	2862	27.7	7.6	28.3	75.3	80.7	575	175
MT	Lake	3.82	213	27.8	7	21.9	75.9	80.6	3973	1211
TX	Aransas	3.71	223	27.8	8.6	26.5	73.9	81.3	8	2
CA	San Bernardino	3.57	241	27.8	8.1	21.7	74.3	79.5	2666	813
GA	Union	2.94	316	27.8	9.7	23	74.9	80.1	2362	720
FL	Duval	2.31	410	27.8	11	26.2	72.5	78	36	11
WA	Spokane	1.33	665	27.8	7.9	20.2	76.2	80.5	2388	728
VA	York	1.27	702	27.8	9.1	22.1	78.3	81.3	33	10
MD	Calvert	0.65	984	27.8	8.8	23.1	75	79.7	79	24
VA	Radford	0.27	1244	27.8	9.3	22.8	74.5	79.7	1861	567
ME	Waldo	0.20	1306	27.8	8.1	22.2	75.4	80.8	357	109
MD	Harford	0.04	1410	27.8	8.3	24.5	75.6	80.6	320	98
WV	Monongalia	-0.07	1504	27.8	9.6	24.9	75.4	80.1	1280	390
TX	Lavaca	-0.08	1515	27.8	8.7	26.5	74.2	80.6	252	77
GA	Henry	-0.53	1833	27.8	10.6	23.5	74	78.7	784	239
OH	Cuyahoga	-0.63	1899	27.8	9.5	25	74	79.7	852	260
WI	Iron	-0.70	1945	27.8	7.5	21.4	75.3	80.7	1531	467
MT	Dawson	-1.01	2138	27.8	6.7	29.7	75.3	80.5	2575	785
NJ	Camden	-1.15	2216	27.8	9.2	27.9	74	79.7	86	26
NE	Knox	-1.32	2289	27.8	7.2	29.5	75.3	81.4	1595	486
MN	Douglas	-2.23	2663	27.8	6.8	19	78	82.8	1385	422
IN	Wayne	-2.54	2794	27.8	7.6	27.6	73.4	79.6	1048	319
MN	Nicollet	-2.58	2805	27.8	7.5	17	78	82.1	987	301
IL	Cumberland	-2.80	2860	27.8	8.2	29.9	75.3	80.2	602	184
MN	Watonwan	-2.85	2877	27.8	7.2	21.7	76.3	81.8	1106	337
NY	Genesee	-2.94	2893	27.8	8.7	23.7	76.3	81.2	834	254
IL	Bureau	-3.05	2913	27.8	7.5	28.1	75.9	80.7	708	216
MN	Lk of the Woods	-3.09	2924	27.8	7.1	21.6	75.3	81.1	1134	345
MN	Pipestone	-4.13	3079	27.8	7.4	19.2	75.1	81.8	1714	522

ST	COUNTY	USDA	AMEN	OBES	DIAB	INACT	M AGE	W AGE	ALT ft	ALT m
AZ	Mohave	5.84	68	27.9	9.5	28	72	78.5	3769	1149
OR	Columbia	4.98	125	27.9	7.7	18.9	75.5	80.8	761	232
ID	Boise	3.40	257	27.9	7.3	19	75.8	80.4	5531	1686
TX	Crosby	2.45	381	27.9	8.9	29.6	72.9	78.7	2925	892
NE	Garden	2.14	444	27.9	7.8	29.8	76.1	80.2	3804	1159
NC	Yancey	1.37	647	27.9	7.8	26.5	74.5	79.8	3365	1026
GA	Hall	0.96	830	27.9	10.5	21.9	74.7	79.7	1136	346
MO	Cole	0.96	832	27.9	8.8	26.1	75.7	80.5	696	212
KY	Campbell	0.39	1147	27.9	9.6	26.3	73.7	79.6	679	207
NY	Putnam	0.37	1170	27.9	7	22.5	78.6	82.6	649	198
NC	Stokes	0.02	1422	27.9	8.3	25	73.1	79.5	976	297
VA	Salem	0.01	1439	27.9	9	22.4	75	80.6	1087	331
IL	Monroe	-0.06	1491	27.9	7.8	29.2	76.8	80.7	510	156
VT	Franklin	-0.30	1677	27.9	7.2	24.4	76.4	81.1	671	205
NC	Union	-0.34	1702	27.9	8.3	22.4	75.2	79.8	566	173
GA	Dade	-0.39	1743	27.9	10	23.2	71.7	78.3	1293	394
NE	Platte	-0.60	1881	27.9	6.9	23.6	77.2	82.1	1620	494
NE	Deuel	-0.61	1886	27.9	6.5	28.2	76.1	81.4	3731	1137
WI	Vernon	-0.66	1922	27.9	7.2	22.9	75.2	80.4	1061	324
IL	Calhoun	-0.75	1970	27.9	8.1	32.3	74.5	79.5	557	170
WI	St. Croix	-1.37	2309	27.9	7	17	77.8	82.2	1065	324
IN	Franklin	-1.45	2351	27.9	11	25.5	74.7	80.7	902	275
IL	Hancock	-1.63	2438	27.9	8	29	76	81.2	632	193
MN	Aitkin	-1.74	2483	27.9	7.6	20.2	76.2	81.6	1274	388
NE	Cedar	-2.01	2587	27.9	6.9	28.6	76.5	82	1486	453
NY	Schenectady	-2.06	2603	27.9	8.7	24.3	76	81.2	713	217
MN	Carlton	-2.15	2636	27.9	8.1	19.1	74.9	81	1195	364
OH	Knox	-2.89	2885	27.9	10.1	25.9	74.8	79.8	1114	340
NE	Butler	-3.37	2981	27.9	6.3	27.7	75.5	81.1	1543	470
CA	Shasta	5.69	75	28	7.1	18.9	73.9	79.1	2997	913
CA	Sacramento	3.65	230	28	8.3	19	75.6	81	103	32
TX	Gillespie	2.59	362	28	8.2	25.7	76.4	81.6	1832	558
AR	Benton	2.39	389	28	7.2	27.8	76.8	81.8	1230	375
WA	Whitman	2.23	429	28	8.2	21	77.1	80.8	2076	633
FL	Santa Rosa	1.94	487	28	10	24.6	75.6	79.8	146	45
SC	Greenville	1.83	515	28	9.4	24.3	74.1	79.9	1081	329
NC	Pamlico	1.00	814	28	9.8	25.2	73	78.5	13	4
MI	Charlevoix	0.94	841	28	8.9	21.2	76.8	81.4	798	243
PA	Westmoreland	0.88	871	28	8.6	26.9	75.8	80.9	1312	400
GA	Bryan	0.70	959	28	9.6	24.6	73.7	78.9	43	13
KS	Mitchell	0.32	1203	28	8.5	24.3	75.5	80.1	1509	460
VA	Norton	0.25	1258	28	9	24	71.1	77.1	2246	684
PA	Greene	0.22	1287	28	9.1	33.6	74.7	79.8	1196	365
MO	Platte	0.12	1354	28	8.8	28.1	76.8	81.5	889	271
TX	Erath	0.03	1415	28	9.2	25.5	73.9	79.6	1251	381
NJ	Atlantic	-0.04	1476	28	8.8	24.6	73.6	79.8	48	15
VA	King George	-0.17	1579	28	9.5	21.5	74.7	79.7	88	27

HEALTHIEST PLACES TO LIVE

ST	COUNTY	USDA	AMEN	OBES	DIAB	INACT	M AGE	W AGE	ALT ft	ALT m
VT	Rutland	-0.35	1717	28	6.9	22.2	76.1	81.5	1256	383
NE	Nance	-0.42	1771	28	8	29.5	75.6	80.5	1736	529
NC	Guilford	-0.85	2038	28	9.8	23	74.9	80.5	787	240
VA	Spotsylvania	-0.97	2114	28	9.5	20	75.4	80.8	282	86
IN	Gibson	-1.56	2404	28	8.6	26.5	74.8	80	439	134
IA	Mahaska	-1.82	2512	28	7.4	29.4	76.3	81.6	808	246
MI	Hillsdale	-2.40	2738	28	9.1	25.8	75.2	80.5	1057	322
MN	Pope	-2.45	2762	28	7.1	23.4	77.8	81.9	1281	391
SD	Davison	-3.29	2963	28	6.7	27.2	76.2	81.6	1382	421
MN	Olmsted	-3.96	3062	28	7	17.4	78.3	83.7	1172	357
WA	Snohomish	4.68	151	28.1	7.8	19.1	77.3	81.1	2135	651
TX	Culberson	3.62	236	28.1	8.8	26.2	76.3	82	4130	1259
TX	Loving	3.31	272	28.1	8.5	25.4	72.2	78	2954	900
TX	Borden	2.39	391	28.1	8.7	27	72.4	77.8	2542	775
FL	Leon	1.75	537	28.1	9.8	21.2	76.1	80.4	102	31
TX	Sutton	1.47	607	28.1	8.5	26	75.5	81	2252	686
GA	Heard	0.22	1283	28.1	9.9	27.3	71.4	77.1	794	242
MD	Kent	-0.23	1619	28.1	8.8	25.8	74.5	80.6	39	12
VA	Bristol	-0.23	1624	28.1	9	24.7	72.8	79.4	1771	540
NY	Chautauqua	-0.26	1644	28.1	7.6	24.6	75.7	80.4	1376	419
TX	Archer	-0.33	1694	28.1	10	27.4	74.9	81.1	1071	327
IN	Lawrence	-0.35	1710	28.1	11.2	28.8	74	79.5	653	199
GA	Franklin	-0.50	1812	28.1	9.5	24.7	72	78.9	760	232
GA	Clarke	-0.71	1947	28.1	11	20.3	74.3	79.6	722	220
NY	Otsego	-0.77	1991	28.1	7.6	23.9	75.7	81.3	1559	475
VA	Fairfax City	-1.31	2286	28.1	9	26.6	76.6	82.1	390	119
SD	Potter	-1.38	2315	28.1	6.7	26.8	72.9	79.9	1928	588
IL	Putnam	-1.52	2384	28.1	7.9	27	75.9	80.7	591	180
WI	Washington	-2.63	2822	28.1	6.6	21.8	77.6	82.5	982	299
IN	Tippecanoe	-2.79	2857	28.1	9.4	24.2	75.6	80.7	676	206
IA	Linn	-2.83	2865	28.1	7.8	23.4	77.6	81.5	851	259
ND	Griggs	-3.18	2942	28.1	6.5	24.3	75.2	81.1	1449	442
MN	Pennington	-4.97	3099	28.1	8.6	23.1	74.9	81	1121	342
TX	Hudspeth	4.00	199	28.2	8.8	29.2	76.3	82	4437	1352
NC	Graham	3.14	290	28.2	10.1	25.9	72	78.6	2801	854
TX	Bexar	2.63	352	28.2	8.7	22.5	74.9	80.7	818	249
TX	Chambers	1.57	578	28.2	8.7	29.8	74.1	79.8	15	5
NC	Iredell	1.32	668	28.2	8.1	24.7	73.9	80.2	895	273
TX	Knox	0.62	1013	28.2	9.4	26.3	72.6	79	1453	443
TN	Cumberland	0.54	1047	28.2	9.5	25.6	74.7	80.6	1784	544
TX	Comanche	0.36	1179	28.2	8.6	27.1	72.9	79.5	1360	415
NY	Greene	0.31	1211	28.2	8.2	25.1	73.8	80	1420	433
NH	Cheshire	0.26	1248	28.2	7.8	21.3	77.4	81.4	1041	317
TX	Hansford	0.05	1408	28.2	8.8	28.5	74.2	79.8	3137	956
ID	Clark	-0.06	1490	28.2	8.1	22.8	76.2	80.4	6414	1955
IL	Gallatin	-0.19	1584	28.2	7.7	27	73	79.5	391	119
VA	Frederick	-0.38	1739	28.2	8.5	26	75.3	80.5	916	279

ST	COUNTY	USDA	AMEN	OBES	DIAB	INACT	M AGE	W AGE	ALT ft	ALT m
VA	Scott	-0.47	1802	28.2	8.2	30	71.9	78.2	1822	555
WI	Crawford	-0.55	1847	28.2	7.7	22	75.1	80.2	937	286
NY	Franklin	-0.63	1898	28.2	8.2	25.4	75	80.1	1397	426
NY	Washington	-0.64	1907	28.2	8.9	30	76.1	80.2	590	180
IL	Clinton	-0.72	1958	28.2	8	27.3	74.9	81.2	454	138
VA	Colonial Hghts	-0.84	2031	28.2	9	22.3	75	80.5	75	23
GA	Walton	-0.94	2090	28.2	10.3	30.5	74.4	79.6	809	247
IL	Pike	-1.88	2534	28.2	7.6	26	75	80.5	601	183
NE	Cass	-2.12	2626	28.2	8.1	26	76.1	81.2	1165	355
NY	Onondaga	-2.26	2680	28.2	8.4	21.6	76.3	81.3	780	238
WI	Florence	-2.61	2817	28.2	6.9	22.4	75.8	80.6	1391	424
NE	Boyd	-2.64	2825	28.2	6.2	28.7	75.6	80.9	1726	526
MN	Kanabec	-3.04	2911	28.2	7.4	21.3	76.2	80.7	1087	331
WI	Eau Claire	-3.16	2939	28.2	6.5	23.2	77.3	81.9	987	301
MN	Traverse	-3.57	3015	28.2	7.2	21.8	76.5	82.2	1041	317
KS	Nemaha	-3.62	3025	28.2	8.7	25.4	75.1	80.9	1257	383
ND	Cass	-4.84	3096	28.2	7	22.3	77.2	82.9	1008	307
TX	Blanco	4.05	195	28.3	8.6	25.1	76.6	81.3	1334	407
UT	San Juan	3.60	239	28.3	8.7	29	74.9	80.2	5658	1725
SC	Pickens	3.02	307	28.3	9.5	26.6	74.2	79.7	1122	342
NE	Morrill	1.63	565	28.3	9.8	26.6	74.4	80.9	4004	1220
TX	Matagorda	1.54	589	28.3	9.8	27	73.4	77.9	26	8
TX	Stephens	1.38	644	28.3	8.4	27.7	72.6	79.1	1282	391
NM	Harding	1.28	690	28.3	6.2	20.5	75.4	80.3	5044	1537
VA	Poquoson	1.27	701	28.3	8.5	21.9	78.3	81.3	3	1
NC	Alexander	1.17	742	28.3	8.9	24	73.9	78.9	1197	365
OK	Washita	-0.30	1671	28.3	9	28.5	72	78.5	1632	497
WI	Kenosha	-0.45	1789	28.3	7.9	23.3	75.3	80	739	225
PA	Warren	-0.71	1952	28.3	9.5	28.3	75.4	79.9	1623	495
NY	Tioga	-1.05	2164	28.3	7.5	25	76	80.6	1248	380
KS	Lincoln	-1.33	2291	28.3	7.6	24.2	75.2	80.7	1515	462
IL	Moultrie	-1.96	2568	28.3	8.2	28.5	75.1	81	662	202
IN	Parke	-2.30	2690	28.3	9.8	32.5	74.5	80.1	637	194
NE	Hayes	-2.55	2798	28.3	6.5	28.2	76.1	81.4	3023	922
IN	Elkhart	-2.72	2843	28.3	9	25.7	75.6	80.3	817	249
NY	Lewis	-2.79	2859	28.3	8.4	26.1	75.4	81	1300	396
IL	Clay	-3.01	2907	28.3	7.6	29.9	74.4	80	487	148
MN	Morrison	-3.09	2926	28.3	6.8	20.6	75	81.1	1221	372
IA	Howard	-4.16	3080	28.3	6.8	22	76.6	81.4	1271	387
WA	Clallam	6.52	45	28.4	8.2	17.6	76.2	81.6	1501	458
OR	Jefferson	4.99	122	28.4	7.7	21	74.6	79.2	3261	994
WA	Thurston	3.32	270	28.4	8.2	18.5	77	81.3	492	150
WY	Converse	2.86	325	28.4	6.7	23.7	75.9	81.2	5426	1654
TX	McCulloch	2.36	395	28.4	8.9	29.3	73.6	78.3	1681	512
MT	Mineral	1.80	522	28.4	6.9	28.3	76.7	81	4712	1436
AR	Garland	1.64	557	28.4	8.6	26.7	72.5	79.6	704	215
NE	Keith	1.50	599	28.4	6.9	21.7	76.1	80.2	3353	1022

HEALTHIEST PLACES TO LIVE

ST	COUNTY	USDA	AMEN	OBES	DIAB	INACT	M AGE	W AGE	ALT ft	ALT m
VA	Warren	1.07	786	28.4	9.7	23.9	75.2	79.8	860	262
TX	DeWitt	0.50	1075	28.4	9.1	25.2	73.3	79.2	283	86
PA	Allegheny	0.47	1095	28.4	8.4	24.6	74.7	80.2	1043	318
MA	Hampden	-0.08	1508	28.4	9.3	25.7	75.2	80.5	629	192
TX	Shackelford	-0.09	1521	28.4	8.5	26.7	72.6	79.1	1545	471
TX	Bee	-0.36	1727	28.4	9.7	25.9	74.2	79.4	240	73
NE	Dawes	-0.39	1747	28.4	7.1	24.3	75.4	80.3	3827	1166
NY	Niagara	-0.52	1828	28.4	8.1	28.1	74.9	80.1	459	140
NE	Sioux	-0.67	1924	28.4	6.5	27.5	75.4	80.3	4450	1356
NY	Erie	-0.70	1944	28.4	9	25.6	75.3	80.2	936	285
WY	Weston	-0.91	2079	28.4	6.3	26.9	75.9	81.5	4452	1357
VA	Manassas	-0.94	2098	28.4	9.9	24.9	76.5	80.4	249	76
MO	Adair	-1.11	2193	28.4	9.3	31.5	74.8	80.2	896	273
IL	Wabash	-1.68	2458	28.4	7.9	28.8	75.2	80.1	430	131
VA	Clarke	-1.75	2490	28.4	8.8	23.4	75.2	79.8	631	192
MO	Livingston	-2.04	2596	28.4	9.3	32.5	74.2	80.2	770	235
MI	Kalamazoo	-2.10	2616	28.4	9.3	22.3	75.7	80.8	880	268
ND	Foster	-2.53	2793	28.4	7	27.5	75.2	81.1	1531	467
WI	Polk	-2.73	2849	28.4	6.9	19	76.1	81.7	1121	342
MN	Stearns	-2.87	2880	28.4	7.6	19	78.8	83.9	1197	365
MN	Fillmore	-2.93	2890	28.4	6.7	21.7	76.4	82	1194	364
IL	Piatt	-4.21	3084	28.4	7.9	30.2	75.1	81	695	212
IN	Clinton	-4.37	3090	28.4	11.9	26.3	74.6	79.9	844	257
TX	Burnet	4.36	171	28.5	8.4	25.7	76.9	82.3	1159	353
ID	Elmore	2.94	318	28.5	8.5	23.9	75.5	79.9	4737	1444
UT	Millard	2.69	342	28.5	6.6	21	75.2	79.9	5412	1650
FL	Nassau	2.04	461	28.5	8.6	23.6	74.6	79.4	39	12
NC	Burke	1.82	518	28.5	10.1	27.2	73.3	79.3	1492	455
TX	Briscoe	1.76	533	28.5	8.7	25.3	74.6	79.8	2791	851
NC	Dare	1.63	564	28.5	8.4	23.7	75.9	80.4	4	1
NC	Carteret	1.22	725	28.5	8.4	27.2	74.6	79.8	13	4
UT	Emery	0.83	901	28.5	7.3	20.8	75.7	80	5846	1782
TX	Smith	0.72	948	28.5	8.7	25.7	75	81	445	136
OH	Muskingum	0.42	1129	28.5	11	30.3	73.9	79.3	891	272
TX	King	0.40	1144	28.5	8.7	26.3	73.2	78.7	1805	550
TX	Ochiltree	0.39	1153	28.5	8.3	26.4	74.2	79.8	2920	890
TX	Hall	0.27	1241	28.5	9	26.2	72.2	77.9	2059	628
VA	Montgomery	0.27	1243	28.5	7.7	22.3	75.8	79.6	2022	616
VT	Orleans	0.09	1375	28.5	6.9	24.5	75.4	80.3	1319	402
MS	Madison	-0.01	1446	28.5	10.8	25.9	69.9	75.9	283	86
TX	Harris	-0.04	1481	28.5	9	23.3	75.8	80.5	85	26
NY	Fulton	-0.24	1632	28.5	7.9	25.9	75.2	81.1	1222	372
TX	Roberts	-0.41	1766	28.5	8.6	27.7	73.8	79.3	2830	863
OH	Lake	-0.42	1772	28.5	10.6	24.6	76.1	81	765	233
NC	Davie	-0.46	1794	28.5	8.9	27.7	74.7	80.2	749	228
NE	Madison	-0.53	1834	28.5	7.5	23.4	75.6	80.8	1703	519
VA	Henrico	-0.93	2088	28.5	8.7	25.6	75.6	80.3	142	43

ST	COUNTY	USDA	AMEN	OBES	DIAB	INACT	M AGE	W AGE	ALT ft	ALT m
VA	Southampton	-0.94	2101	28.5	11.6	27.2	72	77.8	65	20
KS	Harper	-1.26	2267	28.5	8.8	31.5	75.3	80.1	1374	419
NE	Franklin	-1.56	2408	28.5	7.8	31.8	75.6	80.3	2038	621
IA	Madison	-2.15	2634	28.5	7.4	20.6	76.5	81.5	1072	327
IA	Palo Alto	-2.29	2686	28.5	7.4	24.9	75.7	81.2	1285	392
MN	Becker	-2.34	2706	28.5	7.5	21.1	75.7	81.2	1454	443
OH	Summit	-2.40	2740	28.5	9.4	23.6	74.8	80	1023	312
IA	Buena Vista	-2.44	2756	28.5	7.1	26.4	76.7	81.2	1376	419
IL	Scott	-2.47	2769	28.5	7.9	28.9	75	80.5	530	162
IL	De Witt	-2.52	2790	28.5	7.5	27.9	73.9	79.6	723	220
MN	Faribault	-2.91	2887	28.5	7.2	22.8	76	81.8	1114	340
IL	Vermilion	-3.21	2950	28.5	9	30.1	73.1	78.7	683	208
MN	Mower	-5.18	3103	28.5	7.2	21.8	77.6	82.6	1309	399
CA	Kern	4.84	142	28.6	8.1	23.7	73.5	78.7	2377	724
NV	Esmeralda	4.12	192	28.6	7.4	23.2	72.2	78.8	5670	1728
UT	Uintah	3.53	243	28.6	8.6	27.2	75	80.6	6258	1908
TX	Live Oak	2.67	344	28.6	8.7	28.1	74.6	80.4	246	75
TX	Taylor	2.04	464	28.6	8.9	32.9	73.6	79	2008	612
ID	Cassia	1.81	521	28.6	8.5	22.8	75.6	80.5	5375	1638
TX	Ward	1.46	610	28.6	8.9	29.6	73.4	78.5	2612	796
VA	Gloucester	1.27	696	28.6	8.5	24.3	75	80.7	44	13
VA	Middlesex	1.27	698	28.6	9.2	28.1	72.4	79.2	54	16
TX	Limestone	1.12	766	28.6	9.7	26.6	71	77.7	495	151
MT	Toole	0.97	826	28.6	7.6	26.6	74.6	80.7	3508	1069
TX	Floyd	0.86	886	28.6	9.6	28.7	73.8	79	3140	957
TX	Reagan	0.60	1022	28.6	8.9	28.7	75.9	81.1	2650	808
MD	St. Mary's	0.53	1050	28.6	9.6	23.4	75.5	80.3	75	23
TX	Frio	0.40	1143	28.6	8.5	29.7	72.9	78.7	581	177
VA	New Kent	0.24	1272	28.6	9.8	21.2	78.1	82.5	89	27
TX	Glasscock	0.23	1281	28.6	8.8	27.5	75.9	81.1	2654	809
TX	Irion	0.11	1363	28.6	8.8	27.8	74.3	79.9	2406	733
WI	Sheboygan	-0.37	1732	28.6	7.7	22.4	76.7	81.2	845	257
OH	Erie	-0.91	2077	28.6	9.8	27.6	75.3	80.1	665	203
NE	Gosper	-1.08	2182	28.6	7.6	25.8	75.6	80.9	2452	747
NE	Brown	-1.10	2190	28.6	8	27.1	75.6	81.2	2601	793
NE	Boone	-1.21	2243	28.6	6.9	28.1	75.6	80.5	1904	580
SD	Marshall	-1.65	2447	28.6	8.1	29.2	74.9	81.2	1559	475
PA	Crawford	-1.99	2579	28.6	10.1	24.9	74.8	80.1	1299	396
ND	Wells	-2.27	2682	28.6	6.4	27.4	74.3	81.1	1681	512
IL	Peoria	-2.41	2741	28.6	9.6	25.6	74.5	79.9	651	198
IL	Winnebago	-2.50	2783	28.6	9.1	26.2	75.1	80.8	803	245
MN	Isanti	-2.66	2829	28.6	7.6	18.7	76.7	81.7	956	291
MN	McLeod	-2.93	2891	28.6	6.9	18.6	77.3	82.4	1057	322
IA	Hancock	-4.06	3076	28.6	7.1	23.8	76.6	81.4	1233	376
MN	Wilkin	-6.10	3107	28.6	7.2	25	76.5	82.4	993	303
NC	Mitchell	1.55	585	28.7	9	24.4	72.8	79.1	3130	954
GA	Jasper	1.46	608	28.7	10.8	27.6	73	78.7	545	166

HEALTHIEST PLACES TO LIVE

ST	COUNTY	USDA	AMEN	OBES	DIAB	INACT	M AGE	W AGE	ALT ft	ALT m
AR	Montgomery	1.32	666	28.7	9.1	27	73.2	78.7	906	276
TX	Bell	1.26	707	28.7	10.4	28.3	74.5	79.7	668	203
TX	Tyler	1.18	739	28.7	9.8	28.8	72.4	78.4	203	62
TX	Somervell	1.17	744	28.7	8.7	27.2	73.9	79.6	817	249
WA	Walla Walla	1.06	788	28.7	8.5	16.3	76.4	80.9	1198	365
ID	Oneida	0.17	1322	28.7	7.1	25.7	75.6	80.5	5531	1686
ME	Franklin	0.17	1324	28.7	7.1	21.4	76.1	80.3	1552	473
GA	Bleckley	0.15	1334	28.7	10.6	27.2	70.5	77.1	328	100
GA	Houston	-0.04	1471	28.7	10.5	25.6	74.2	79.6	347	106
NE	Kimball	-0.08	1513	28.7	7.6	24.3	75.8	80.7	4933	1504
VA	Henry	-0.28	1657	28.7	10.4	31.3	71.2	78.3	913	278
TX	Brooks	-0.34	1705	28.7	8.7	28.3	73.4	78.6	187	57
NY	Rensselaer	-0.49	1810	28.7	8	23.3	75.8	80.3	823	251
GA	Barrow	-0.70	1940	28.7	10.9	28	72.5	78.6	863	263
WI	Pepin	-0.71	1956	28.7	7.8	25.1	76.8	81.8	910	277
WI	Monroe	-1.36	2305	28.7	8.2	24.6	74.4	80.1	1050	320
MO	Sullivan	-1.58	2412	28.7	9.3	29.1	73.9	80	927	282
NY	Oneida	-1.65	2445	28.7	8.1	25.7	75.5	80.7	899	274
NE	Holt	-1.67	2454	28.7	7.4	30.8	75.6	80.9	2041	622
OH	Clinton	-2.07	2609	28.7	9.8	31.7	74.7	80	1017	310
IL	Woodford	-2.26	2677	28.7	7.4	23.5	76.6	81.4	706	215
WI	Rusk	-2.32	2698	28.7	7.4	25.4	74.8	80.2	1250	381
IL	Macoupin	-2.36	2715	28.7	8.2	25.4	74.6	80.2	630	192
MN	Freeborn	-2.38	2731	28.7	7	21.5	76.6	81.7	1257	383
IN	Marshall	-2.41	2743	28.7	8.4	28.6	75	81.1	803	245
MN	Kandiyohi	-2.60	2810	28.7	6.5	22.8	77.2	82.5	1176	358
NY	Wyoming	-2.69	2838	28.7	7.8	22.7	74.9	80.5	1479	451
WI	Lincoln	-2.98	2905	28.7	8	23	76	81	1476	450
WI	Outagamie	-3.35	2979	28.7	8.8	21.6	77.8	82.4	774	236
IA	Worth	-3.51	3006	28.7	7.5	24.2	76.5	81.8	1232	375
NE	Keya Paha	-3.69	3033	28.7	7.1	32.7	75.6	80.9	2271	692
MN	Swift	-3.74	3043	28.7	8.2	26.5	76.8	81.7	1076	328
IA	Iowa	-3.84	3051	28.7	6.9	29.1	76.6	81.8	811	247
WA	Clark	4.25	181	28.8	8.2	18.8	77.3	81.4	727	221
FL	Brevard	3.93	204	28.8	9.7	23.7	75.9	81.2	16	5
NC	Haywood	2.23	427	28.8	8.5	22.7	74	80.2	3581	1092
NC	Madison	1.92	490	28.8	8.7	21.4	73.9	79	2649	807
VA	Covington	1.77	528	28.8	9.5	24.9	72.8	79	1397	426
VA	Botetourt	1.15	752	28.8	9	20.7	75.7	80.4	1483	452
TX	Bailey	0.91	855	28.8	8.9	28.2	73.1	78.8	3874	1181
PA	Cameron	0.73	942	28.8	8.8	25.9	75.2	80	1671	509
MO	St. Louis	0.64	989	28.8	8	23.8	76.1	80.8	542	165
MA	Bristol	0.54	1045	28.8	9.9	28.1	75.8	81.4	100	30
TX	Sterling	0.27	1242	28.8	8.5	27.5	73.2	78.8	2482	756
VA	Giles	0.09	1373	28.8	9.7	27.4	72.5	78.8	2479	756
NH	Sullivan	-0.17	1574	28.8	7.8	25	75.6	81.2	1179	359
NY	Cattaraugus	-0.32	1689	28.8	9.1	26	74.5	80	1700	518

ST	COUNTY	USDA	AMEN	OBES	DIAB	INACT	M AGE	W AGE	ALT ft	ALT m
KY	Clark	-0.51	1816	28.8	10.5	29.5	74.1	78.8	900	274
GA	Pierce	-0.63	1893	28.8	10.6	27.6	70.3	77.5	103	32
ND	Slope	-0.78	1997	28.8	6.8	30.3	75.7	81.6	2845	867
NY	Allegany	-0.90	2071	28.8	8.5	25.7	75.6	79.9	1826	557
ND	Burke	-2.07	2608	28.8	7.8	30.1	76.5	81.9	2108	643
IL	Jasper	-2.25	2669	28.8	7.5	30.7	75.3	80.2	528	161
SD	Faulk	-2.32	2696	28.8	6.9	29.2	76.3	82.4	1627	496
IL	Sangamon	-2.47	2768	28.8	8.6	25.6	74.8	80	597	182
IN	Vanderburgh	-2.48	2773	28.8	9.3	27.1	73.8	79.4	424	129
OH	Defiance	-2.60	2813	28.8	9.9	27.5	75.6	80.7	727	222
IA	Black Hawk	-3.07	2917	28.8	8.5	23	76.8	80.8	921	281
MN	Kittson	-4.90	3098	28.8	7.6	22.3	75.3	82.4	904	276
NV	Churchill	5.42	85	28.9	7.3	26	75.1	80.1	4754	1449
FL	Pasco	3.37	261	28.9	8.8	27.4	73.7	80.6	72	22
VA	Grayson	1.20	734	28.9	9.6	26.3	72.3	77.9	3015	919
TX	Upton	1.02	808	28.9	8.7	27.6	73.4	78.5	2743	836
ID	Gooding	0.76	926	28.9	7.8	26.2	74.3	80	3867	1179
GA	Echols	0.73	939	28.9	10.2	24.9	72.2	77.9	142	43
GA	Tattnall	0.54	1044	28.9	10.9	28.1	70.6	77.1	162	49
TX	Dimmit	0.48	1088	28.9	9	26.3	72.2	78.1	609	186
TX	Kent	0.45	1112	28.9	8.5	26.6	72.9	78.9	2113	644
GA	Floyd	0.33	1197	28.9	9.2	28.7	72.1	78.2	755	230
IL	Johnson	0.28	1231	28.9	8.2	29.5	72.8	78.8	506	154
GA	Brantley	0.05	1402	28.9	9.5	28	70.6	77.2	66	20
VA	Waynesboro	-0.12	1544	28.9	9.1	25.3	74	80.9	1356	413
IA	Allamakee	-0.27	1646	28.9	7.7	22.1	76	80.2	974	297
OK	Tulsa	-0.30	1670	28.9	9.3	28.3	73.3	78.2	682	208
NY	Clinton	-0.34	1703	28.9	7.6	24	75.8	80.5	918	280
IL	Jo Daviess	-0.40	1752	28.9	7.5	22.9	76.5	81.6	838	255
PA	Lehigh	-0.40	1759	28.9	9.3	24.1	76.2	81.8	589	179
MO	Grundy	-0.57	1860	28.9	8	26.2	73.9	80	835	254
OH	Mahoning	-1.72	2478	28.9	9.3	26.8	73.3	79.6	1087	331
IL	White	-1.82	2513	28.9	8.1	30.7	73.5	79.5	403	123
IN	Scott	-1.92	2552	28.9	10.8	31.5	72	77.9	626	191
NE	Sarpy	-2.03	2590	28.9	7.7	20.8	77.6	80.9	1121	342
NE	Antelope	-2.49	2781	28.9	8	27.3	75.3	81.4	1872	570
IN	Fountain	-2.68	2833	28.9	9.5	28.7	74.3	79.5	649	198
SD	Jerauld	-2.91	2888	28.9	5.5	29.8	75.8	81.4	1641	500
IA	Kossuth	-4.47	3092	28.9	6.7	32.2	77.1	82.7	1182	360
NV	Pershing	4.23	184	29	7.7	26	74.7	80.1	4891	1491
MT	Pondera	3.45	251	29	7	28.2	74.4	80.2	4062	1238
GA	Fannin	2.78	334	29	9.9	23.5	72.9	79.3	2109	643
FL	Flagler	2.70	339	29	9	22.4	76.7	83.1	21	6
TX	Haskell	2.04	463	29	8.7	26.6	72.6	79	1535	468
GA	Chatham	1.76	530	29	10.9	23.4	73	78.4	11	3
MS	Tishomingo	1.66	553	29	10.3	29.5	70.8	77.8	527	161

HEALTHIEST PLACES TO LIVE

ST	COUNTY	USDA	AMEN	OBES	DIAB	INACT	M AGE	W AGE	ALT ft	ALT m
TX	Fayette	1.04	801	29	8.6	26	74.1	79.9	362	110
VA	Rockbridge	0.64	997	29	8.7	27.4	74.3	80.4	1606	489
PA	Washington	0.40	1141	29	9.3	24.5	75.1	80.6	1139	347
GA	Morgan	0.37	1163	29	11.1	24.5	73.2	78.5	609	186
TX	Armstrong	0.36	1178	29	8.6	26.9	74.6	79.8	3125	952
ID	Butte	0.07	1386	29	8	23.2	76.2	80.4	5977	1822
VA	Staunton	-0.12	1543	29	9.1	24.2	73.7	79.7	1527	465
WV	Greenbrier	-0.20	1602	29	10.2	29.7	73.3	78.7	2627	801
IN	Brown	-0.29	1661	29	9.6	24.8	75.8	81	756	230
GA	Whitfield	-0.36	1720	29	10.7	27.9	72.5	78.6	842	257
TX	Lipscomb	-0.43	1775	29	8.7	30.1	73.8	79.3	2604	794
TX	Delta	-0.59	1877	29	9.2	28.2	73.8	80	453	138
PA	Berks	-0.73	1964	29	7.9	23.6	76	81.5	566	172
IN	Johnson	-1.16	2219	29	9.9	27.6	76	80.3	778	237
MO	Marion	-1.48	2365	29	7.9	30.2	74	79.2	621	189
MN	Le Sueur	-2.17	2641	29	6.9	21	77.6	81.9	1016	310
MO	Stoddard	-2.43	2753	29	8.7	39.4	71.8	78.2	343	105
KS	Rush	-2.57	2804	29	7.6	25.7	75.2	80.6	2082	635
IL	Boone	-3.32	2969	29	7.3	26	76.5	80.6	864	263
IA	Jefferson	-3.35	2975	29	7.9	22.1	76.9	80.9	741	226
IL	Livingston	-3.95	3060	29	8.3	30.9	74	79.3	683	208
NE	Wayne	-4.02	3071	29	6.8	25.8	76.5	82	1611	491
OR	Linn	3.65	231	29.1	7.7	20.1	75.2	80.1	2071	631
ID	Benewah	3.10	295	29.1	8.7	28.1	74.6	80.2	3123	952
WY	Sweetwater	2.63	354	29.1	7.1	24.4	74.8	80.5	6869	2094
UT	Juab	1.91	496	29.1	7.2	21.2	75.4	80.2	5528	1685
GA	Camden	1.88	501	29.1	11.2	24.1	74.2	79.5	15	5
WA	Columbia	1.84	514	29.1	9	17.4	77.1	80.8	2805	855
TX	Colorado	1.72	542	29.1	9.3	29	73.5	79.3	237	72
VA	Harrisonburg	1.25	713	29.1	9.2	25.5	75.6	80.5	1357	414
MO	Morgan	1.22	723	29.1	8.6	35	73.5	79.6	884	269
VA	Mathews	1.11	774	29.1	9	24.4	75	80.7	4	1
TX	Martin	0.91	856	29.1	8.6	26.4	72.4	77.8	2779	847
SC	Horry	0.88	872	29.1	10.2	24.4	73.7	79.8	50	15
PA	Clearfield	0.81	910	29.1	9	23.7	74.8	80.8	1636	499
VA	Buena Vista	0.64	994	29.1	8.8	23.7	74.3	80.4	999	304
GA	Atkinson	0.24	1261	29.1	10.1	29.5	69.4	76.5	212	65
GA	Polk	0.21	1295	29.1	11.1	26.4	70.4	76.9	914	279
TX	Motley	-0.22	1616	29.1	8.9	27.3	73.2	78.7	2330	710
WI	Grant	-0.46	1797	29.1	7.6	19.5	76.2	80.8	931	284
WI	Bayfield	-0.56	1856	29.1	7.1	21.2	76.2	80.9	1117	340
TN	Rutherford	-0.85	2039	29.1	10.6	27.4	75.2	79.5	678	207
TX	Jim Hogg	-1.01	2141	29.1	8.7	27	73.4	78.6	542	165
IA	Wapello	-1.40	2321	29.1	8.7	25.5	75.1	80.8	782	238
IA	Sac	-1.45	2350	29.1	7.1	24.9	76.3	81.2	1331	406
KS	Scott	-1.50	2377	29.1	7.2	23.1	75.9	81.2	2984	910

ST	COUNTY	USDA	AMEN	OBES	DIAB	INACT	M AGE	W AGE	ALT ft	ALT m
KS	Ness	-1.54	2398	29.1	8.2	24.8	75.2	80.6	2379	725
WI	Dunn	-1.54	2400	29.1	6.5	23.9	76.3	81.6	983	300
NE	Cheyenne	-1.68	2462	29.1	6.8	24	75.8	80.7	4268	1301
IL	Bond	-2.01	2583	29.1	8.6	30.8	74.1	79.5	537	164
ND	Oliver	-2.18	2646	29.1	7.4	24.7	77.4	83	2030	619
IL	Christian	-2.19	2648	29.1	8.3	25.9	73.6	80.2	617	188
IA	Greene	-2.37	2723	29.1	6.8	26.3	76.2	82	1106	337
LA	Lafayette	-2.47	2770	29.1	7.8	25.1	73.3	78.7	29	9
SD	Minnehaha	-2.58	2807	29.1	6.9	23.6	77.1	82.3	1544	471
IL	Wayne	-2.61	2815	29.1	7.3	26	74.6	80.3	435	132
IL	Warren	-3.17	2940	29.1	8.1	26.8	75.1	79.6	715	218
NE	Seward	-3.21	2951	29.1	8	23	76.7	81.5	1499	457
SD	Hanson	-3.42	2990	29.1	6.2	25.8	76.2	81.6	1338	408
NE	Fillmore	-4.00	3069	29.1	6.9	26.7	75.9	80.7	1636	499
CA	Fresno	6.03	60	29.2	9.3	21	75.2	80.2	3364	1025
TX	Val Verde	5.20	101	29.2	9	25.4	75.5	81	1686	514
FL	Osceola	4.50	163	29.2	9.3	26	76	80.8	60	18
FL	Hernando	3.71	222	29.2	8.6	24.8	74.3	81.1	73	22
TX	Kenedy	3.14	291	29.2	8.8	26.8	73.8	78.4	28	8
FL	Clay	2.01	466	29.2	10	24.1	74.8	79.1	89	27
TX	Starr	1.99	477	29.2	8.5	28.9	74.1	80	359	109
TX	Galveston	1.87	507	29.2	9.5	24.6	73.4	78.7	12	4
AR	Logan	1.75	536	29.2	10.1	30.2	72.5	78.7	666	203
TX	Goliad	1.61	567	29.2	9	25.6	73.3	79.8	199	61
TX	Scurry	1.44	622	29.2	8.3	29.1	73.2	79.3	2357	718
TX	Washington	1.43	626	29.2	8.8	27.1	73.7	80.2	304	93
WA	Asotin	1.22	727	29.2	9	22.8	75.4	81.6	2773	845
TX	Webb	1.12	767	29.2	9.1	27.7	75.3	81.8	588	179
PA	Monroe	0.94	843	29.2	9	25.6	75.6	80.4	1241	378
VA	Lexington	0.64	995	29.2	9.5	23.7	74.3	80.4	1055	322
IL	Randolph	0.63	999	29.2	7.4	25.3	73.8	79.2	464	141
TX	Stonewall	0.61	1019	29.2	9	28	72.9	78.9	1750	533
AR	Sharp	0.49	1078	29.2	8.9	32.1	72.7	79.4	560	171
AL	Marshall	0.37	1162	29.2	10.9	31.5	71.5	77.5	880	268
MN	Lake	0.24	1265	29.2	7.4	22.2	76.3	81.7	1560	475
PA	Montour	0.11	1361	29.2	9.4	28.1	75.4	80.5	688	210
DE	Sussex	0.05	1401	29.2	9.3	24.8	74.8	80.8	31	9
VA	Stafford	-0.12	1542	29.2	8.4	20.4	76.2	79.5	212	65
IN	Martin	-0.19	1585	29.2	8.6	30	74.2	79.8	571	174
IL	Saline	-0.41	1763	29.2	8.3	31.6	72.4	78.7	421	128
TX	Mills	-0.43	1776	29.2	8.5	25.2	73.8	79.5	1462	446
TX	Montague	-0.57	1866	29.2	8.7	28.7	73.2	79.6	971	296
TX	Sherman	-0.65	1917	29.2	8.6	27.7	73.7	78.9	3524	1074
KY	Warren	-0.68	1928	29.2	9.5	28.7	73.9	80	574	175
ND	Billings	-0.76	1982	29.2	6.9	26.3	75.7	82.2	2591	790
KY	Oldham	-0.85	2036	29.2	9.3	27.5	76.4	80.7	694	211
IA	Clayton	-1.01	2134	29.2	6.5	28.3	76.1	81.5	968	295

HEALTHIEST PLACES TO LIVE

ST	COUNTY	USDA	AMEN	OBES	DIAB	INACT	M AGE	W AGE	ALT ft	ALT m
NE	Loup	-1.42	2335	29.2	7.5	27.1	75.6	81.2	2424	739
KY	Barren	-1.47	2361	29.2	11.8	30.4	73.4	78.6	725	221
KS	Harvey	-1.71	2474	29.2	7.5	23.6	76	80.9	1445	440
ND	Stark	-1.74	2486	29.2	7.8	27.1	75.7	81.6	2498	761
SD	McPherson	-1.98	2577	29.2	6.4	25.8	74.1	80.3	1827	557
IL	Morgan	-2.25	2670	29.2	7.4	28.6	74.6	79.5	613	187
IL	Lawrence	-2.34	2703	29.2	7.8	28.8	73.7	79.3	454	138
IN	Jennings	-2.48	2772	29.2	9	28.1	73.2	79.2	699	213
IN	St. Joseph	-2.51	2788	29.2	8.9	26.7	74.4	80.8	770	235
IL	Coles	-2.99	2906	29.2	7.3	24.8	74.7	80.1	677	206
MN	Redwood	-3.67	3031	29.2	6.9	21	76	81.1	1073	327
WA	Wahkiakum	3.25	277	29.3	9.1	20.1	74.8	80.3	676	206
ID	Idaho	3.17	284	29.3	7.6	24	75.8	80.6	5119	1560
TX	Edwards	3.15	287	29.3	8.9	27.4	73.7	79.9	2129	649
TX	San Saba	2.92	320	29.3	8.9	29.8	76.4	81.6	1445	440
WA	Kitsap	2.61	358	29.3	7.3	18	77.7	80.9	295	90
TX	Refugio	2.56	366	29.3	9.1	28.2	73.3	79.8	42	13
GA	Putnam	2.34	402	29.3	11.3	24.2	73	78.7	490	149
GA	White	1.55	583	29.3	9.2	23	74.6	79.7	1737	529
OK	Love	1.34	658	29.3	11.2	31.7	73	78.8	804	245
GA	Murray	1.16	745	29.3	10.4	31.4	70.8	77.8	1107	338
GA	Jones	0.98	822	29.3	10.4	29.4	73.1	79.3	468	143
MO	St. Charles	0.86	881	29.3	8	24.4	77.5	81.1	531	162
PA	Lancaster	0.45	1109	29.3	8.1	21.3	76.8	81.4	462	141
TX	Wilson	0.44	1120	29.3	9.6	26.4	74.3	79.6	458	140
PA	Indiana	0.40	1140	29.3	8.5	29.3	76.2	81	1426	435
KS	Geary	0.39	1146	29.3	9.1	29.9	74.4	80.2	1272	388
VA	Westmoreland	0.25	1259	29.3	10.4	28.9	73	79.5	68	21
VA	Wythe	0.11	1364	29.3	9.2	24.5	73.2	78.6	2474	754
NY	Warren	0.00	1441	29.3	8.2	19.8	76.7	81.4	1285	392
NC	Davidson	-0.09	1519	29.3	8.9	29.1	73	78.8	761	232
NH	Strafford	-0.10	1529	29.3	8.3	22.9	76.5	81	423	129
GA	Coweta	-0.28	1651	29.3	9.9	23.7	74.1	79.1	839	256
TX	Hamilton	-0.65	1916	29.3	8.5	29	73.8	79.5	1200	366
KS	Sedgwick	-0.70	1941	29.3	9.1	23.1	74.3	79.8	1361	415
SD	Perkins	-0.73	1965	29.3	7.3	30.6	74.8	80.5	2611	796
NE	Cuming	-0.77	1990	29.3	6.6	28.4	75.7	81.6	1438	438
IL	Perry	-1.20	2233	29.3	8.3	29.8	73.4	79.1	462	141
KS	Comanche	-1.26	2266	29.3	7.7	28.8	75.4	80	1937	590
IL	Cass	-1.94	2561	29.3	8.2	29.1	74.8	80	533	162
IL	Marion	-2.18	2644	29.3	6.7	29.3	73.6	79.5	535	163
NE	Saunders	-2.60	2812	29.3	7.1	24.8	76.6	81.5	1290	393
MN	Lyon	-2.70	2840	29.3	7.1	22.5	76.9	81.6	1306	398
IA	Buchanan	-3.24	2954	29.3	7.8	25.7	76.2	81.3	987	301
TX	Pecos	4.40	168	29.4	8.9	28.1	73.2	78.7	3133	955
NV	Humboldt	3.87	208	29.4	7	24.4	74.7	80.1	5085	1550
TX	Real	3.48	248	29.4	9	26.9	73.7	79.9	2043	623

ST	COUNTY	USDA	AMEN	OBES	DIAB	INACT	M AGE	W AGE	ALT ft	ALT m
FL	Sumter	2.84	326	29.4	9.4	19.5	74.4	80.2	74	23
FL	Escambia	2.34	400	29.4	10.5	25.5	73.6	79	150	46
TX	Hays	2.18	438	29.4	8.6	26.3	77	80.8	978	298
FL	Okaloosa	2.01	467	29.4	8.9	22.2	75.6	80.2	172	52
ID	Canyon	1.82	517	29.4	8.5	22.6	75.1	80.3	2490	759
TX	Denton	1.40	633	29.4	9.4	24.6	77.3	80.9	643	196
TX	Lynn	1.32	669	29.4	9.2	27.7	72.9	78.7	3083	940
VA	Williamsburg	1.15	754	29.4	9.8	23.7	78.1	82.5	55	17
SC	York	0.45	1111	29.4	9	25.5	74	79.2	618	188
TX	Swisher	0.42	1131	29.4	9.1	29	74.6	79.8	3452	1052
TX	Van Zandt	0.42	1132	29.4	9.5	29.5	73.6	79.2	466	142
OK	Garvin	0.38	1158	29.4	9.9	33.7	71.6	78.1	1004	306
TX	Wheeler	0.31	1212	29.4	9.1	28	73.2	78.9	2454	748
NE	Howard	0.30	1215	29.4	6.4	28.9	76.2	80.7	1917	584
TX	Eastland	0.24	1270	29.4	9.1	27.2	72.9	79.5	1514	462
TX	Schleicher	0.08	1382	29.4	8.6	26.5	73.6	78.3	2370	722
TX	Hale	-0.07	1503	29.4	8.6	28.5	73.8	79	3407	1038
VA	Pittsylvania	-0.30	1676	29.4	10.2	26.8	72.5	79.3	703	214
TX	Clay	-0.36	1728	29.4	8.7	31.5	73.2	79.6	954	291
WV	Putnam	-0.43	1778	29.4	10.4	27.7	75.5	79.3	792	241
IN	Ohio	-0.49	1809	29.4	9.5	28.2	74.7	79.5	712	217
NY	Wayne	-0.51	1817	29.4	8.7	23.3	75.6	80.7	434	132
PA	Erie	-0.57	1864	29.4	8.6	28.8	75.3	80.3	1158	353
KY	Calloway	-0.58	1868	29.4	10.8	24	74.7	79.7	493	150
NY	Orleans	-0.58	1872	29.4	8	27.5	75.5	80.6	476	145
WI	Douglas	-0.66	1921	29.4	7.4	20.9	74.6	80.6	1061	323
TX	Throckmorton	-0.79	2006	29.4	8.6	27.4	72.6	79	1363	416
MO	Putnam	-0.90	2069	29.4	7.7	28.5	74.8	80.2	964	294
OK	Woods	-1.14	2211	29.4	8.4	30.4	74.4	79.7	1573	479
WI	Winnebago	-1.37	2310	29.4	7.7	19.4	76.6	81.5	788	240
SD	Campbell	-1.45	2354	29.4	6.7	33	74.1	80.3	1807	551
IA	Ringgold	-1.90	2544	29.4	6.9	26.1	76.4	80.9	1174	358
IA	Decatur	-2.04	2592	29.4	6.6	25.3	75.5	80.8	1054	321
OH	Portage	-2.17	2642	29.4	8.6	28.3	75.8	80.1	1098	335
NE	Washington	-2.35	2711	29.4	7.3	21.7	77	81.2	1200	366
OH	Richland	-2.88	2883	29.4	9.3	27	74.8	79.4	1195	364
IN	Warren	-3.25	2956	29.4	10.2	29.9	74.8	80.6	701	214
MN	Lac qui Parle	-3.43	2993	29.4	7.7	19.8	76.5	82.2	1068	326
IL	Stark	-3.87	3052	29.4	7.6	28.1	74.9	80.3	721	220
MN	Koochiching	-4.20	3083	29.4	8.1	19.8	75.3	81.1	1215	370
TX	Kerr	4.52	161	29.5	9.2	22.1	75.5	81.5	2005	611
TX	Kinney	3.80	215	29.5	8.6	27	74.2	80.1	1240	378
UT	Tooele	2.83	330	29.5	9.6	22.1	76.1	79.5	4788	1459
TX	Tom Green	2.62	356	29.5	9.1	25.5	74.3	79.9	2080	634
MO	Wayne	2.18	436	29.5	9.2	30.1	71.8	78.2	578	176
TX	Calhoun	1.86	510	29.5	8.8	24.9	73.8	78.9	12	4
TX	Willacy	1.85	511	29.5	8.8	28.1	73.8	78.4	23	7

HEALTHIEST PLACES TO LIVE

ST	COUNTY	USDA	AMEN	OBES	DIAB	INACT	M AGE	W AGE	ALT ft	ALT m
TX	Austin	1.38	642	29.5	9	25.9	74.5	80.2	240	73
OK	Cleveland	1.06	787	29.5	9.4	26.1	75	79.8	1144	349
MO	Dade	0.95	837	29.5	8.8	26.4	73.7	79	1024	312
MI	Benzie	0.75	934	29.5	8.8	23	75.7	80.9	777	237
TN	Washington	0.67	974	29.5	10.2	28.6	72.5	79.6	1700	518
KS	Chautauqua	0.23	1276	29.5	7.7	24.7	73	79.9	958	292
GA	Worth	0.06	1396	29.5	10.2	26.4	71.8	78.3	331	101
TX	Foard	0.03	1416	29.5	9.6	28.3	73.2	78.7	1497	456
NE	Valley	-0.06	1495	29.5	8	28.6	76.2	80.7	2202	671
OH	Clermont	-0.06	1496	29.5	9	24.4	75.6	79.5	819	249
TN	Bradley	-0.17	1578	29.5	11.6	30.2	73.3	79.2	848	258
VA	Winchester	-0.38	1742	29.5	9.3	24.5	73.9	80.6	748	228
GA	Coffee	-0.49	1807	29.5	11.3	32.2	70.2	78	254	77
WI	Ashland	-0.63	1903	29.5	7.8	20.4	74.4	80.9	1281	390
PA	Bedford	-0.67	1926	29.5	9.4	25.9	75.2	80.6	1458	444
NY	Broome	-0.84	2029	29.5	8.4	23.6	75.5	81.2	1317	401
PA	Jefferson	-0.93	2087	29.5	10.7	28.8	74.9	80.3	1569	478
KS	Gray	-0.96	2107	29.5	8.7	25.8	75.3	80.2	2738	834
KS	Miami	-1.15	2213	29.5	8.1	25.2	75.9	80.2	985	300
WI	Brown	-1.36	2304	29.5	7.9	20.1	77.4	82	746	227
NE	Custer	-1.40	2324	29.5	6.8	29.3	75.6	81.2	2616	797
MO	Pettis	-2.05	2600	29.5	8.4	31.8	74.7	79.7	825	251
IN	LaGrange	-2.36	2716	29.5	8.8	24.3	74.1	79.7	907	276
IA	Clarke	-2.42	2746	29.5	6.7	28	75.5	80.8	1095	334
ND	Dickey	-2.96	2900	29.5	7.5	28.4	75.8	82	1534	468
MN	Steele	-3.05	2915	29.5	6.6	21.2	77.7	82.5	1215	370
NE	Thayer	-3.12	2931	29.5	7.6	27.5	75.9	80.7	1563	476
IL	McDonough	-3.19	2945	29.5	7.4	27.4	76.1	80.5	667	203
IA	Floyd	-4.03	3072	29.5	7.3	24.6	76.5	81.1	1072	327
CA	San Joaquin	4.77	145	29.6	8.5	21.4	74.9	80.1	158	48
NM	Chaves	3.87	207	29.6	7.5	25.9	73	79.7	4233	1290
ID	Shoshone	3.64	233	29.6	7.8	26.9	74.6	80.2	4239	1292
NM	San Juan	2.83	329	29.6	8.5	24.1	73.9	80.1	6047	1843
TX	San Patricio	1.97	479	29.6	9.9	27.8	73.7	79.9	60	18
VA	Franklin	1.92	493	29.6	9.4	24.4	74.6	80.2	1198	365
ID	Bannock	1.73	540	29.6	8.8	20.3	75.9	80.3	5633	1717
TX	Palo Pinto	1.45	616	29.6	9.2	26.2	72.6	79.1	1042	318
TX	Castro	1.23	719	29.6	8.8	29.1	73.7	79.3	3770	1149
AR	Washington	1.22	720	29.6	9.1	24.9	74.9	80.1	1399	426
TX	Childress	1.02	805	29.6	9.4	25.9	72.2	77.9	1765	538
TX	Atascosa	0.90	860	29.6	8.5	28	74.6	80.4	434	132
TX	La Salle	0.71	956	29.6	8.6	26.8	72.9	78.7	429	131
TX	Andrews	0.68	966	29.6	8.9	27.1	73.9	78.9	3177	968
TX	Medina	0.68	968	29.6	9.2	24.9	75.3	79.8	960	292
TX	Zavala	0.49	1083	29.6	8.7	27.4	72.2	78.1	691	211
MO	Moniteau	0.39	1151	29.6	9.2	32	74.4	79.9	802	244
TX	Hockley	0.37	1172	29.6	8.6	30.6	72.9	78.7	3485	1062

ST	COUNTY	USDA	AMEN	OBES	DIAB	INACT	M AGE	W AGE	ALT ft	ALT m
PA	Lawrence	0.24	1268	29.6	9.5	27.7	74.5	80.6	1093	333
SD	Hughes	0.07	1394	29.6	8.4	21.3	76.2	81.5	1718	524
NE	Buffalo	0.04	1412	29.6	7	23.1	76.7	81.7	2185	666
NC	Randolph	-0.01	1447	29.6	9.6	29.5	73.6	79.7	649	198
GA	Telfair	-0.36	1719	29.6	11.5	27	70.1	76	205	62
VA	Fluvanna	-0.51	1819	29.6	9.6	21.3	76	80.3	387	118
IN	Porter	-0.54	1838	29.6	9.1	25.8	76.2	80.5	693	211
IN	Harrison	-0.78	1996	29.6	9.5	28.4	75.1	80.2	673	205
SC	Dorchester	-1.11	2197	29.6	10.1	26.5	74.1	79.4	62	19
IL	Franklin	-1.19	2230	29.6	8.8	28.9	72.2	78.6	435	133
WV	Monroe	-1.38	2316	29.6	11.7	30.1	72.6	79.2	2308	704
OH	Greene	-1.97	2574	29.6	9.3	22.7	76.5	80.5	966	294
OH	Trumbull	-2.12	2627	29.6	9.4	29.2	73.7	79.5	973	297
IL	La Salle	-2.75	2850	29.6	8.1	25.7	74.4	80.1	658	201
SD	Aurora	-2.83	2871	29.6	6.5	34.1	74.9	81.2	1573	479
IA	Pocahontas	-2.95	2895	29.6	8	24.5	75.9	81.1	1243	379
IL	Douglas	-3.50	3004	29.6	7.1	27.8	74.6	80.3	659	201
IN	Grant	-3.54	3009	29.6	10.2	31.4	73	79.2	842	257
OR	Polk	3.28	274	29.7	7.6	18.9	77.7	82.2	862	263
TX	San Jacinto	2.18	439	29.7	9.4	29.6	71.7	78.4	214	65
TX	Nacogdoches	2.12	448	29.7	9.3	26.5	72.6	78.8	330	101
AR	Boone	1.98	478	29.7	9.9	30.6	74.1	79.6	1169	356
CT	Windham	1.28	687	29.7	8.3	25.2	75.4	80.7	471	143
GA	Crawford	0.97	824	29.7	10.5	27.5	70.6	76.6	473	144
MO	Washington	0.86	882	29.7	9	27.8	70.4	77.3	933	284
PA	Carbon	0.67	971	29.7	9.3	26.3	73.6	79.5	1244	379
TX	Orange	0.44	1119	29.7	10	33.9	71.5	78	12	4
MO	Osage	0.42	1125	29.7	8.7	26.8	74.3	79.8	715	218
PA	Luzerne	0.30	1217	29.7	8.8	29.7	73.3	79.8	1268	386
OK	Oklahoma	0.24	1267	29.7	9.9	30.1	73.2	78.8	1143	348
TX	Ellis	0.24	1271	29.7	8.9	25.2	75	78.9	533	162
LA	Orleans	0.14	1339	29.7	11.7	28.8	68.4	79.5	3	1
PA	Northampton	-0.04	1478	29.7	7.1	23.7	76.5	81.8	578	176
VA	King William	-0.06	1497	29.7	9.4	28.1	73.3	79	89	27
GA	Pike	-0.63	1894	29.7	10.4	25.4	72.1	77.9	825	251
MO	Atchison	-0.76	1980	29.7	8.5	27	76.2	80.7	998	304
NE	Blaine	-0.81	2017	29.7	7	28.4	75.6	81.2	2651	808
VA	Manassas Park	-0.94	2099	29.7	9.5	25.9	76.5	80.4	235	72
VA	Fredericksburg	-0.97	2113	29.7	9.7	25	73.5	80.6	103	31
MT	Chouteau	-0.98	2118	29.7	7.9	27.7	74.4	80.2	3231	985
WI	Sauk	-1.01	2143	29.7	8	23.5	76.2	81.9	981	299
PA	Fulton	-1.20	2237	29.7	8.9	26	74.6	80.4	1118	341
IL	Madison	-1.69	2465	29.7	9.6	27.3	74.5	79.5	512	156
IL	St. Clair	-1.81	2507	29.7	8.8	28.7	72.2	78.5	466	142
IN	Washington	-2.13	2629	29.7	9.1	32.5	73.7	79	761	232
NE	Adams	-2.36	2720	29.7	7.3	23.5	76.8	81.8	1949	594
IL	Brown	-2.39	2733	29.7	8.5	28.2	74.4	79.5	625	191

ST	COUNTY	USDA	AMEN	OBES	DIAB	INACT	M AGE	W AGE	ALT ft	ALT m
OH	Hancock	-2.63	2821	29.7	8.4	24.5	76.5	81.3	805	245
OH	Wood	-2.80	2861	29.7	8.4	25	76.4	81.3	677	206
IL	Hamilton	-2.97	2902	29.7	7.8	30.4	73	79.5	441	134
IL	DeKalb	-3.58	3017	29.7	7.9	25.4	77	81	832	254
ND	Towner	-3.99	3067	29.7	7.1	24.6	75	81.2	1562	476
TX	Bandera	5.83	70	29.8	9.1	28.9	76.4	81.2	1684	513
FL	Citrus	3.43	253	29.8	9.6	25.1	73.1	80.8	53	16
AZ	Pinal	3.36	263	29.8	9	23.6	75.3	80.7	2340	713
AR	Baxter	2.64	348	29.8	8	30.3	73.4	79.8	746	227
FL	Gulf	2.25	422	29.8	10.3	27.1	72	77.7	17	5
OK	Texas	2.01	468	29.8	8.6	30.6	74.4	79.8	3171	966
TX	Crane	1.34	660	29.8	9.4	28	73.4	78.5	2566	782
TX	Coryell	1.01	812	29.8	10.8	28.2	74.9	79.8	953	291
VA	Galax	0.67	976	29.8	8.8	24.4	72.3	77.9	2487	758
TX	Guadalupe	0.58	1033	29.8	8.2	23.9	76.5	81.1	564	172
TX	Maverick	0.52	1057	29.8	9	29	74.2	80.1	794	242
TN	Davidson	0.33	1200	29.8	9.5	26.9	73.3	79.2	579	177
TX	Fannin	0.22	1289	29.8	9.2	30.9	72.9	78.4	595	181
TX	Hardeman	0.14	1344	29.8	8.8	26.9	72.2	77.9	1518	463
TX	Cottle	-0.19	1591	29.8	9	28.5	73.2	78.7	1808	551
IL	Pope	-0.22	1612	29.8	7.9	28	72.4	78.7	507	155
AL	Lee	-0.24	1626	29.8	11.3	27.9	73.9	78.6	615	187
NE	Dodge	-0.55	1843	29.8	7.9	29	75.2	81.5	1301	397
GA	Lamar	-0.57	1857	29.8	10.8	26.8	72.1	77.9	746	227
TN	Wilson	-0.82	2020	29.8	9.3	28.6	74.7	78.9	664	203
NE	McPherson	-0.90	2070	29.8	7.9	28.1	76.1	80.2	3326	1014
MI	Marquette	-1.09	2186	29.8	7.9	20.9	76.3	80.4	1246	380
ND	Divide	-2.06	2602	29.8	6.5	30.5	76.5	81.9	2146	654
IA	Clinton	-2.35	2707	29.8	7.3	28.7	75.5	80.7	726	221
OH	Shelby	-2.44	2758	29.8	9.6	29.2	75.4	80.3	994	303
MO	Lawrence	-2.46	2765	29.8	8.4	28.5	73.3	79.4	1239	378
OH	Morrow	-2.67	2831	29.8	9	31.6	74.5	79.1	1167	356
PA	Mercer	-2.78	2855	29.8	10.1	23.9	74.7	80.2	1211	369
MN	Sibley	-3.10	2929	29.8	6.9	23.1	76.6	81.5	1012	308
OH	Fayette	-3.20	2948	29.8	9.9	30.4	73.2	78.6	970	296
OH	Seneca	-3.37	2982	29.8	9	28.5	74.8	79.9	811	247
IN	Boone	-3.68	3032	29.8	8.5	29.8	76.6	80.9	918	280
CA	Madera	6.00	61	29.9	8.5	20.4	74.6	80.2	3089	942
WY	Carbon	5.41	86	29.9	7.5	31.2	75.2	80	7294	2223
ID	Owyhee	2.10	452	29.9	8.7	28.4	75.5	79.9	4773	1455
GA	McDuffie	1.96	481	29.9	11.6	26.9	70.1	76.3	441	134
TX	McMullen	1.76	534	29.9	8.9	27	72.9	78.7	330	101
TX	Crockett	1.64	560	29.9	8.7	26.2	73.4	78.5	2438	743
NC	Brunswick	1.12	765	29.9	8.6	25.6	74.4	80	40	12
MD	Washington	0.85	889	29.9	9.8	27.7	74.6	79.7	639	195
VA	Amherst	0.83	902	29.9	10.4	24.9	73.2	79.4	1129	344
TX	Young	0.51	1067	29.9	9.6	26.6	73.3	78.8	1179	359

ST	COUNTY	USDA	AMEN	OBES	DIAB	INACT	M AGE	W AGE	ALT ft	ALT m
TX	Yoakum	0.21	1302	**29.9**	8.5	28	73.9	78.9	3661	1116
WI	Juneau	-0.43	1777	**29.9**	7.9	22.8	74.1	80.1	949	289
WI	Iowa	-0.98	2120	**29.9**	8.2	23.6	76.6	81.5	1006	307
IA	Pottawattamie	-1.03	2148	**29.9**	7.3	26.7	74.9	80	1188	362
KS	Stevens	-1.18	2227	**29.9**	9.7	26.4	74.6	79.4	3101	945
KS	Sheridan	-1.21	2240	**29.9**	7.7	25.7	76.3	81.5	2727	831
SD	Union	-1.78	2500	**29.9**	5.9	23.7	77.4	82.7	1253	382
IL	Richland	-2.20	2651	**29.9**	8.2	29.2	74.4	80	474	145
OH	Paulding	-2.67	2832	**29.9**	8.9	29.3	74.4	80.2	714	218
IL	Stephenson	-3.75	3045	**29.9**	8	27.9	75.5	80.8	871	265
MN	Clay	-4.17	3081	**29.9**	7.9	22.3	77.3	82.6	1022	312
NV	Lyon	5.70	74	**30**	7.4	25.3	74.5	79.9	5207	1587
OR	Coos	5.53	83	**30**	8	20.5	74	79.3	932	284
TX	Uvalde	4.26	180	**30**	9.1	27	73.7	79.9	1190	363
TX	Kleberg	3.15	288	**30**	8.7	26.8	73.6	79.6	48	15
NV	White Pine	3.04	305	**30**	7.5	24	74.9	80.3	6825	2080
ID	Power	2.04	462	**30**	7.5	24.1	75.6	80.5	5178	1578
GA	Bibb	1.81	520	**30**	11.8	28.2	70	76.9	383	117
ID	Franklin	1.68	546	**30**	8.2	23.3	76.2	80.9	5829	1777
AR	Izard	1.44	619	**30**	8.4	30.4	72.5	78.7	654	199
AR	Sebastian	1.10	775	**30**	9.7	33.9	73.6	79.3	633	193
TX	McLennan	0.76	932	**30**	9.3	24.9	73.4	79.2	572	174
SC	Spartanburg	0.52	1055	**30**	9.9	27.5	72	78.4	769	234
TX	Hidalgo	0.46	1101	**30**	10.2	23.8	77.8	83.4	129	39
MD	Garrett	0.35	1186	**30**	10.1	29.5	75	80.2	2460	750
TN	Sumner	0.25	1257	**30**	10	28.1	74.9	79.4	691	211
OH	Carroll	0.01	1431	**30**	9.1	23.6	75	80.2	1128	344
TX	Collingsworth	0.01	1436	**30**	9	27.6	73.2	78.9	2137	651
SD	Haakon	-0.30	1673	**30**	7.1	27.5	76.6	81.5	2287	697
IA	Appanoose	-0.51	1815	**30**	7.1	28.8	75	80.2	952	290
KY	Nelson	-0.63	1896	**30**	10.3	28.5	73.9	80.4	639	195
ND	Bowman	-1.01	2139	**30**	7.5	29.5	75.7	81.6	2974	906
MI	Schoolcraft	-1.05	2163	**30**	9.3	24.8	74.7	80	745	227
KY	Harrison	-1.72	2477	**30**	11.6	33.5	72.5	78	808	246
SD	Codington	-1.73	2481	**30**	6.3	26.6	76.2	82.2	1813	553
ND	Stutsman	-1.79	2504	**30**	7.7	26.9	75.2	81.3	1674	510
IL	Fayette	-1.97	2570	**30**	7.7	30.9	73.6	79.2	550	168
OH	Preble	-1.97	2575	**30**	9.9	28.5	74.7	79.8	1035	315
OH	Miami	-2.33	2702	**30**	10.2	28.4	75.5	80.3	953	290
MN	Anoka	-2.41	2744	**30**	7.7	20.8	78.3	82.4	909	277
IA	Dallas	-2.56	2800	**30**	8.1	23.9	77	81.9	992	302
NY	Montgomery	-2.63	2820	**30**	7.4	27.9	74.3	80.7	712	217
MN	Todd	-2.84	2872	**30**	7.4	25.8	75.7	81.1	1335	407
IA	Webster	-3.20	2947	**30**	8.6	30.4	75.1	80.2	1131	345
IA	Jones	-3.45	2996	**30**	7.4	24.7	76.1	81.4	879	268
IA	Wright	-3.56	3011	**30**	7	28	76	81.9	1179	359
TX	Jasper	2.25	424	**30.1**	10.1	33.7	72.9	78.2	155	47

HEALTHIEST PLACES TO LIVE

ST	COUNTY	USDA	AMEN	OBES	DIAB	INACT	M AGE	W AGE	ALT ft	ALT m
ID	Minidoka	1.42	627	30.1	9.5	25.6	74.2	79.6	4374	1333
TX	Wood	1.37	648	30.1	9	28.8	73.3	80.3	442	135
TX	Rains	0.78	923	30.1	9	27.1	73.6	78.9	454	138
SC	Anderson	0.71	953	30.1	10.7	28.8	71.8	79	756	231
OH	Guernsey	0.55	1042	30.1	9.7	30.8	73.4	79.4	962	293
PA	Lycoming	0.33	1199	30.1	8.5	27.5	74.9	80	1290	393
AL	Cleburne	0.21	1293	30.1	11.1	32.8	71.8	78	1050	320
NC	Yadkin	0.20	1308	30.1	9.4	27.6	73.5	79.3	934	285
GA	Early	0.16	1329	30.1	12.2	29.5	69.6	75.8	225	69
AR	Independence	0.09	1370	30.1	10.1	32.3	73.5	78.9	433	132
GA	Wheeler	0.07	1385	30.1	10.9	26.3	71.3	76.5	179	55
IL	Hardin	0.07	1387	30.1	8	26	73	79.5	482	147
GA	Long	-0.04	1472	30.1	11.2	25.3	70.6	77.8	63	19
TX	Cochran	-0.12	1540	30.1	9.1	27.9	73.1	78.8	3784	1153
ME	Kennebec	-0.14	1556	30.1	8.2	22.5	75.7	80.4	287	87
NC	Durham	-0.26	1643	30.1	9.4	20.8	74.4	80.1	369	112
MI	Van Buren	-0.61	1885	30.1	9.2	27.3	73.9	79.6	737	225
NY	Monroe	-0.75	1973	30.1	8.5	20.4	76.9	81.4	492	150
TN	Dickson	-0.83	2024	30.1	10.4	31.5	72.4	78.8	706	215
KY	McCracken	-0.87	2049	30.1	9.6	28.4	73.6	79.1	375	114
IN	Morgan	-0.88	2056	30.1	9.2	27.2	74.6	79.2	729	222
TN	Lawrence	-0.89	2065	30.1	10.7	32.2	71.5	78.6	876	267
SD	Hamlin	-1.37	2308	30.1	7.5	28.3	74.9	80.6	1738	530
WI	Green Lake	-1.58	2413	30.1	8	23.9	76.3	81	857	261
MO	Bates	-1.65	2444	30.1	8.9	27.4	73.8	79.5	848	259
MI	Delta	-1.94	2562	30.1	8.7	24.3	76.5	80.9	733	224
ND	Williams	-2.01	2586	30.1	7.3	30.8	76.5	81.9	2205	672
MI	Kent	-2.28	2685	30.1	8.9	21.3	76.5	81	796	243
MI	Crawford	-2.37	2725	30.1	8.3	23.4	74.1	79.2	1218	371
IN	Marion	-2.51	2787	30.1	10.5	26.1	72.6	78.7	794	242
OH	Ashland	-2.84	2873	30.1	10.1	28.6	75.7	80.5	1122	342
IA	Henry	-2.95	2894	30.1	8	24.2	76	81.4	690	210
WI	Langlade	-3.13	2934	30.1	7.6	22.3	75.1	80.9	1535	468
OH	Fulton	-3.29	2962	30.1	11.1	26.1	75.8	81.1	734	224
IA	O'Brien	-4.23	3086	30.1	7.5	24.2	75.9	81.8	1455	443
CA	Stanislaus	7.21	30	30.2	8.2	23.9	74.8	79.4	491	150
OR	Curry	6.47	46	30.2	7.6	21.6	74.8	80.2	1633	498
AZ	Yuma	4.24	183	30.2	8.7	23.2	78	83.8	878	268
FL	Highlands	4.14	191	30.2	9.8	26.6	75.5	81.6	74	23
TX	Nueces	3.33	267	30.2	9.8	23.7	74.3	80.5	55	17
TX	Zapata	2.36	397	30.2	8	27.9	74.1	80	436	133
MO	Barry	1.95	485	30.2	8.7	31.6	72.7	79.2	1319	402
NC	Avery	1.95	486	30.2	9.1	20.7	73.1	79.5	3536	1078
NC	Wilkes	1.88	502	30.2	10	30.7	72.9	79	1490	454
TX	Panola	1.35	654	30.2	9.7	26.3	72.1	78.9	287	88
VA	Northampton	1.29	685	30.2	11.3	28.7	71.5	77.6	18	6
TX	Hardin	1.04	802	30.2	10.6	29.2	73.5	78.3	71	22

ST	COUNTY	USDA	AMEN	OBES	DIAB	INACT	M AGE	W AGE	ALT ft	ALT m
MO	Miller	0.83	897	30.2	8.4	30	73.6	78.9	787	240
NC	Onslow	0.74	935	30.2	9.9	24	74.5	79.6	42	13
MO	Greene	0.62	1010	30.2	8.5	25.2	74.7	80.7	1226	374
TX	Brazos	0.59	1025	30.2	9.1	22.9	77.1	80.4	284	87
MI	Grand Traverse	0.37	1168	30.2	7.5	19.5	77.7	82	905	276
MD	Worcester	0.34	1191	30.2	8.3	23.2	75.3	80.7	23	7
GA	Pulaski	0.28	1230	30.2	10.7	30.4	70.9	77.1	278	85
KY	Madison	-0.10	1525	30.2	9.7	30.3	73.8	79.5	888	271
VA	Russell	-0.38	1741	30.2	10.4	33.4	71.3	77.5	2239	682
GA	Peach	-0.64	1904	30.2	12.4	28.5	70.6	76.3	435	133
NC	Lee	-0.68	1930	30.2	10.3	23.5	73.3	80	324	99
PA	Union	-1.08	2185	30.2	9	24.4	76	80.5	956	291
IA	Taylor	-1.44	2344	30.2	7.2	23.5	76.4	80.9	1204	367
WI	Calumet	-1.49	2375	30.2	6.9	18.6	78.3	82.3	853	260
IN	Posey	-1.53	2392	30.2	9.3	26.7	75.1	80.9	402	123
ND	Golden Valley	-1.55	2401	30.2	6.6	30.2	75.7	82.2	2696	822
KY	Kenton	-1.62	2435	30.2	10.1	27.1	73.5	78.6	767	234
IA	Union	-1.83	2518	30.2	7.2	27.6	76.5	81.5	1219	371
NE	Dundy	-1.93	2559	30.2	8.2	30.4	76.1	81.4	3287	1002
ND	Ward	-2.01	2585	30.2	8.1	27.4	75.7	81.4	1934	589
IL	Washington	-2.23	2660	30.2	7.6	27.3	75.3	80.6	482	147
MN	Otter Tail	-2.41	2745	30.2	6.7	22.7	76.5	82.4	1355	413
MI	Iron	-2.88	2881	30.2	9.2	23	75.1	80.9	1538	469
MN	Beltrami	-2.89	2884	30.2	7.4	21.3	74.6	81	1261	384
WI	Shawano	-3.40	2986	30.2	8.1	25.4	76.3	81	979	298
IL	McLean	-3.57	3013	30.2	7.6	24.7	76.6	80.9	767	234
ND	Sargent	-3.61	3024	30.2	8	29.1	75.8	82	1239	378
ND	Nelson	-3.72	3040	30.2	7.2	28.1	75.2	81.1	1487	453
OR	Marion	3.51	244	30.3	8.1	19	75.8	80.6	1553	473
WY	Uinta	3.32	271	30.3	7	23.1	75.7	80.9	7249	2210
GA	Gilmer	2.33	403	30.3	10.2	24.4	72.6	78.5	1839	560
TN	Sevier	1.76	532	30.3	10.5	28.2	73.6	79.6	1978	603
OK	Johnston	1.67	550	30.3	10.7	33	71.1	78.1	847	258
GA	Upson	1.37	645	30.3	11.3	26.7	70.5	76.3	660	201
TX	Oldham	1.19	735	30.3	9	28.4	72.4	79.1	3697	1127
TX	Duval	0.96	835	30.3	8.8	26.3	73.4	78.6	487	148
TN	Hardin	0.44	1118	30.3	9.4	33.9	71.5	78.1	507	154
WV	Ohio	-0.13	1552	30.3	10.8	28.9	74.2	79.8	1084	331
VA	Shenandoah	-0.77	1994	30.3	8.8	27.1	74.8	80.4	1240	378
KS	Rooks	-0.94	2092	30.3	8.7	25.8	75.7	82	2013	614
IA	Guthrie	-1.19	2229	30.3	6.6	25.8	76.2	82	1206	368
IL	Fulton	-1.77	2498	30.3	7.3	29.9	73.9	79.8	604	184
NE	Nuckolls	-1.85	2526	30.3	6.8	27.6	76.8	81.8	1719	524
MN	Jackson	-2.05	2599	30.3	6.6	22.2	77.5	82.9	1435	437
WI	Marinette	-2.16	2640	30.3	7.1	25.3	75.1	81.2	906	276
IL	Clark	-2.35	2708	30.3	8.1	30.3	74.5	80.5	590	180
MI	Clare	-2.36	2717	30.3	8.9	30.4	72.7	79	1069	326

ST	COUNTY	USDA	AMEN	OBES	DIAB	INACT	M AGE	W AGE	ALT ft	ALT m
MN	Waseca	-2.36	2719	30.3	7.7	23	77.5	81.3	1124	343
IL	Will	-2.41	2742	30.3	8.6	25	77	80.9	661	202
IA	Plymouth	-2.69	2836	30.3	7.3	28.7	76.4	81.8	1329	405
OH	Williams	-2.97	2904	30.3	9.2	23.7	75.8	80.7	832	254
IN	Newton	-3.42	2988	30.3	9.8	28.6	74	79.3	671	205
IL	Edgar	-3.65	3029	30.3	8.1	28.4	73.8	79.7	666	203
IA	Benton	-3.66	3030	30.3	7	25	77.7	82	893	272
TX	Reeves	2.84	327	30.4	9.5	27.3	73.2	78.7	2981	909
TX	Concho	2.30	413	30.4	8.7	25.6	73.6	78.3	1859	566
MO	Stone	2.24	426	30.4	8.9	26.7	75.1	81.2	1138	347
TX	Nolan	2.11	451	30.4	9.3	28.3	72.1	78	2353	717
TX	San Augustine	1.96	482	30.4	10.3	29.7	71.8	78.2	272	83
KS	Norton	1.57	576	30.4	8.2	24.8	76.3	81.5	2342	714
TX	Karnes	1.38	643	30.4	9.3	28.4	72.1	79.1	353	108
TX	Hood	1.35	653	30.4	8.6	23.9	75.7	80	872	266
VA	Patrick	1.27	700	30.4	9.7	24.9	73.4	78.9	1577	481
IL	Williamson	1.05	792	30.4	7.4	31.1	73.2	79.2	466	142
TX	Deaf Smith	0.94	845	30.4	8.6	28	72.4	79.1	4046	1233
FL	Holmes	0.89	862	30.4	12.9	32.7	71.8	78	131	40
TX	Wilbarger	0.88	874	30.4	9.2	25.9	73.2	78.7	1231	375
TX	Donley	0.86	885	30.4	9.3	27.5	74.6	79.8	2672	814
PA	Wyoming	0.68	965	30.4	8.5	24.3	74.8	80.7	1256	383
GA	Hart	0.62	1006	30.4	9.6	24.4	72	78.4	742	226
IL	Union	0.57	1034	30.4	7.7	31.5	72.9	79.7	503	153
NC	Chowan	0.51	1062	30.4	10.8	28.1	73	78.8	18	5
TX	Jack	0.35	1190	30.4	9.5	27.3	74.9	81.1	1091	332
GA	Berrien	0.32	1202	30.4	10.5	29.1	71.1	77.6	256	78
TX	Upshur	0.28	1236	30.4	10.3	34.9	72.3	78.4	383	117
TX	Jackson	-0.02	1458	30.4	8.9	26.1	73.7	79.7	57	17
MO	Cooper	-0.08	1510	30.4	9.1	25.7	74.4	79.9	743	227
PA	Juniata	-0.34	1704	30.4	9.4	26.6	74.6	80.8	865	264
KS	Haskell	-0.61	1883	30.4	9.3	27.2	75.3	80.2	2917	889
NE	Banner	-0.75	1972	30.4	7.9	26.9	75.8	80.7	4655	1419
TX	Victoria	-0.82	2021	30.4	9.2	24.9	74.5	80.1	87	27
WI	Jackson	-0.87	2054	30.4	8.4	24.1	74.8	79.6	983	300
IN	Jefferson	-0.89	2061	30.4	8.8	30	74.4	79.9	738	225
MI	Otsego	-0.89	2062	30.4	8.5	23.6	76	80.4	1219	371
WV	Lewis	-0.98	2121	30.4	11.1	31.9	72	78.5	1216	371
MI	Kalkaska	-1.11	2192	30.4	10	25	74.8	80	1121	342
GA	Schley	-1.42	2331	30.4	11.3	27.3	70.9	77	483	147
WV	Upshur	-1.52	2391	30.4	12.5	30.1	73.3	78.7	1807	551
MO	Worth	-1.56	2407	30.4	8.6	28.3	74.9	80.2	1035	315
SD	Bon Homme	-1.59	2421	30.4	7.5	30.1	75	80.9	1432	437
KY	Jessamine	-1.99	2578	30.4	11.4	30.6	74.3	79.5	886	270
IN	Spencer	-2.20	2652	30.4	9.4	25.2	75.3	80.3	434	132
IN	Vermillion	-2.30	2691	30.4	10.9	26.8	73.8	79.2	599	182
IL	Crawford	-2.44	2757	30.4	7.9	31.1	74.9	79.6	503	153

ST	COUNTY	USDA	AMEN	OBES	DIAB	INACT	M AGE	W AGE	ALT ft	ALT m
IL	Mercer	-2.47	2767	30.4	7.5	25	75.9	80.9	677	206
MN	Sherburne	-2.88	2882	30.4	7.9	22.4	77.3	80.8	979	298
MN	Clearwater	-2.96	2899	30.4	7.5	21	74.9	81	1427	435
IN	Decatur	-3.09	2922	30.4	9.4	24.5	74.3	80.2	885	270
MN	Norman	-5.37	3105	30.4	8.1	21.2	75.7	81.2	984	300
IN	Tipton	-5.40	3106	30.4	9.3	28.2	75.7	80.7	872	266
TX	Lampasas	2.81	331	30.5	8.4	25.5	75.4	79.8	1231	375
ID	Gem	2.45	380	30.5	7.1	25.2	75.8	80.4	3598	1097
ID	Nez Perce	1.41	629	30.5	9.6	22.8	76.1	80.7	2558	780
VA	Bedford City	1.39	639	30.5	10	23.8	75.8	80.9	973	297
MO	Carter	1.23	717	30.5	9.3	29.7	70.4	77.3	726	221
TN	Hamilton	1.16	746	30.5	9.5	26.7	73.4	79.5	978	298
TX	Terry	1.11	773	30.5	9.4	30.9	73.1	78.8	3337	1017
ID	Lewis	0.99	818	30.5	8	24.1	75.8	80.6	3403	1037
TX	Dallas	0.64	993	30.5	10.2	25.3	75.1	80.3	511	156
TN	Knox	0.62	1012	30.5	10.3	27.3	74.3	79.5	1009	307
KY	Pulaski	0.61	1015	30.5	10.2	32.2	72.5	78.9	1012	308
TX	Menard	0.51	1066	30.5	8.6	26.3	76.4	81.6	2101	640
TX	Dickens	0.38	1160	30.5	9.1	27	73.2	78.7	2395	730
MI	Alcona	0.35	1187	30.5	9.3	24	75.2	79.6	853	260
TX	Fisher	0.30	1218	30.5	8.5	28.3	72.9	78.9	1997	609
TX	Liberty	0.08	1381	30.5	9.1	31.3	71	77.3	71	22
GA	Walker	-0.40	1751	30.5	10	34.9	71.3	78	1078	329
VA	Greene	-0.44	1781	30.5	8.7	23.2	74.7	80.1	1167	356
KS	Lyon	-0.48	1804	30.5	8.1	24.7	75.5	79.5	1207	368
TX	Wharton	-0.99	2124	30.5	9.8	27.6	73.2	79.2	101	31
GA	Madison	-1.05	2161	30.5	10.1	24	72.5	78.7	740	225
GA	Oglethorpe	-1.15	2212	30.5	10.1	23.7	71.7	78.1	598	182
KY	Daviess	-1.20	2234	30.5	10.1	27.8	74.3	79.7	429	131
MO	Ralls	-1.20	2236	30.5	8.5	27.9	74.4	80.1	679	207
IL	Henderson	-1.29	2277	30.5	8	26.2	75.9	80.9	630	192
IA	Woodbury	-1.51	2381	30.5	8.4	29.1	75.4	80.5	1230	375
MN	Winona	-1.61	2430	30.5	7.2	19.5	77.3	82.2	1063	324
IA	Montgomery	-1.67	2450	30.5	7.7	24.4	76.2	81.1	1161	354
IN	Pike	-1.75	2487	30.5	9.2	28.1	74.8	80	479	146
IL	Mason	-1.86	2528	30.5	7.6	28.6	74.4	79.5	502	153
NE	Webster	-1.88	2536	30.5	8.5	31.1	76.8	81.8	1880	573
IN	Bartholomew	-2.38	2728	30.5	9.8	25.9	75.3	80.4	677	206
PA	Potter	-2.42	2749	30.5	9.1	26.9	75.2	80	1996	608
IA	Clay	-2.52	2789	30.5	6.8	26.5	77	81.6	1391	424
IA	Poweshiek	-3.42	2987	30.5	7.5	24.8	77.4	80.8	920	280
MN	Polk	-3.76	3047	30.5	7.7	26	75.3	81.4	1012	308
MO	Ste. Genevieve	2.06	458	30.6	9.1	33	74.8	80.2	679	207
NV	Elko	2.05	460	30.6	7.2	24.7	75	79.7	6144	1873
TN	Claiborne	1.57	577	30.6	10.3	34.4	71.1	77.7	1478	451
NC	Caldwell	1.51	597	30.6	9.1	26.7	72.9	78.7	1503	458
GA	Monroe	1.13	759	30.6	10.6	26	73.1	78.1	542	165

HEALTHIEST PLACES TO LIVE

ST	COUNTY	USDA	AMEN	OBES	DIAB	INACT	M AGE	W AGE	ALT ft	ALT m
TX	Cass	0.63	1002	30.6	9.9	32.3	71.7	78.4	319	97
MI	Antrim	0.58	1030	30.6	8.1	22.6	76.2	80.9	895	273
SC	Richland	0.56	1037	30.6	11.2	26.4	73.1	78.8	256	78
TX	Falls	0.34	1196	30.6	10.6	29.6	70.9	76.7	430	131
MO	Howell	0.31	1209	30.6	10.1	29	72.2	79	1058	322
LA	Jackson	0.20	1303	30.6	9.3	32.4	71.5	77.1	230	70
ND	Dunn	0.20	1309	30.6	8.8	31.3	75.7	82.2	2259	689
PA	Huntingdon	0.15	1337	30.6	9.3	30.6	74.6	79.8	1136	346
OH	Belmont	0.13	1349	30.6	9.9	28.5	73.5	79.4	1107	337
OK	Wagoner	0.05	1406	30.6	11.2	33.8	74.8	80	599	183
MO	Holt	-0.15	1560	30.6	8.8	26.9	76.2	80.7	939	286
PA	Mifflin	-0.19	1589	30.6	9.3	28.3	74.7	80.3	1072	327
SC	Cherokee	-0.31	1683	30.6	11	30.7	70.1	76.7	690	210
WI	Columbia	-0.52	1831	30.6	7.3	26.3	76.7	81.6	914	278
MO	Macon	-0.55	1842	30.6	8.8	29.1	73.8	79.8	830	253
IN	Jackson	-0.57	1858	30.6	8.9	32.4	74.7	79.4	626	191
SD	Gregory	-0.64	1910	30.6	7.8	29.5	75	80.8	1919	585
SD	Harding	-0.65	1915	30.6	6.7	30.2	74.8	80.5	3077	938
VA	Bland	-0.85	2040	30.6	9.4	24.9	72.5	78.8	2705	825
MI	Alger	-0.91	2073	30.6	8.7	24	74.7	80	858	262
OH	Ashtabula	-0.92	2084	30.6	9.1	30.7	73.7	79.1	891	272
OH	Holmes	-0.95	2105	30.6	8.9	26.7	73.5	78.5	1079	329
MI	St. Clair	-1.25	2263	30.6	9.3	24	75.5	79.8	697	213
MI	Tuscola	-1.63	2439	30.6	9	26.4	74.7	79.7	709	216
ND	Adams	-1.82	2515	30.6	7.5	26.2	75.7	81.6	2654	809
IN	Noble	-1.93	2557	30.6	9.4	27.2	74.4	79.9	929	283
IA	Lee	-1.95	2564	30.6	7.3	26.7	74.5	80.1	646	197
MI	Cass	-2.14	2632	30.6	8.5	27.4	74.6	79.6	846	258
MN	Murray	-2.21	2654	30.6	7	18.9	75.8	82.1	1611	491
WI	Washburn	-2.26	2681	30.6	8.5	21	75.6	81.2	1178	359
IN	Ripley	-2.40	2737	30.6	8	29.5	74.9	79.8	933	284
MN	Brown	-3.07	2919	30.6	7.4	22.1	77.4	82	1019	310
IA	Washington	-3.28	2961	30.6	7	22.9	76.4	82	727	222
IA	Humboldt	-4.05	3073	30.6	7.4	24.7	75.9	81.1	1140	347
WA	Pierce	4.62	153	30.7	9.2	20.2	75.5	80.4	2244	684
WA	Pend Oreille	3.33	269	30.7	7.7	19.7	74.5	80	3454	1053
TX	Parmer	1.93	489	30.7	8.6	28.2	73.7	79.3	4052	1235
MD	Allegany	1.26	705	30.7	12.3	31	74	79.7	1252	382
TX	Gaines	0.84	894	30.7	9.2	29.2	73.9	78.9	3320	1012
FL	Suwannee	0.70	958	30.7	9.8	29.1	72.4	78.2	96	29
TX	Hartley	0.51	1065	30.7	9.8	27.8	73.7	78.9	3947	1203
MO	Franklin	0.38	1156	30.7	8.3	26.7	74.2	79.4	667	203
TX	Callahan	0.33	1201	30.7	8.4	24	73.1	79.5	1801	549
TN	Grundy	0.02	1425	30.7	9.9	31.8	68.8	77.9	1706	520
GA	Screven	-0.02	1452	30.7	11.9	29.5	70.1	76.4	149	45
GA	Carroll	-0.11	1532	30.7	12.7	24.7	72.6	77.8	1035	315
OH	Fairfield	-0.17	1576	30.7	9.7	27.3	75.6	79.8	938	286

ST	COUNTY	USDA	AMEN	OBES	DIAB	INACT	M AGE	W AGE	ALT ft	ALT m
GA	Haralson	-0.39	1744	30.7	10.4	27.8	71.4	77.7	1166	355
WA	Franklin	-0.39	1749	30.7	9.5	20.5	75.4	79.2	931	284
GA	Douglas	-0.45	1783	30.7	10.3	25.8	73.4	77.5	987	301
PA	Lebanon	-0.66	1920	30.7	9	22.7	75.7	80.9	612	187
IN	Greene	-0.77	1988	30.7	10.9	27.8	74.2	79.4	591	180
TN	Marshall	-0.89	2066	30.7	9.6	32.9	72.4	79.1	818	249
GA	Chattooga	-1.08	2179	30.7	10.1	27.6	70.1	76.9	899	274
NC	Cabarrus	-1.08	2181	30.7	9.4	23.1	74.2	79	644	196
ND	Kidder	-1.40	2323	30.7	7.3	29.6	75.2	81.3	1852	564
VA	Charlotte	-1.49	2374	30.7	9.8	25.6	71.1	78.1	491	150
IA	Adair	-1.59	2416	30.7	8	28.7	76.1	82.6	1276	389
OH	Adams	-1.84	2521	30.7	9.1	33.6	72.2	77.8	850	259
ND	Sheridan	-1.89	2543	30.7	7.3	29.5	74.3	81.1	1865	568
WI	Fond du Lac	-1.92	2556	30.7	7.3	25	76.5	81.4	940	287
IA	Davis	-1.96	2567	30.7	7.2	27.9	74.7	80.9	841	256
IL	Adams	-2.10	2615	30.7	8.7	32.8	74.4	80.7	648	197
KY	Fayette	-2.39	2734	30.7	9.7	24.7	75.4	80.3	944	288
NE	Jefferson	-2.42	2748	30.7	8.1	30.6	75.9	80.7	1434	437
OH	Franklin	-2.43	2754	30.7	10.5	25.5	73.7	79	833	254
IN	Clark	-2.49	2780	30.7	8.7	31.3	73.3	78.8	606	185
IA	Calhoun	-2.73	2846	30.7	7.9	27.7	76.3	81.2	1198	365
MO	Nodaway	-2.85	2878	30.7	8.2	30.5	76.2	80.7	1049	320
WI	Marathon	-3.30	2966	30.7	7.9	26	77.8	82.6	1307	398
MN	Wadena	-3.74	3044	30.7	7.8	21.7	76	81.5	1358	414
WA	Mason	5.20	102	30.8	7.9	20.6	75.3	79.8	1052	321
GA	Butts	1.86	508	30.8	11.8	25.7	71.9	76.9	630	192
TX	Winkler	1.31	675	30.8	9.4	27.4	72.2	78	2914	888
PA	Pike	1.26	706	30.8	9	23.9	77.3	82.3	1234	376
AL	Jackson	1.25	708	30.8	12	29.3	71.2	77.6	1051	320
OK	Ellis	1.11	771	30.8	9.4	32.8	74.4	79.8	2298	700
TX	Bastrop	0.94	844	30.8	9.5	26.3	74	79.3	465	142
GA	Brooks	0.35	1183	30.8	12.6	30.3	70.1	76.7	191	58
KY	Boone	0.29	1222	30.8	9.4	28.3	75.4	79.6	751	229
LA	Livingston	0.07	1389	30.8	9.7	30	72.3	78.6	32	10
KS	Pottawatomie	-0.09	1517	30.8	8.7	24.2	75.8	80.8	1223	373
NH	Coos	-0.09	1520	30.8	8	27.8	74.3	80.4	1857	566
GA	Charlton	-0.36	1718	30.8	10.8	29.8	70.6	77.2	96	29
VA	Caroline	-1.22	2249	30.8	10.5	23.5	71.7	78.9	162	49
MI	Macomb	-1.24	2258	30.8	9.4	24.6	75.6	80.5	680	207
IA	Carroll	-1.70	2470	30.8	6.2	27.9	76.7	82	1311	400
MO	Lafayette	-1.70	2472	30.8	8.4	26.8	73.9	79.9	804	245
NE	Red Willow	-1.76	2495	30.8	7.6	24.2	76	81	2551	777
IN	Henry	-2.61	2816	30.8	9.1	30.1	73.2	79.3	1051	320
SD	Miner	-3.45	2997	30.8	6.3	33.9	76.2	81.6	1489	454
OH	Putnam	-3.70	3036	30.8	8.8	26.8	76.3	81.6	732	223
MT	Glacier	4.69	150	30.9	11.5	30.8	74.4	80.2	4812	1467
ME	Washington	2.69	341	30.9	9.5	29.8	73.1	80.1	277	84

HEALTHIEST PLACES TO LIVE

ST	COUNTY	USDA	AMEN	OBES	DIAB	INACT	M AGE	W AGE	ALT ft	ALT m
TX	Marion	1.40	634	30.9	10.3	28.9	71.7	78.4	266	81
OK	Harper	0.51	1063	30.9	10	34.6	74.4	79.8	1982	604
NC	Caswell	0.45	1105	30.9	12.1	27.9	71.7	78.1	577	176
TN	Moore	0.37	1171	30.9	9.8	28.6	72.8	79	988	301
KY	Grayson	0.21	1297	30.9	11.7	32.8	71.9	77.8	638	194
OK	Lincoln	0.13	1350	30.9	10.4	39.8	72.4	78.5	935	285
GA	Emanuel	-0.16	1564	30.9	11.2	26.8	69.3	75.6	260	79
KS	Meade	-0.16	1565	30.9	8.4	23.9	75.4	80	2527	770
MT	Richland	-0.22	1615	30.9	6	28.9	75.3	80.5	2283	696
WV	Pocahontas	-0.42	1773	30.9	10.8	27.4	73.3	78.6	3215	980
AR	Madison	-0.43	1774	30.9	9.8	28.2	73	79.4	1651	503
OH	Vinton	-0.64	1909	30.9	9.9	29.3	71.9	78.5	834	254
KY	Hardin	-0.69	1934	30.9	11.5	29.7	75.2	80.2	718	219
MI	Huron	-0.74	1968	30.9	7.8	22.6	75.1	80	682	208
NY	Steuben	-0.76	1983	30.9	9.7	25	75.4	80.8	1602	488
KS	Clay	-0.80	2007	30.9	8.1	26.9	75.8	81.2	1291	394
KS	Montgomery	-0.81	2014	30.9	9.1	30.3	73	79.9	826	252
IN	Floyd	-1.04	2156	30.9	8.7	24.1	74.9	79.3	709	216
IA	Harrison	-1.06	2169	30.9	7.2	27.2	75	80.4	1171	357
NE	Rock	-1.06	2173	30.9	7.8	29.5	75.6	80.9	2391	729
NY	Seneca	-1.08	2183	30.9	8	31.1	75.4	80.4	608	185
ND	Morton	-1.30	2283	30.9	7.1	26	74.6	80.6	2049	624
ND	McLean	-1.41	2327	30.9	7.3	29.4	75.8	80.8	1966	599
OK	Major	-1.49	2373	30.9	8.9	32.4	74.4	79.7	1421	433
MI	Menominee	-1.61	2429	30.9	8.3	25.6	76.2	81	799	243
MI	Gogebic	-1.69	2468	30.9	8.4	24.7	75	80.7	1481	451
NE	Burt	-1.73	2480	30.9	8.1	31.5	74.2	79.8	1226	374
IN	LaPorte	-1.87	2532	30.9	9.7	25.9	73.7	80.1	729	222
NE	Phelps	-2.21	2657	30.9	6.8	25.2	75.6	80.9	2324	708
OH	Montgomery	-2.23	2664	30.9	10.9	24.6	73.9	79.6	902	275
IA	Osceola	-3.19	2944	30.9	6.5	23.9	75.8	81.2	1542	470
IL	Kankakee	-3.30	2964	30.9	8.2	27.9	73.3	79	646	197
MI	Ingham	-3.38	2983	30.9	8.3	22.4	76.1	80.4	914	279
ND	Grand Forks	-5.01	3100	30.9	7.4	23	76.5	81.4	1015	309
CA	Yuba	4.97	126	31	7.3	24.8	72.1	78.9	1073	327
NV	Nye	4.97	128	31	7.9	28.7	72.2	78.8	5823	1775
OK	Pushmataha	1.75	538	31	10.9	33.8	70.2	77.5	808	246
TX	Jones	1.55	586	31	9.6	29.3	72.9	78.9	1690	515
OK	Stephens	1.13	761	31	8.6	28.7	73.4	78.8	1101	336
IL	Alexander	0.95	836	31	9.3	29.8	69.9	77	392	119
GA	Lanier	0.94	840	31	11.7	29.4	69.4	76.5	200	61
TX	Lee	0.88	873	31	9.4	28.7	74.6	80.2	409	125
VA	Carroll	0.67	975	31	10	28.5	73	79	2470	753
GA	Wilkes	0.65	981	31	12.3	28.4	70.8	76.8	500	153
VA	Isle of Wight	0.51	1068	31	11.4	26.9	72.8	78.9	53	16
SD	Butte	0.43	1123	31	7	30.5	74.8	80.5	3019	920
GA	Candler	0.39	1145	31	10.3	27.5	70.1	77.7	214	65

ST	COUNTY	USDA	AMEN	OBES	DIAB	INACT	M AGE	W AGE	ALT ft	ALT m
TX	Brown	0.35	1189	31	8.9	27.2	72.4	78.9	1522	464
TN	Decatur	0.34	1195	31	10.5	34.4	70.6	78.2	474	144
LA	Bossier	0.25	1252	31	11.7	26.4	73.4	79.1	209	64
TX	Houston	0.11	1362	31	10.1	26.3	72.3	77.8	302	92
MD	Baltimore	-0.37	1729	31	11.7	30.6	66.7	75.6	436	133
GA	Bacon	-0.47	1799	31	10	33.8	68.8	76.4	181	55
AR	Union	-0.50	1811	31	10.1	27.3	71.2	77.6	170	52
ME	Penobscot	-0.52	1824	31	9.7	25.5	75	80.1	440	134
AR	Lafayette	-0.59	1874	31	10.5	31.8	70.2	77.1	252	77
KS	Kingman	-0.77	1989	31	8.5	29.7	75.3	80.1	1575	480
MO	Monroe	-0.94	2094	31	9.6	27.1	74.4	80.1	722	220
MO	Clinton	-1.49	2369	31	9.9	29	74.2	80.1	981	299
WI	Lafayette	-1.53	2397	31	7.2	21.5	75.8	81.2	954	291
WI	Forest	-2.56	2803	31	8.7	24.2	75.8	80.6	1594	486
WI	Rock	-2.62	2819	31	8	23.7	75.8	80.5	887	270
IN	DeKalb	-2.81	2863	31	8.8	26.3	75.4	80.4	884	269
MI	Midland	-3.09	2923	31	8.1	21.6	77.1	81.2	669	204
IN	Montgomery	-3.35	2977	31	9.4	30.1	74.9	80.3	803	245
OH	Hardin	-3.57	3016	31	10.5	26.4	73.7	79.8	968	295
CA	Tulare	5.65	76	31.1	7.9	24.5	74.1	79.4	4352	1326
SC	Oconee	3.55	242	31.1	10	24.5	74	79.9	1094	333
WA	Benton	1.58	575	31.1	8.7	19.8	77.4	80.6	958	292
GA	Newton	1.45	612	31.1	10.8	26	72.6	78.1	700	213
TX	Carson	1.21	731	31.1	9.2	25.5	74.6	79.8	3349	1021
TX	Hunt	1.05	795	31.1	10.3	30.4	73.1	78.7	541	165
TX	Wichita	0.80	914	31.1	10.6	30.3	72.5	78.7	1046	319
TX	Gray	0.79	917	31.1	10.3	37.6	73.2	78.9	3006	916
AL	Cherokee	0.64	986	31.1	11.2	34.6	71.3	77.9	756	231
PA	Beaver	0.64	992	31.1	9.2	26.6	74.6	80.4	1053	321
AR	Saline	0.49	1077	31.1	10	25.2	74.7	79.8	537	164
OK	Payne	0.42	1130	31.1	9.6	28.1	76.2	79.9	938	286
TX	Leon	0.36	1181	31.1	9.7	30.3	73.8	79.3	346	105
MO	Howard	0.29	1224	31.1	8.4	31.5	75.2	79.9	712	217
GA	Irwin	0.23	1274	31.1	10.9	25.4	70.8	76.6	314	96
MO	Maries	0.20	1307	31.1	9.2	29.4	74.3	79.8	885	270
GA	Bulloch	0.19	1315	31.1	12.2	26.1	73.2	78.9	158	48
TX	Johnson	0.12	1357	31.1	10.1	29.1	74.2	78.8	791	241
TX	Dawson	-0.24	1633	31.1	9.8	28.8	73.1	78.8	2954	900
VA	Danville	-0.30	1675	31.1	10.1	28.7	70.2	76.9	516	157
WI	Manitowoc	-0.37	1731	31.1	7	22.2	77	81.6	775	236
PA	Franklin	-0.57	1865	31.1	8.6	24.9	76.1	81.4	893	272
OH	Coshocton	-0.64	1908	31.1	9.5	29.5	74.5	79.6	946	288
GA	Marion	-0.86	2042	31.1	11	26.4	71.9	78.2	563	172
MO	Andrew	-1.01	2136	31.1	8.5	24.3	74.8	79.6	979	298
KS	Gove	-1.79	2502	31.1	9	27.7	76.3	81.5	2676	816
KS	Ellis	-2.31	2693	31.1	7.5	24.3	76.6	81.6	2039	621
MO	Audrain	-2.43	2752	31.1	8.4	31.1	73.6	79.3	790	241

HEALTHIEST PLACES TO LIVE

ST	COUNTY	USDA	AMEN	OBES	DIAB	INACT	M AGE	W AGE	ALT ft	ALT m
IN	Putnam	-2.71	2842	31.1	10.1	29.8	75.8	79.7	795	242
NE	Hamilton	-2.83	2870	31.1	6.9	27.8	77.1	81.3	1798	548
WI	Barron	-2.86	2879	31.1	6.9	23.7	75.8	81.2	1199	365
OH	Madison	-3.07	2920	31.1	11.3	32.6	74.9	79.5	985	300
MI	Eaton	-3.14	2935	31.1	8.5	22.4	76	80.4	892	272
IA	Chickasaw	-3.65	3028	31.1	7.1	26.4	76.3	81	1137	346
WI	Clark	-4.34	3089	31.1	6.8	24.1	75.7	81.2	1166	355
NM	Eddy	4.97	127	31.2	9.9	26.9	73.8	80.1	3739	1140
GA	Baldwin	2.09	453	31.2	11.6	27.8	72.1	77.7	388	118
TN	Anderson	1.36	650	31.2	10.5	31.5	73.7	79.2	1299	396
SC	Lexington	0.99	821	31.2	9.1	25.4	74.5	80	389	119
TX	Camp	0.71	955	31.2	10.4	26.6	71.3	78.3	353	107
NC	Rutherford	0.45	1106	31.2	9.9	29.8	71.4	78	1114	340
TX	Parker	0.14	1345	31.2	9.8	29.7	74.4	79.3	974	297
MD	Cecil	0.10	1366	31.2	8.9	27.9	73.8	79.4	181	55
GA	Montgomery	0.07	1384	31.2	10.5	26.7	71.3	76.5	227	69
MI	Alpena	0.07	1390	31.2	8	21	75.4	81.2	745	227
MO	Chariton	0.06	1397	31.2	9.7	28.8	75.2	79.9	695	212
WV	Pleasants	-0.12	1546	31.2	11	29.7	73.3	79	860	262
GA	Ware	-0.17	1571	31.2	12.1	33.7	69.7	76.6	139	42
KS	Leavenworth	-0.35	1712	31.2	9.1	24.8	75.2	80	938	286
KS	Kearny	-0.36	1721	31.2	8.7	24.9	74.6	79.4	3161	963
WI	Racine	-0.51	1820	31.2	7.8	24.6	75.7	80.6	759	231
GA	Gordon	-0.52	1822	31.2	9.7	28.4	72	78.5	762	232
WV	Berkeley	-0.55	1848	31.2	10.5	29.2	73.4	78.7	642	196
IA	Jackson	-0.85	2035	31.2	6.6	23.5	76	80.8	794	242
KS	Stanton	-1.59	2418	31.2	8.5	25.5	75.9	81.2	3367	1026
OH	Butler	-1.65	2446	31.2	11.3	26	74.9	79	788	240
MO	Gentry	-1.76	2493	31.2	9.5	28.2	74.9	80.2	951	290
KS	McPherson	-1.81	2509	31.2	8.4	24	76.7	81.3	1501	458
IN	Sullivan	-2.07	2605	31.2	8.8	32.1	73.1	79	507	154
KS	Kiowa	-2.08	2611	31.2	7.8	24.4	75.4	80	2185	666
NE	Pawnee	-2.50	2785	31.2	8	31.5	75.4	80.8	1276	389
IN	Fulton	-3.13	2932	31.2	9	25.9	73.3	79.3	791	241
OH	Meigs	-3.23	2953	31.2	9.6	31.2	71.9	78.5	759	231
MI	Clinton	-3.49	3003	31.2	9	24.9	77	81.5	768	234
IA	Grundy	-4.86	3097	31.2	7.4	23.4	77.1	81.4	1036	316
OR	Douglas	6.78	39	31.3	9.2	20.6	74.1	80.7	2109	643
TX	Sabine	2.13	447	31.3	8.8	28.1	71.8	78.2	243	74
AL	Elmore	2.11	449	31.3	11.8	31.5	73.1	78.8	382	117
GA	McIntosh	2.00	470	31.3	11.4	28.8	70.6	77.8	14	4
TX	Hutchinson	1.90	498	31.3	8.9	26.2	73.8	79.3	3060	933
TX	Newton	1.44	621	31.3	10	30.4	71.1	77.4	167	51
MO	Cedar	1.24	715	31.3	9.1	27.8	73.9	80	907	276
TN	Loudon	1.14	755	31.3	10.7	28.7	74.2	80	911	278
OK	Washington	0.96	834	31.3	9	29	75.1	80.3	729	222
TX	Wise	0.87	878	31.3	8.6	29.1	73.8	79	879	268

ST	COUNTY	USDA	AMEN	OBES	DIAB	INACT	M AGE	W AGE	ALT ft	ALT m
WY	Campbell	0.79	919	31.3	7.9	27.5	75.9	81.5	4501	1372
MI	Leelanau	0.73	941	31.3	8.5	26.6	78.6	82.8	731	223
OK	Custer	0.46	1100	31.3	9.6	34.6	73.3	79.7	1729	527
TN	Perry	0.43	1124	31.3	9.7	30.2	70.6	78.2	602	183
TN	Hancock	0.38	1159	31.3	10.9	34.9	71.2	77.2	1515	462
TX	Red River	-0.11	1537	31.3	10	31.3	72.5	78.1	400	122
MO	Phelps	-0.16	1566	31.3	8.4	27.5	74.4	79.2	990	302
KY	Boyle	-0.23	1618	31.3	11.1	29.9	73.9	79	958	292
AL	Limestone	-0.42	1767	31.3	10	30.9	73	79	690	210
PA	Perry	-0.45	1788	31.3	10	26.2	74.9	79.8	841	256
KY	Christian	-0.63	1895	31.3	11.1	33.2	72.7	78.6	568	173
PA	Snyder	-0.63	1900	31.3	9.9	24	75.1	81.2	855	261
OK	Woodward	-0.65	1914	31.3	9.6	31.5	74.5	80.4	1941	591
OH	Lucas	-0.87	2051	31.3	10.3	27.5	73.4	78.8	629	192
KS	Dickinson	-0.96	2106	31.3	8.3	25.9	75.1	81.2	1272	388
MO	Saline	-1.00	2130	31.3	9.4	28.7	74	78.6	720	219
AL	Madison	-1.25	2260	31.3	11.2	24.9	74.7	79.3	795	242
NY	Jefferson	-1.27	2270	31.3	8.7	26.8	75.8	80.7	544	166
WI	Richland	-1.29	2279	31.3	7.8	24	76.2	81.1	953	290
KS	Cloud	-1.49	2367	31.3	9.7	23	75.8	81.2	1444	440
KY	McLean	-1.52	2386	31.3	11.2	34.1	72.4	78.9	416	127
IL	Grundy	-2.11	2618	31.3	7.5	34.8	75.8	80.5	584	178
IA	Lucas	-2.61	2814	31.3	6.7	28.3	75	80.2	979	298
SD	Hand	-3.20	2949	31.3	6.8	31.9	75.8	81.4	1652	504
SD	Turner	-3.48	3002	31.3	6.5	30.7	76.9	81.5	1384	422
ND	Cavalier	-3.52	3007	31.3	7	27	75	81.2	1549	472
IL	Iroquois	-4.00	3068	31.3	7.8	30.4	74.6	79.5	665	203
MN	Dodge	-5.08	3101	31.3	7.2	19.6	77.5	82.3	1259	384
TX	Mitchell	2.47	376	31.4	9.7	28.5	72.1	78	2180	665
TX	Moore	2.46	378	31.4	8.9	30.3	73.7	78.9	3503	1068
TX	Rusk	1.88	503	31.4	9.8	27.6	73	78.9	403	123
MO	St. Francois	1.70	544	31.4	9.4	27.2	72.1	77.6	922	281
TX	Waller	1.28	691	31.4	9.8	30.1	73.8	78.8	203	62
AR	Pike	1.15	749	31.4	9.7	27.6	73.1	79.3	586	179
VA	Dickenson	0.61	1020	31.4	9.6	29	70.2	77.4	1896	578
WV	Morgan	0.41	1137	31.4	11	29.2	74.1	80	888	271
GA	Colquitt	0.26	1245	31.4	11	28.2	70.9	77.2	282	86
NE	Sherman	0.26	1247	31.4	6.7	29.3	76.2	80.7	2157	657
AL	Franklin	0.16	1328	31.4	13.3	36.4	70.7	77.1	744	227
PA	Somerset	0.01	1434	31.4	9	26.8	74.6	80.8	2193	668
GA	Effingham	-0.10	1524	31.4	10.5	25.7	74.4	78.8	70	21
MS	Lamar	-0.26	1642	31.4	9.2	28.8	74	78.9	307	93
KS	Woodson	-0.36	1722	31.4	9.1	31.1	74	79.6	1037	316
PA	Philadelphia	-0.46	1796	31.4	11.1	29.6	69.2	77.6	114	35
MI	Allegan	-0.52	1825	31.4	8.5	23.3	76	80.9	711	217
GA	Meriwether	-0.59	1875	31.4	11.9	26.5	69.4	76	827	252
KS	Marion	-0.81	2013	31.4	8	27.7	75.1	81.2	1426	435

HEALTHIEST PLACES TO LIVE

ST	COUNTY	USDA	AMEN	OBES	DIAB	INACT	M AGE	W AGE	ALT ft	ALT m
PA	Venango	-0.86	2046	31.4	7.9	27.2	74.5	80.1	1376	419
VA	Richmond City	-0.93	2089	31.4	11.4	28	69.2	78.6	160	49
WV	Mingo	-1.12	2205	31.4	11.7	40	68.7	75.9	1249	381
MO	Mississippi	-1.39	2317	31.4	9.7	37.3	69.9	76.9	305	93
MI	Chippewa	-1.40	2322	31.4	10	22.9	75.9	80.7	722	220
IL	Pulaski	-1.43	2338	31.4	9.8	29.3	69.9	77	367	112
KS	Thomas	-1.58	2411	31.4	8.1	20.8	76	80.6	3170	966
IL	Massac	-1.69	2466	31.4	8.8	29.5	72.8	78.8	394	120
IN	Warrick	-1.81	2508	31.4	9.5	22.8	76.2	79.7	437	133
IA	Crawford	-1.89	2539	31.4	7	30.8	75.4	81.7	1361	415
IA	Emmet	-2.10	2614	31.4	7.4	27.2	75.7	81.2	1304	397
TX	Howard	2.23	428	31.5	9.1	28.9	72.4	77.8	2525	769
TX	Jim Wells	1.45	615	31.5	8.7	26	72.8	79.8	215	66
TX	Jefferson	1.04	803	31.5	10.7	30.2	72.4	78.4	12	4
KY	Mason	0.40	1139	31.5	10.5	29.8	72.9	79.1	831	253
GA	Toombs	0.24	1262	31.5	11.8	31.6	70.6	77.5	197	60
TX	Madison	0.22	1290	31.5	10	27	72.8	78.4	278	85
PA	Elk	0.07	1393	31.5	9.4	28.4	74.9	80.7	1769	539
TN	Cheatham	-0.23	1623	31.5	9.3	32.1	73.5	78.8	588	179
PA	Tioga	-0.25	1639	31.5	8.6	25.9	75.8	80.4	1709	521
IN	Dubois	-0.34	1697	31.5	8.3	24	75.5	80.9	534	163
LA	E Baton Rouge	-0.73	1963	31.5	11.1	25.9	72.3	78	59	18
AR	White	-0.84	2025	31.5	9.4	27.8	73.2	78.8	352	107
ND	Mercer	-1.60	2425	31.5	8.1	27.1	75.8	80.8	2015	614
KY	Woodford	-2.04	2595	31.5	9.6	27.3	75.5	80.1	811	247
IA	Marion	-2.28	2684	31.5	7.2	23.7	75.7	81.1	832	254
WI	Chippewa	-2.36	2722	31.5	8.3	17.4	76.7	81	1064	324
LA	West Carroll	-2.79	2858	31.5	11.2	32.1	70.1	76.2	95	29
KS	Jackson	-2.85	2876	31.5	8.2	26.3	75.8	80.8	1115	340
IN	Wells	-3.73	3041	31.5	8.7	25.9	75.7	81.4	820	250
ID	Clearwater	2.33	404	31.6	7.6	24.9	75.8	80.6	3881	1183
AZ	Navajo	1.91	494	31.6	12.3	24.9	71.4	79.5	6016	1834
VA	Lancaster	1.33	664	31.6	9.9	28.6	72.5	78.7	44	13
TX	Gonzales	0.68	967	31.6	9.5	28.2	72.1	79.1	342	104
ID	Jerome	0.63	998	31.6	8.2	19.5	74.7	80.3	3996	1218
TX	Robertson	0.63	1005	31.6	10.1	28.2	72.8	78.4	379	116
TN	Humphreys	0.61	1018	31.6	11.4	30.7	72.1	78.5	565	172
MO	Ripley	0.48	1087	31.6	8.9	34.4	70.7	77.8	519	158
SC	Kershaw	0.27	1239	31.6	9.7	27.1	73	78.9	297	90
OH	Harrison	-0.01	1449	31.6	11.6	28.8	73.7	79	1102	336
NC	Rowan	-0.10	1528	31.6	10.8	29.2	73.4	79.3	746	227
LA	Grant	-0.20	1597	31.6	10.8	32.1	71.3	78.1	139	42
MO	Montgomery	-0.31	1680	31.6	9.3	28.5	73.7	79.1	732	223
GA	Spalding	-0.33	1690	31.6	10.9	27.6	71.2	77	818	249
OH	Lorain	-0.33	1692	31.6	10.4	27.5	75.6	80.3	774	236
NC	Harnett	-0.52	1827	31.6	9.5	27.6	72.6	78.2	247	75
GA	Webster	-0.55	1839	31.6	12.3	27.1	69.6	75.8	455	139

ST	COUNTY	USDA	AMEN	OBES	DIAB	INACT	M AGE	W AGE	ALT ft	ALT m
KY	Washington	-0.58	1869	31.6	11.2	29.4	73.3	79.6	757	231
PA	York	-0.58	1873	31.6	8.9	22.6	76.1	81.6	595	182
MS	Oktibbeha	-0.62	1892	31.6	11.4	26.9	73.9	79.3	301	92
MI	Oscoda	-1.37	2307	31.6	9.8	26.7	75.2	79.6	1136	346
NE	Hall	-1.83	2519	31.6	8	26.1	75.1	80.8	1931	589
IL	Greene	-2.24	2666	31.6	8.5	31	74.5	79.5	545	166
WI	Burnett	-2.24	2668	31.6	7.7	22.8	75.5	81.1	994	303
IA	Muscatine	-2.37	2724	31.6	6.7	23.8	75.7	80.7	670	204
MN	Mahnomen	-3.09	2925	31.6	9.1	27	74.9	81	1365	416
OH	Darke	-3.31	2968	31.6	9.4	30.6	75	81.2	1037	316
MN	Chippewa	-3.42	2989	31.6	7.3	20.7	76.8	81.7	1036	316
IA	Marshall	-3.70	3034	31.6	7.3	24.2	74.4	81.7	985	300
IA	Hamilton	-3.74	3042	31.6	7.2	23.6	76.7	82.4	1127	344
OH	Marion	-3.93	3057	31.6	10.4	30.4	74	78.8	928	283
ND	Ransom	-4.21	3085	31.6	7.5	28.2	75.9	81.3	1199	365
MN	Roseau	-4.30	3088	31.6	6.7	22.2	75.9	81.3	1092	333
FL	Okeechobee	4.70	149	31.7	9.4	31	72.2	78.7	44	13
TX	Coke	3.73	219	31.7	8.4	29.9	73.2	78.8	2127	648
NM	Lea	1.79	525	31.7	7.8	29.8	73.2	78.9	3784	1153
AL	Mobile	1.52	590	31.7	11.6	30.2	70.7	77.8	123	38
TX	Lamb	1.31	674	31.7	8.5	26.5	72.1	78.6	3636	1108
AR	Searcy	1.26	704	31.7	10.1	31.9	73.1	79.2	1137	346
OK	Osage	1.17	743	31.7	10.1	34.1	74.4	80	932	284
MO	St. Clair	1.11	769	31.7	9	30.7	72.8	79	816	249
MI	Emmet	0.93	848	31.7	7.9	21.5	77.7	81.6	794	242
NC	Richmond	0.89	865	31.7	10.7	29.8	70.7	77.1	335	102
TN	Marion	0.83	899	31.7	9.4	35.6	71.2	77.8	1321	403
PA	Northumberland	0.72	946	31.7	8.1	29.6	74.3	80.2	774	236
MO	Dent	0.61	1016	31.7	8.6	29.6	72.8	78.6	1189	362
AR	Fulton	0.51	1060	31.7	9.3	28.1	72.5	78.7	737	225
KS	Wabaunsee	0.40	1138	31.7	7.7	24.8	75.3	80.4	1253	382
TX	Freestone	0.40	1142	31.7	9.5	28.1	73.4	79.1	385	117
MO	Warren	0.14	1340	31.7	8.9	28.2	75.3	80.2	706	215
NE	Box Butte	-0.02	1456	31.7	8.2	25.4	75.4	80.3	4169	1271
MO	Carroll	-0.14	1557	31.7	7.9	25.6	74.5	80.4	737	225
WI	Door	-0.15	1563	31.7	6.7	19.8	78.2	82.7	676	206
KS	Hamilton	-0.59	1876	31.7	7.8	25.9	75.9	81.2	3446	1050
VA	Louisa	-0.68	1933	31.7	9.9	29.1	73.4	80.2	362	110
MO	Ray	-0.72	1961	31.7	9.4	30.9	74.8	79.6	849	259
TN	Lewis	-0.80	2011	31.7	10.3	36	71.1	77.6	842	257
MO	Douglas	-0.88	2059	31.7	9.3	28.1	72.5	79.3	1142	348
KS	Smith	-0.94	2093	31.7	7.3	30.9	75.7	82	1830	558
PA	Forest	-1.09	2188	31.7	10	24.4	74.9	80.7	1570	479
KY	Montgomery	-1.12	2201	31.7	10.2	31.6	72.3	79.1	929	283
OH	Stark	-2.50	2786	31.7	9.8	25.8	75.6	80.4	1108	338
NE	Pierce	-2.58	2806	31.7	7.2	32.6	75.3	81.4	1718	524
TN	Cannon	-2.75	2851	31.7	9.6	31.8	71.5	78.4	980	299

HEALTHIEST PLACES TO LIVE

ST	COUNTY	USDA	AMEN	OBES	DIAB	INACT	M AGE	W AGE	ALT ft	ALT m
IN	Carroll	-2.83	2866	**31.7**	9.2	26	75.3	80.8	680	207
OH	Wayne	-3.22	2952	**31.7**	8.9	23.5	75.4	80.4	1071	326
MI	Shiawassee	-3.48	3001	**31.7**	9.5	25.6	75.2	80.5	787	240
CA	Merced	4.51	162	**31.8**	7.6	20.3	75	79.9	368	112
OK	Cimarron	1.56	580	**31.8**	9.1	34.7	74.4	79.8	4139	1262
GA	Liberty	1.46	609	**31.8**	13.1	27	73	78.1	35	11
LA	Ouachita	0.51	1061	**31.8**	12.3	29.5	72.1	77.8	102	31
PA	Schuylkill	0.49	1082	**31.8**	8.8	31.7	73.2	79.5	1052	321
TX	Morris	0.41	1136	**31.8**	10.7	29.4	71.3	78.3	350	107
GA	Evans	0.28	1229	**31.8**	12.2	28.6	70.1	77.7	141	43
TN	Scott	0.28	1235	**31.8**	10.2	36.4	70.7	77.1	1514	461
NE	Lincoln	0.25	1254	**31.8**	8	27.4	76.1	81.4	2983	909
KY	Muhlenberg	0.21	1298	**31.8**	9.9	31.9	71.6	77.8	481	146
LA	W Baton Rouge	-0.01	1444	**31.8**	11.5	29.3	71.7	77.2	15	5
SC	Chester	-0.04	1480	**31.8**	11.3	33	70.2	77.9	490	149
WV	Kanawha	-0.12	1545	**31.8**	11.3	30.4	72	78.3	1015	309
ME	Aroostook	-0.14	1555	**31.8**	10.5	32.4	74.6	80.1	855	261
OK	Alfalfa	-0.17	1577	**31.8**	9.7	32.1	74.4	79.7	1267	386
MO	McDonald	-0.20	1599	**31.8**	8.6	31.2	71.9	77.8	1100	335
VA	Campbell	-0.38	1738	**31.8**	9.5	23.5	74.7	80.1	692	211
VA	Lynchburg	-0.38	1740	**31.8**	10.7	29.3	74.3	79.2	743	226
MO	Webster	-0.45	1786	**31.8**	8.6	25.3	73.5	79.7	1411	430
VA	Appomattox	-0.69	1938	**31.8**	10.8	26.4	73.1	79.7	658	201
KS	Chase	-0.88	2058	**31.8**	8.1	22.5	74.7	80.4	1361	415
VA	Orange	-0.89	2067	**31.8**	9.7	24.5	75.1	80.1	420	128
KY	Wolfe	-1.00	2129	**31.8**	10.6	33	68.2	76.2	1063	324
MI	Luce	-1.21	2241	**31.8**	9.1	26.6	75	80.3	780	238
LA	Ascension	-1.22	2247	**31.8**	9.7	28.5	73.3	78.9	9	3
MO	New Madrid	-1.52	2388	**31.8**	10	30.3	69.9	76.9	283	86
OH	Clark	-2.03	2591	**31.8**	10.4	29.1	73.5	78.5	1050	320
NY	St. Lawrence	-2.11	2619	**31.8**	9.3	30.5	74.5	79.1	804	245
OH	Sandusky	-2.54	2795	**31.8**	10.6	26.3	74.6	79.7	650	198
IN	Miami	-2.83	2867	**31.8**	10.3	30.2	74.2	79.9	775	236
OH	Huron	-3.09	2927	**31.8**	10.1	31.7	74.6	79.4	883	269
SD	Hutchinson	-3.33	2971	**31.8**	6.4	27.5	74.9	81.2	1391	424
ND	Bottineau	-3.44	2994	**31.8**	8.1	26.1	74.4	80.2	1584	483
SD	Douglas	-3.59	3020	**31.8**	6.7	31.6	74.9	81.2	1564	477
IL	Ford	-4.02	3070	**31.8**	7.9	29.4	74.6	79.5	748	228
MN	Red Lake	-6.40	3108	**31.8**	7.2	19.8	75.3	81.4	1089	332
AR	Van Buren	2.41	387	**31.9**	9.1	33	73.5	79.7	978	298
TN	Union	1.35	652	**31.9**	9.9	31.6	71.1	77.9	1227	374
OK	Le Flore	1.31	671	**31.9**	10.4	36.9	71.3	78.1	830	253
NC	Surry	1.24	716	**31.9**	11.2	26.7	72.8	79	1231	375
PA	Dauphin	1.07	783	**31.9**	9.3	27.2	74.8	80.1	681	208
OK	Delaware	0.72	945	**31.9**	11.1	34.9	73.3	79	945	288
AL	Jefferson	0.51	1058	**31.9**	11.7	28.8	71	77.8	575	175
PA	Clinton	0.47	1096	**31.9**	8	28.4	74.3	79.8	1438	438

ST	COUNTY	USDA	AMEN	OBES	DIAB	INACT	M AGE	W AGE	ALT ft	ALT m
MI	Keweenaw	0.44	1115	31.9	8.9	25.1	75.2	80.1	847	258
KY	Carroll	0.37	1164	31.9	10.5	34.4	72.8	78.6	645	196
LA	Jefferson	0.18	1319	31.9	11.1	28.6	72.4	79.5	4	1
LA	Pointe Coupee	0.17	1323	31.9	10.9	29.9	71.7	78.1	24	7
VA	Suffolk	0.17	1326	31.9	11.2	26.4	72.6	78	42	13
MO	Laclede	-0.11	1535	31.9	8.8	33.8	73.4	78.8	1138	347
OH	Licking	-0.55	1844	31.9	11.2	24.9	75.1	79.6	1030	314
VA	Madison	-0.76	1986	31.9	8.3	24.2	74.7	80.1	1015	309
PA	Blair	-0.86	2045	31.9	9.1	29.3	73.4	80	1538	469
MI	Montmorency	-0.92	2081	31.9	8.9	24.4	74.7	80.4	960	293
NC	Granville	-0.94	2095	31.9	10.9	26.6	71.8	78.4	424	129
SD	Day	-1.21	2244	31.9	6.9	28.5	74.9	81.2	1739	530
MO	Mercer	-1.24	2259	31.9	8.7	33	74.8	80.2	965	294
MO	Knox	-1.47	2362	31.9	8.6	29.4	73.8	79.8	774	236
SD	Jones	-1.48	2366	31.9	6.9	30.6	76.6	81.5	2070	631
OH	Highland	-1.49	2371	31.9	9.3	33.6	73.1	78.9	983	299
NY	Herkimer	-1.59	2420	31.9	8	26.1	75.4	79.8	1534	468
IN	Steuben	-1.61	2427	31.9	10.9	27.3	75.2	80.5	999	305
TN	Weakley	-1.62	2436	31.9	10.1	34.9	72.9	78.4	399	121
KS	Wichita	-1.80	2506	31.9	8.8	28.7	75.9	81.2	3295	1004
IN	Knox	-1.98	2576	31.9	8.9	32.9	73.5	79.9	462	141
MO	DeKalb	-2.33	2700	31.9	8.4	29.8	74.8	79.6	967	295
WI	Price	-2.66	2830	31.9	7.8	24.3	75.3	80.7	1534	468
ND	Pierce	-2.72	2844	31.9	7.4	31.6	74.3	81.1	1576	480
SD	Brown	-2.72	2845	31.9	6.8	29.5	76.3	82.4	1337	408
ND	Ramsey	-3.10	2930	31.9	6.8	24.9	75	81.2	1493	455
NV	Mineral	5.71	73	32	9.9	28.2	72.2	78.8	5872	1790
TX	Ector	2.50	370	32	9.5	27.8	72.2	78	3018	920
AR	Pope	2.29	414	32	9	25.3	75.1	79	857	261
GA	Wilkinson	1.54	587	32	11.8	27.2	70.6	76.1	345	105
TN	Grainger	1.45	614	32	10.4	32.9	71.2	77.2	1289	393
TN	Johnson	0.74	937	32	10.8	31.2	70.8	77.4	2915	888
NC	Tyrrell	0.67	970	32	11.1	28	71.6	77.6	5	1
MI	Mason	0.60	1021	32	8.6	26.7	75.5	80.5	693	211
NC	Camden	0.42	1127	32	9.8	25.4	72.9	78.2	10	3
WA	Skamania	-0.04	1482	32	7.4	20.4	76.3	81	2892	881
GA	Twiggs	-0.11	1533	32	12.2	29.4	70.5	77.1	390	119
WV	Wood	-0.19	1593	32	11.7	31	74.9	79.5	794	242
MO	Dallas	-0.20	1598	32	8.1	28.6	73.1	78.7	1093	333
KS	Decatur	-0.83	2023	32	9.5	26.1	76	80.6	2648	807
KS	Pratt	-1.42	2332	32	7.5	29.2	75.4	80.6	1923	586
KS	Wallace	-1.45	2352	32	8	27.6	75.9	81.2	3620	1103
KS	Ottawa	-1.67	2451	32	7.7	31.2	75.5	80.1	1345	410
VA	Prince Edward	-1.67	2455	32	9.9	29	71.5	77	462	141
AR	Jackson	-1.85	2523	32	11	35.8	70.6	76.9	255	78
MO	Schuyler	-1.90	2547	32	9.1	28.4	74.8	80.2	892	272
KY	Robertson	-1.91	2549	32	10.8	33.9	72.3	78.5	782	238

HEALTHIEST PLACES TO LIVE

ST	COUNTY	USDA	AMEN	OBES	DIAB	INACT	M AGE	W AGE	ALT ft	ALT m
MI	St. Joseph	-2.40	2739	32	9.5	25.5	73.5	79.8	848	258
KY	Green	-3.72	3039	32	11.4	36.2	71.9	77.9	711	217
MN	Renville	-3.90	3054	32	7.4	23	76.2	80.9	1066	325
IN	Rush	-3.97	3063	32	9.9	30.2	74.5	80.1	951	290
OK	Atoka	3.20	281	32.1	11.3	28.9	71.3	77.3	660	201
TX	Angelina	1.92	492	32.1	9.5	28.8	73.1	78.7	230	70
TN	Pickett	1.67	551	32.1	10.3	31.6	71.2	77.1	1055	321
TN	DeKalb	1.23	718	32.1	10	29	71.5	78.4	872	266
TX	Garza	1.11	772	32.1	9.1	28.6	73.2	79.3	2518	768
AR	Pulaski	0.85	887	32.1	10	28.6	72.1	78.9	335	102
LA	Cameron	0.77	924	32.1	10.2	25	72.6	78	3	1
LA	Caddo	0.65	983	32.1	11.5	30.4	70.8	77.6	212	65
NE	Dawson	0.56	1036	32.1	8.4	26.4	75.6	80.9	2519	768
AL	Blount	0.23	1273	32.1	11.5	35.1	72.5	78.8	788	240
GA	Rockdale	0.14	1338	32.1	10.9	27.2	74.4	78.9	785	239
OK	Canadian	-0.10	1530	32.1	10.6	29.2	75.7	79.9	1350	412
ME	Androscoggin	-0.32	1687	32.1	8.7	26.5	75.2	79.9	345	105
WI	Milwaukee	-0.40	1760	32.1	9.9	26.6	73.9	79.7	700	213
WI	Jefferson	-1.63	2442	32.1	7.9	21.8	76.8	82.5	848	259
KY	Magoffin	-1.67	2452	32.1	11.8	41.1	70.8	76.9	1076	328
MD	Caroline	-1.68	2459	32.1	11.1	29.2	73.2	78.7	40	12
ND	Emmons	-1.81	2510	32.1	7.5	28.6	74.6	80.6	1893	577
IA	Shelby	-2.01	2582	32.1	7.6	24.1	77	81.6	1335	407
KS	Anderson	-2.42	2747	32.1	7.4	25.8	75.2	80.6	1049	320
IN	Starke	-2.85	2875	32.1	9.9	33.8	72.1	77.8	700	213
IN	Jasper	-3.57	3014	32.1	9.9	29.1	74.9	80.6	681	208
NC	Hyde	1.48	603	32.2	11.3	30.1	71.6	77.6	5	2
VA	Page	0.94	846	32.2	8.9	26.4	73.9	80	1402	427
TX	Milam	0.72	947	32.2	9.8	30.1	73.3	78.2	406	124
AL	Cullman	0.64	987	32.2	11.9	28.7	71.9	78.4	750	229
NC	Pender	0.52	1054	32.2	10.7	23.7	74.3	79.5	37	11
OK	Rogers	0.23	1280	32.2	10.3	30.8	75	79.2	674	205
OH	Athens	-0.01	1448	32.2	11.4	28.7	73.7	79.3	806	246
AR	Faulkner	-0.08	1505	32.2	10.8	28.8	73.5	79.8	428	130
LA	St. Charles	-0.10	1527	32.2	10.1	28.8	73.6	79.3	4	1
GA	Wayne	-0.12	1539	32.2	9.6	31.3	70.9	77.3	85	26
AR	Sevier	-0.13	1547	32.2	12	32.7	71.8	77.9	435	132
MO	Henry	-0.46	1793	32.2	9	30	73.7	78.9	796	242
AL	Coffee	-0.66	1918	32.2	12.5	28.2	73.4	79	328	100
TN	Wayne	-0.71	1955	32.2	9.6	29.4	71.1	77.6	785	239
OH	Pike	-0.79	2005	32.2	10.5	35.2	71.4	78.4	833	254
IA	Fremont	-0.81	2012	32.2	7.1	29.8	76.2	81.1	1028	313
OH	Gallia	-1.02	2146	32.2	10.4	38	72.1	79.3	732	223
KS	Labette	-1.05	2162	32.2	9.3	31.4	73.8	79	867	264
PA	McKean	-1.11	2196	32.2	9.1	27.7	74.3	80	1917	584
VA	Culpeper	-1.15	2217	32.2	9.8	23.9	74.7	79.6	380	116
NC	Wilson	-1.23	2253	32.2	11.2	30.9	71.1	77.6	128	39

ST	COUNTY	USDA	AMEN	OBES	DIAB	INACT	M AGE	W AGE	ALT ft	ALT m
KS	Graham	-1.28	2273	32.2	8.2	23.6	76.3	81.5	2345	715
KS	Sherman	-1.34	2293	32.2	9.7	26.9	76	80.6	3657	1115
IN	Union	-1.51	2382	32.2	9.5	25.3	74.7	80.7	973	296
AR	Columbia	-1.63	2437	32.2	11.8	29	71.8	77.7	271	83
TN	Robertson	-1.92	2555	32.2	11.5	33.1	72.8	78.5	664	202
MO	Daviess	-2.06	2601	32.2	9.1	27.4	74.9	80.2	870	265
NE	Otoe	-2.36	2721	32.2	7.7	27.2	76.6	80.9	1149	350
SD	Grant	-2.49	2782	32.2	8.7	28.9	76.2	82.2	1441	439
NM	Cibola	3.04	302	32.3	11.2	26	73.4	80.4	7096	2163
SD	Fall River	1.89	500	32.3	8.3	21.5	71.1	78.5	3596	1096
WA	Yakima	1.48	604	32.3	8.9	24	75	80.1	2834	864
TX	Trinity	1.45	617	32.3	9.8	31.4	71.7	78.4	248	76
TN	Jefferson	1.39	636	32.3	10.5	31.4	73	78.7	1151	351
AR	Scott	1.02	804	32.3	9.4	32	73.2	78.7	933	284
NC	Currituck	0.88	868	32.3	9.1	23.5	73.7	79.6	6	2
TN	Henderson	0.82	904	32.3	9.1	31.5	71.3	77.3	500	152
KY	McCreary	0.73	940	32.3	12.4	40.8	69	76.2	1159	353
WA	Lincoln	0.56	1039	32.3	7.2	21.5	75.7	80.4	2148	655
MD	Charles	0.55	1041	32.3	10	24.7	74.7	79.2	113	34
TX	Caldwell	0.51	1064	32.3	8.8	24.8	73.5	79.4	497	151
MS	Lafayette	0.50	1072	32.3	10.3	28.9	72.5	79.4	389	119
OK	Muskogee	0.45	1107	32.3	11	35.4	71.9	78.3	597	182
KY	Harlan	0.37	1165	32.3	13.8	34.8	68.4	76.2	2095	638
LA	St. Bernard	0.37	1167	32.3	10.8	31.7	70.6	76.1	3	1
TX	Gregg	0.21	1301	32.3	10.2	29.6	71.8	78.7	332	101
KS	Elk	0.13	1348	32.3	9.8	26.5	73	79.9	1109	338
LA	West Feliciana	-0.27	1647	32.3	12	29.8	71.7	77.2	137	42
MO	Crawford	-0.28	1653	32.3	8	28.4	73.1	79.2	928	283
MO	Newton	-0.36	1723	32.3	10.2	30.5	74.7	80	1135	346
TN	Morgan	-0.52	1829	32.3	9.9	29	71.5	77.7	1496	456
KY	Todd	-0.98	2116	32.3	10.2	35.9	72.5	78.1	623	190
AR	Bradley	-1.06	2168	32.3	11.9	32	72	78.3	169	52
IA	Van Buren	-1.07	2175	32.3	7.4	24.3	76.9	80.9	705	215
IN	Daviess	-1.70	2471	32.3	9.7	26.3	74.2	79.8	494	150
SD	Lake	-1.86	2529	32.3	6.9	26.6	76.8	82.3	1704	519
WV	Doddridge	-2.52	2791	32.3	11.1	36.3	73	78.9	1051	320
IN	Whitley	-2.56	2802	32.3	7.7	20.1	75.2	80.6	871	265
IL	Macon	-2.79	2856	32.3	7.9	27	74	80.1	665	203
ND	Richland	-3.81	3049	32.3	6.4	27.8	76.8	82.2	1022	311
KY	Simpson	-3.98	3065	32.3	11.5	35.4	73.1	79.3	668	204
IN	Benton	-4.71	3095	32.3	9.8	33	74.8	80.6	757	231
GA	Greene	2.34	401	32.4	11.6	25.8	73.2	78.5	568	173
MO	Taney	1.63	563	32.4	8.8	29.3	74.5	79.9	966	295
TN	Smith	0.87	877	32.4	10.8	31.5	71.3	77.6	692	211
WA	Grant	0.62	1014	32.4	8.7	22.9	75.5	79.7	1400	427
MO	Pulaski	0.54	1046	32.4	9.5	27.5	74.6	79.5	984	300
MO	Gasconade	0.47	1094	32.4	8.5	31.1	73.7	79.1	774	236

HEALTHIEST PLACES TO LIVE

ST	COUNTY	USDA	AMEN	OBES	DIAB	INACT	M AGE	W AGE	ALT ft	ALT m
KS	Clark	0.22	1285	32.4	7.9	27.8	75.4	80	2162	659
GA	Richmond	0.02	1417	32.4	11.2	27.3	69.7	77.2	290	89
WV	Taylor	-0.01	1450	32.4	11	35.2	73.8	78.8	1341	409
VA	Mecklenburg	-0.03	1468	32.4	10.8	27.8	70.9	78	360	110
GA	Jenkins	-0.22	1611	32.4	11.5	26.7	70.1	76.4	208	63
MS	DeSoto	-0.24	1631	32.4	10	30.3	73.9	78.8	293	89
PA	Clarion	-0.30	1672	32.4	9.9	28.5	74.9	80.3	1396	426
IN	Perry	-0.38	1734	32.4	8.6	29	74	79.5	548	167
KY	Ballard	-0.55	1840	32.4	10.5	32.4	73.6	79.1	367	112
MI	Baraga	-0.55	1841	32.4	10.4	23.1	75.1	80.9	1336	407
WI	Buffalo	-1.17	2226	32.4	7.9	23.3	76.8	81.8	947	289
MT	Hill	-1.22	2248	32.4	7.3	28.8	74.6	80.7	2969	905
WV	Harrison	-1.36	2306	32.4	11.7	31.2	72.7	79.3	1190	363
KS	Logan	-1.43	2340	32.4	8.9	29.4	76.3	81.5	3090	942
KY	Clay	-1.46	2357	32.4	13.2	35.4	69.2	76.1	1178	359
MI	Lake	-1.68	2460	32.4	10	24.5	74.1	78.9	969	295
NC	Lenoir	-1.71	2475	32.4	11.4	33.2	70.6	77.8	77	24
IL	Jefferson	-1.74	2482	32.4	9	29.4	74.3	79.7	489	149
TN	Hickman	-2.18	2647	32.4	10.5	31.8	71.7	79	679	207
IN	Kosciusko	-2.25	2671	32.4	9.2	26.3	75.2	80.8	853	260
WI	Waupaca	-2.48	2779	32.4	7.4	21.6	74.3	80.2	873	266
IA	Delaware	-3.45	2995	32.4	6.9	27.4	77.4	81.7	1016	310
AZ	Graham	5.20	98	32.5	9.6	27.3	74.6	79.5	4541	1384
NC	Swain	2.97	311	32.5	12.1	28.5	72	78.6	3171	966
TX	Burleson	1.40	632	32.5	9.8	30.8	74.7	79.4	319	97
NE	Scotts Bluff	1.11	770	32.5	8.7	27	74.4	80.9	4149	1265
TX	Walker	1.07	785	32.5	9.6	27.9	73.9	78.8	277	84
AL	Etowah	0.96	829	32.5	11.8	33.3	70.5	77.2	766	233
NC	Cleveland	0.76	929	32.5	11.6	29.2	71.8	78.2	889	271
AL	Randolph	0.71	949	32.5	12.6	33.8	70.8	77.4	916	279
VA	Richmond	0.64	996	32.5	9.9	29.2	72.5	78.7	82	25
KS	Butler	0.58	1029	32.5	8.3	23.5	75.8	80.3	1396	425
TX	Navarro	0.57	1035	32.5	9.1	30.3	72.3	78.9	402	122
TN	Greene	0.14	1343	32.5	10.1	33	72.6	77.8	1548	472
KS	Russell	0.12	1351	32.5	8	27.3	75.2	80.7	1751	534
SC	Lancaster	0.09	1372	32.5	11	31.4	72.9	79.1	519	158
GA	Appling	0.06	1395	32.5	11.1	31.4	70.8	76.9	174	53
DE	Kent	-0.07	1498	32.5	11	27.9	73.5	79.5	33	10
OK	Logan	-0.27	1648	32.5	10.2	29.8	74.5	79.8	1036	316
OK	Harmon	-0.46	1795	32.5	9.8	34.4	72	77.9	1687	514
MO	Clark	-0.52	1826	32.5	8.6	30.6	74	80.2	644	196
NE	Stanton	-0.61	1887	32.5	6.5	30.8	75.7	81.6	1609	490
TN	Obion	-0.71	1954	32.5	11.4	35.2	71.8	77.9	354	108
MI	Ontonagon	-0.72	1960	32.5	9.3	20.9	75	80.7	1110	338
AR	Prairie	-0.86	2041	32.5	9.5	30.2	70.9	77.3	200	61
IA	Adams	-1.00	2126	32.5	7	24.1	76.4	80.9	1214	370
MO	Harrison	-1.19	2231	32.5	9	30.3	74.9	80.2	974	297

ST	COUNTY	USDA	AMEN	OBES	DIAB	INACT	M AGE	W AGE	ALT ft	ALT m
OK	Garfield	-1.25	2265	32.5	8.4	28.9	73.9	79.3	1167	356
MO	Jackson	-1.49	2370	32.5	8.9	25.4	73.2	79.2	894	272
VA	Amelia	-1.52	2390	32.5	9.4	25	72.4	78.7	303	92
LA	Acadia	-1.56	2405	32.5	8.9	31.6	70	76.7	27	8
SD	Clay	-1.87	2533	32.5	6.4	23.6	77.4	82.7	1230	375
KY	Scott	-1.89	2541	32.5	10.1	31.7	74.9	80.4	871	265
MO	Barton	-1.93	2558	32.5	9.6	27.7	73.9	80	944	288
IA	Monroe	-2.36	2714	32.5	7.2	34.4	74.7	80.9	887	270
SD	Moody	-2.96	2901	32.5	7.3	27	76.8	82.3	1629	497
OH	Wyandot	-3.19	2946	32.5	10.6	30.5	75.3	80.2	847	258
ND	Walsh	-3.95	3061	32.5	6.6	27.3	75.8	81.4	1124	343
WA	Pacific	4.85	141	32.6	10.2	22.1	74.8	80.3	581	177
AZ	La Paz	4.24	182	32.6	9.2	31.2	73.9	81	1370	418
TX	Shelby	2.45	382	32.6	10	31.6	71.3	77.6	296	90
OK	Kiowa	1.99	476	32.6	10.5	34.5	72.4	78.7	1502	458
OK	Pittsburg	1.64	558	32.6	11	33.8	72.2	78.4	739	225
AR	Stone	1.55	582	32.6	9.3	33.8	73.5	79.7	885	270
NC	Montgomery	1.37	646	32.6	10.7	27.5	71.8	78	522	159
GA	Lincoln	1.13	758	32.6	11.4	28.7	70.8	76.8	394	120
OK	Beaver	0.70	962	32.6	8.8	31.2	74.4	79.8	2568	783
WV	Hancock	0.39	1154	32.6	11.7	27.3	73.9	79	998	304
OK	Dewey	0.16	1332	32.6	10	32.7	73.3	79.7	1873	571
LA	Winn	-0.04	1473	32.6	10.3	36.8	69.7	76.8	165	50
GA	Baker	-0.07	1499	32.6	13	27.5	70.1	77.2	176	54
GA	Ben Hill	-0.10	1523	32.6	12	29.9	70.1	76	297	90
KY	Ohio	-0.21	1607	32.6	12.2	35.3	72.8	78.3	489	149
LA	Rapides	-0.21	1608	32.6	12.4	30.5	72	77.5	119	36
VA	Buckingham	-0.31	1684	32.6	10.9	28.1	71.3	76.9	500	152
SC	Abbeville	-0.61	1889	32.6	11.5	31.6	72	78.1	575	175
NE	Colfax	-0.72	1962	32.6	7.9	28.2	75.5	81.1	1498	457
MO	Butler	-0.84	2028	32.6	8.6	31.7	70.7	77.8	372	113
AL	Lamar	-0.85	2034	32.6	11.1	34.4	71.7	77.3	397	121
KY	Carlisle	-1.03	2150	32.6	11.1	29.5	73.6	79.1	383	117
OH	Logan	-1.38	2314	32.6	10.8	29.7	74.5	79.4	1114	340
LA	Beauregard	-1.45	2353	32.6	10.8	30.2	72.2	77.7	114	35
IA	Page	-1.83	2517	32.6	8.5	28.2	76.3	80.7	1107	337
WV	McDowell	-1.88	2538	32.6	14.2	42.1	66.3	74.7	1869	570
MI	Mecosta	-1.94	2563	32.6	9.6	25.5	75.3	80.6	1002	306
IN	Vigo	-2.12	2623	32.6	8.7	27.8	73.6	79.2	540	165
IA	Franklin	-4.18	3082	32.6	7.8	26.5	76.6	81.4	1174	358
ND	Traill	-5.12	3102	32.6	6.3	29.8	76.5	81.4	943	287
WA	Grays Harbor	3.94	203	32.7	10.3	23.7	73.7	79	515	157
FL	Marion	2.59	361	32.7	9.9	26.9	73.9	80.9	81	25
TN	Clay	1.29	684	32.7	10.5	28.6	71.2	77.1	783	239
MO	Hickory	1.22	722	32.7	8.6	26.4	72.8	79	947	289
TX	Anderson	1.07	784	32.7	10.7	32	69.8	77.8	378	115
GA	Troup	0.93	847	32.7	11.9	28.9	71.4	77.1	725	221

HEALTHIEST PLACES TO LIVE

ST	COUNTY	USDA	AMEN	OBES	DIAB	INACT	M AGE	W AGE	ALT ft	ALT m
GA	Stephens	0.53	1048	32.7	10.4	27.1	71.7	78.1	910	277
VA	Essex	0.48	1090	32.7	10.8	27.4	72.4	79.2	87	26
MO	Pike	0.46	1099	32.7	10.2	31.5	73.8	78.8	668	204
GA	Clinch	0.31	1207	32.7	11.1	29.9	72.2	77.9	150	46
TN	Putnam	0.24	1269	32.7	9.5	28.1	73.4	79	1182	360
IN	Orange	0.21	1296	32.7	10.4	35.4	73.5	78.9	675	206
TX	Hopkins	0.17	1325	32.7	10.2	28.8	73.6	78.9	477	145
LA	La Salle	-0.02	1453	32.7	10.9	30.9	71.8	77.4	126	38
GA	Chattahoochee	-0.35	1708	32.7	12	27.2	71.9	78.2	409	125
VA	Tazewell	-0.56	1855	32.7	10.2	36.1	70.8	78.4	2697	822
MO	Oregon	-0.76	1981	32.7	9.6	32.7	71.9	78.7	767	234
VA	Smyth	-1.55	2403	32.7	8.2	23.3	71.7	78.1	2679	816
VA	Nottoway	-1.57	2410	32.7	10.3	27.2	71.6	77.6	372	114
KS	Republic	-1.61	2428	32.7	8.3	26.5	76.3	81.7	1537	468
KY	Owsley	-1.67	2453	32.7	11	33.6	68.2	76.1	1025	313
IN	Dearborn	-2.04	2594	32.7	9.5	28	75.3	80.6	796	243
SD	Clark	-2.27	2683	32.7	6.9	28.7	74.9	80.6	1705	520
WI	Adams	-2.43	2755	32.7	7.9	24.9	74.7	80	984	300
IN	Delaware	-2.60	2809	32.7	9.4	29.3	73.6	78.9	938	286
ND	McHenry	-3.30	2965	32.7	7.8	36.1	74.4	80.2	1541	470
ND	Pembina	-5.18	3104	32.7	8	29.7	75.8	81.4	888	271
OK	Comanche	2.29	416	32.8	9.8	31.3	73.2	78.4	1309	399
TX	Polk	1.84	513	32.8	9.4	29.2	69.8	78.6	237	72
FL	Gilchrist	1.21	728	32.8	10	28	71.3	78.8	58	18
GA	Quitman	1.05	791	32.8	12.3	30.7	69.6	75.8	331	101
AR	Perry	0.89	861	32.8	10	33.1	72.5	78.1	557	170
OK	Coal	0.88	869	32.8	10.3	31.9	71.1	78.1	684	208
MS	Jackson	0.85	890	32.8	11.3	28.7	72.1	77.7	45	14
TX	Hill	0.83	900	32.8	9.3	31.2	72.7	79.1	631	192
WV	Hardy	0.82	905	32.8	11.2	26.8	73.9	79.3	1742	531
TX	Bowie	0.79	916	32.8	9.7	29.4	72.4	78.4	316	96
OK	Greer	0.74	936	32.8	10.2	33.9	72.4	78.7	1653	504
KY	Gallatin	0.63	1000	32.8	11.1	37.2	72.6	78.7	644	196
KY	Clinton	0.62	1007	32.8	10.2	36.1	70.2	77.3	961	293
MI	Presque Isle	0.18	1320	32.8	9.1	23.3	74.7	80.4	746	228
NC	Vance	0.05	1404	32.8	12.1	32	69.5	76.5	384	117
SC	Aiken	-0.04	1479	32.8	10	25.1	73.6	79.2	363	111
KS	Cheyenne	-0.14	1554	32.8	7.6	20.4	76	80.6	3450	1052
LA	Assumption	-0.22	1613	32.8	10.9	30	71.1	77.8	5	2
WV	Tucker	-0.29	1663	32.8	10.5	35.5	72.8	79.2	2776	846
TN	Trousdale	-0.30	1674	32.8	10.4	34.7	71	77.4	640	195
KS	Finney	-0.35	1711	32.8	9.1	25.8	75.3	80.2	2834	864
KY	Fulton	-0.46	1791	32.8	11	36	72.6	78.2	331	101
TN	Montgomery	-0.51	1818	32.8	12.4	30.5	74.3	79.1	538	164
GA	Catoosa	-0.54	1836	32.8	10	29	73.3	79.2	857	261
TN	Bledsoe	-0.56	1854	32.8	11.1	34.6	72.7	79.1	1601	488
KS	Ford	-0.84	2026	32.8	9.2	28.6	75.4	80	2492	759

ST	COUNTY	USDA	AMEN	OBES	DIAB	INACT	M AGE	W AGE	ALT ft	ALT m
VA	Franklin City	-0.94	2097	32.8	10.3	30.5	72.8	78.9	31	10
VA	Sussex	-1.11	2198	32.8	11.5	29.9	70.5	75.4	95	29
GA	Miller	-1.12	2200	32.8	12.5	32.1	70.1	77.2	167	51
MS	Alcorn	-1.30	2281	32.8	10.7	33.8	71.9	77.9	490	149
NC	Wayne	-1.41	2326	32.8	10.9	31.4	71.6	77.6	126	38
KS	Shawnee	-1.76	2492	32.8	8.9	23.4	74.6	80.4	1007	307
IN	Allen	-2.97	2903	32.8	9.9	25.3	75.4	80.6	793	242
MI	Isabella	-3.10	2928	32.8	8.5	24.2	75.5	80.4	859	262
OR	Wasco	3.38	260	32.9	7.6	19.4	75.9	80.8	2497	761
TN	Hamblen	1.52	594	32.9	11.7	32.7	72.4	78.3	1247	380
GA	Seminole	0.87	875	32.9	11.7	25.8	70.1	77.2	137	42
FL	Lafayette	0.84	892	32.9	11.5	29.9	72.4	78.2	65	20
GA	Cook	0.70	960	32.9	11.5	27.8	70	76.4	246	75
VA	Norfolk	0.48	1091	32.9	10.9	26.6	70.9	77.5	9	3
GA	Grady	0.16	1330	32.9	11.5	29.5	70.8	78	229	70
OK	Hughes	-0.05	1484	32.9	11.7	31.2	71.6	77.3	825	251
GA	Wilcox	-0.29	1660	32.9	11	31.9	70.9	77.1	302	92
MI	Berrien	-0.30	1667	32.9	9.4	27.6	74.8	79.8	680	207
MS	Pearl River	-0.91	2074	32.9	11.6	28.8	71.8	78	184	56
KS	Hodgeman	-0.94	2091	32.9	9	27.1	75.2	80.6	2386	727
NE	Hitchcock	-0.97	2111	32.9	7.5	31	76	81	2858	871
KS	Osborne	-1.07	2176	32.9	9	25.3	75.7	82	1751	534
KS	Cowley	-1.25	2261	32.9	8.5	28.4	73.1	79.9	1249	381
WI	Trempealeau	-1.42	2337	32.9	7.6	24.9	75.4	81.2	930	283
AR	Cleveland	-1.59	2415	32.9	10.7	27.5	72	78.3	224	68
ND	McIntosh	-2.21	2655	32.9	6.7	31.4	75.2	81.3	2052	626
NE	Gage	-2.26	2679	32.9	8.2	27	76.3	80.9	1366	416
MO	Shelby	-2.29	2687	32.9	10	28.4	73.8	79.8	764	233
IL	Knox	-2.43	2751	32.9	8	31	74.2	79.3	714	218
MI	Branch	-2.45	2760	32.9	9.2	28.9	74.7	79.6	949	289
WI	Waushara	-2.61	2818	32.9	8.1	23.2	75.2	80.6	945	288
NE	Saline	-3.04	2912	32.9	7.4	27.2	76.9	81.8	1466	447
SD	Beadle	-3.25	2958	32.9	6	29.3	75.8	81.4	1331	406
IA	Cedar	-3.28	2960	32.9	7.1	24	76.9	82.2	798	243
ND	Steele	-3.56	3012	32.9	6.9	26.3	75.2	81.1	1266	386
OK	Bryan	2.03	465	33	10.2	31	72.7	78	615	188
OK	Haskell	2.00	473	33	10	33.9	72.3	78.8	617	188
FL	Jackson	1.76	529	33	12.3	31	72.5	77.9	124	38
MO	Benton	1.47	605	33	9.4	29.7	73	78.8	856	261
GA	Clay	1.34	657	33	14.2	28.8	69.6	75.8	300	91
TX	Cherokee	1.25	712	33	10.3	29.6	71.9	79	391	119
AL	Morgan	1.09	778	33	10.2	26.6	72.9	78.9	703	214
TN	Stewart	0.98	823	33	10.2	32.6	72.4	78.3	509	155
AL	Lauderdale	0.90	858	33	12.2	32	73.3	79.7	639	195
TX	Titus	0.84	895	33	9	27.1	72.5	78.1	358	109
TX	Cooke	0.63	1003	33	9.8	27.2	74.8	80.6	839	256
KY	Crittenden	0.46	1097	33	9.9	37.8	72.3	77.9	477	145

HEALTHIEST PLACES TO LIVE

ST	COUNTY	USDA	AMEN	OBES	DIAB	INACT	M AGE	W AGE	ALT ft	ALT m
KY	Bath	0.32	1204	33	12.1	34.6	71	77.5	844	257
MS	Calhoun	0.23	1277	33	12.2	36	70.6	77.9	346	105
WV	Cabell	0.11	1365	33	12.9	30.4	71.3	78.2	751	229
TN	Maury	-0.19	1590	33	10.6	30	72.8	78.5	730	222
KY	Franklin	-0.34	1698	33	10.1	31.1	74.3	78.7	730	223
OK	Nowata	-0.36	1725	33	10.3	29	73.2	79	760	232
LA	Evangeline	-0.56	1851	33	10.5	30	69.8	75.5	69	21
KY	Larue	-1.22	2246	33	11.6	30.9	72.4	78.2	781	238
TN	Van Buren	-1.32	2290	33	10.2	32.9	71.6	78.2	1547	471
ND	Logan	-2.59	2808	33	7.7	32	75.2	81.3	2002	610
OH	Henry	-2.68	2834	33	9.5	28.6	75.6	81	689	210
IN	Blackford	-3.27	2959	33	10	28.7	74.2	79.5	868	265
AZ	Apache	3.45	249	33.1	13.1	27.5	70.8	80	6554	1998
NC	Person	1.33	662	33.1	11	27	72.2	78.3	565	172
KY	Whitley	1.15	750	33.1	12.9	34.1	70.7	77	1194	364
KS	Trego	0.81	907	33.1	7.6	28.7	76.3	81.5	2346	715
OH	Noble	0.63	1001	33.1	9.4	27.5	74.4	79.8	964	294
OK	Tillman	0.41	1135	33.1	10.9	32.5	71.7	78.1	1189	362
OH	Washington	0.21	1299	33.1	9.9	22.5	74.7	79.5	822	251
AR	Little River	-0.06	1489	33.1	10.4	31	72	78	315	96
SD	Stanley	-0.15	1562	33.1	7.5	30.6	76.6	81.5	1868	570
LA	Concordia	-0.18	1583	33.1	10.7	32.2	69.9	76.7	44	14
WV	Marshall	-0.34	1706	33.1	10.2	34.7	73.8	80.2	1108	338
KS	Reno	-0.42	1770	33.1	9.4	22.2	75.4	80.6	1602	488
NE	Greeley	-0.60	1880	33.1	7.6	28.3	76.2	80.7	2052	625
NC	Cumberland	-0.71	1951	33.1	12.4	29.8	72.6	78.4	147	45
KS	Morton	-1.59	2417	33.1	8.1	29.8	74.6	79.4	3429	1045
MO	Cass	-1.68	2461	33.1	9.8	27.1	75	79.4	921	281
SD	Deuel	-1.68	2463	33.1	6.5	26.7	76.2	82.2	1771	540
NE	Richardson	-1.91	2550	33.1	8.3	31.5	75.4	80.8	1022	312
IA	Audubon	-1.94	2560	33.1	7.8	26.5	76.1	82.6	1380	421
AR	Craighead	-2.24	2665	33.1	10.9	32	72.3	78.5	257	78
MO	Jasper	-2.26	2678	33.1	8.2	26.5	73.1	78.9	991	302
IN	Hendricks	-3.61	3022	33.1	8.9	23.4	76.9	80.8	888	271
KY	Taylor	0.45	1102	33.2	10.5	26.8	73.2	78.7	837	255
NJ	Cumberland	0.38	1157	33.2	10.2	30.7	72.7	78.6	47	14
TN	Unicoi	0.36	1177	33.2	10.4	30.3	71.4	78.6	2735	834
GA	Tift	0.33	1198	33.2	12.1	28.9	72.1	78.2	328	100
OH	Perry	0.20	1310	33.2	9.9	31.9	72.8	79.6	944	288
TN	Overton	0.20	1313	33.2	9.6	33.8	71.2	77.1	1187	362
SC	Saluda	0.02	1424	33.2	11	31.7	72.6	78.2	484	147
KY	Butler	-0.06	1492	33.2	11.5	30.6	72.8	77.8	515	157
WV	Tyler	-0.22	1617	33.2	10.9	28.1	73	78.9	938	286
AL	Marion	-0.31	1678	33.2	10.6	34.5	71	77.7	635	193
AR	Conway	-0.42	1768	33.2	10.3	29.1	72.5	78.1	492	150
GA	Macon	-0.54	1837	33.2	13.7	26.6	69.2	76.2	375	114
MO	Polk	-0.62	1891	33.2	10	27.2	73.7	79	1050	320

PEGGY FORNEY

ST	COUNTY	USDA	AMEN	OBES	DIAB	INACT	M AGE	W AGE	ALT ft	ALT m
TN	White	-0.76	1985	33.2	10.1	34.6	71.6	78.2	1207	368
LA	Jefferson Davis	-1.04	2157	33.2	12	31	72.6	78	22	7
NC	Hoke	-1.26	2269	33.2	12.7	29.4	71	76.9	278	85
SD	Walworth	-1.45	2355	33.2	8.8	30.5	74.1	80.3	1916	584
NE	Furnas	-1.63	2441	33.2	8.2	25.7	75.6	80.3	2287	697
SD	Yankton	-1.76	2496	33.2	7.2	23.4	76.9	81.5	1333	406
NE	Nemaha	-1.88	2535	33.2	7.3	29	75.4	80.8	1049	320
AR	Clay	-2.30	2689	33.2	10.6	32.6	70.3	78.1	300	91
MI	Osceola	-2.35	2709	33.2	9.1	26.6	74.1	78.9	1194	364
NE	Johnson	-2.60	2811	33.2	7.8	28.9	75.4	80.8	1243	379
MI	Ionia	-3.07	2918	33.2	9.8	23.4	75.1	80	799	244
AR	Marion	2.74	336	33.3	10.4	25.9	75.1	79.4	849	259
AR	Crawford	1.44	618	33.3	8.2	29.4	72.7	78.6	930	284
TN	Blount	1.25	711	33.3	9.5	26.4	74.1	79.6	1420	433
KY	Wayne	0.89	863	33.3	11.3	40.6	71.6	77.8	1049	320
KY	Bracken	0.50	1070	33.3	11.1	30.3	72.3	78.5	798	243
LA	Vermilion	0.44	1114	33.3	10.4	27.6	71.9	78.5	6	2
OK	Okfuskee	0.34	1194	33.3	11.1	36.3	71.6	77.3	837	255
NE	Frontier	0.29	1226	33.3	7	30.7	76	81	2645	806
NC	Rockingham	0.10	1369	33.3	10	29.6	71.7	77.9	703	214
MD	Wicomico	-0.70	1942	33.3	10.4	27.5	73	78.9	31	9
MI	Wexford	-0.76	1979	33.3	8.4	27.3	74.9	79.9	1181	360
AL	Houston	-0.79	2000	33.3	11.2	32.5	73.3	79.5	219	67
KY	Garrard	-1.23	2250	33.3	11.1	35.2	74.5	78.8	918	280
VA	Dinwiddie	-1.34	2296	33.3	10.4	24.1	71.3	78.6	220	67
OH	Ottawa	-1.41	2330	33.3	9.5	24	75.1	79.9	589	180
KS	Rawlins	-1.50	2376	33.3	7.8	26.3	76	80.6	3060	933
NE	Thomas	-1.61	2431	33.3	7.2	27.7	75.6	81.2	2979	908
MI	Lapeer	-2.12	2624	33.3	8.3	25.8	76.1	80.1	862	263
OH	Pickaway	-2.21	2658	33.3	10.6	29.9	74.1	79.2	768	234
WI	Marquette	-2.25	2675	33.3	7.1	25.5	74.9	80.2	840	256
NC	Greene	-2.33	2701	33.3	11.3	29.2	70.4	76.7	79	24
IN	White	-2.73	2847	33.3	8.6	27.6	74.5	80.7	693	211
KS	Washington	-2.95	2896	33.3	8.2	22.5	76.3	81.7	1393	425
ND	Benson	-3.08	2921	33.3	9.7	33	74.3	81.1	1549	472
IN	Adams	-3.55	3010	33.3	7.9	24.6	75.9	80.8	810	247
NC	Jackson	2.62	355	33.4	11.1	24.1	74.6	79.6	3365	1026
TN	Polk	1.67	552	33.4	11.2	33.2	70.9	77.7	1365	416
MO	Reynolds	1.41	630	33.4	9.2	32.8	70.4	77.3	950	290
TX	Grimes	0.74	938	33.4	9.4	25.7	73.1	78.5	299	91
AL	Colbert	0.70	957	33.4	11.7	33.7	71.9	78.3	589	180
KY	Lee	0.53	1049	33.4	11.1	35.5	68.2	76.2	946	288
NC	Pasquotank	0.43	1122	33.4	10.9	25.9	73.7	78.3	8	3
KY	Breckinridge	0.35	1184	33.4	11.2	31.3	72.8	78.9	618	188
MS	Newton	0.34	1192	33.4	11.4	33	71.8	77.9	426	130
OK	Blaine	-0.20	1601	33.4	9.8	30.8	73.6	79.4	1486	453
OH	Tuscarawas	-0.33	1693	33.4	9.8	28.4	75.3	80.3	1019	311

HEALTHIEST PLACES TO LIVE

ST	COUNTY	USDA	AMEN	OBES	DIAB	INACT	M AGE	W AGE	ALT ft	ALT m
KS	Atchison	-0.76	1978	33.4	7.8	29.5	75.2	79.9	1033	315
KY	Jackson	-0.82	2019	33.4	11.3	36	70.3	76.9	1216	371
TN	Coffee	-0.89	2064	33.4	11.1	25.6	72.3	78.5	1093	333
KS	Grant	-0.97	2110	33.4	8.5	20.1	74.6	79.4	3056	931
NE	Hooker	-1.64	2443	33.4	7.3	26.7	76.1	80.2	3386	1032
MI	Missaukee	-1.95	2565	33.4	9.7	25.1	75.1	79	1213	370
MI	Lenawee	-2.31	2694	33.4	8.5	23.8	76.2	79.8	828	252
OH	Champaign	-2.35	2712	33.4	9.2	25.7	74.2	79.1	1117	341
IA	Hardin	-3.63	3027	33.4	7	29.6	76	81.1	1113	339
FL	Polk	3.98	201	33.5	10.9	25.3	74.3	80	117	36
ID	Bingham	1.91	495	33.5	10.8	22.8	75.4	80.4	5125	1562
VA	Newport News	1.27	699	33.5	11.2	29.2	73.1	79.1	10	3
MO	Wright	0.87	876	33.5	8	34	72.1	78.8	1320	402
KY	Edmonson	0.62	1008	33.5	12.5	28.1	72.8	77.8	627	191
VA	Hopewell	0.26	1250	33.5	11	29.1	71.7	77.5	98	30
ND	McKenzie	-0.05	1483	33.5	8.3	28.6	75.7	82.2	2249	685
VA	Martinsville	-0.28	1658	33.5	10.8	27.6	71.2	78.3	897	274
KY	Henderson	-0.72	1959	33.5	10.4	26.9	73.6	78.7	399	122
VA	Emporia	-0.78	1998	33.5	11.5	28.7	70.5	75.4	103	31
AL	Conecuh	-1.00	2125	33.5	14.1	34.9	69.6	77.2	323	98
KY	Allen	-1.50	2378	33.5	10.6	28.6	71.5	77.9	689	210
IA	Wayne	-1.90	2545	33.5	6.7	25.1	74.7	80.9	1042	318
KS	Franklin	-1.97	2571	33.5	9.2	27.1	75.7	79.6	986	300
MO	Johnson	-2.00	2581	33.5	10.1	29.5	74.6	80.1	830	253
IA	Keokuk	-3.95	3059	33.5	6.6	24.3	76.6	81.8	784	239
IA	Fayette	-4.09	3077	33.5	6.4	24.1	76.1	80.8	1100	335
MO	Perry	2.29	415	33.6	9.4	25.8	74.8	80	553	169
NC	McDowell	2.21	430	33.6	10.6	29.4	73.2	79.2	1811	552
VA	Accomack	1.16	747	33.6	10.5	29.2	71.5	77.6	19	6
OK	Caddo	0.95	839	33.6	10.4	32.6	72	78.5	1416	432
MO	Iron	0.81	909	33.6	9.1	28	70.4	77.3	1078	328
VA	Charles City	0.59	1026	33.6	11.3	30.2	72	77.8	63	19
KY	Jefferson	0.32	1205	33.6	10.5	28.5	73.4	79.2	556	169
KY	Trimble	0.31	1208	33.6	11	34.1	73	78.9	728	222
PA	Sullivan	0.01	1435	33.6	9.2	27.4	74.8	80.7	1774	541
KS	Morris	-0.40	1753	33.6	8.9	24.7	74.7	80.4	1410	430
MS	Lee	-0.86	2044	33.6	11.7	30.5	70.9	77	335	102
NC	Alamance	-0.96	2108	33.6	10.1	27.7	74.2	79.4	643	196
OK	Grant	-1.01	2140	33.6	9.1	29	74.7	80.3	1122	342
NC	Nash	-1.39	2318	33.6	10.7	28.3	71.9	78.5	187	57
KY	Nicholas	-1.43	2341	33.6	11.4	34.9	72.5	78	851	259
KS	Stafford	-1.52	2385	33.6	8.7	31.1	74.9	80.1	1901	579
VA	Buchanan	-1.61	2432	33.6	12.3	30.8	69	76.7	1876	572
WV	Randolph	-1.61	2433	33.6	11.3	32.7	73.3	79.2	2938	896
MI	Montcalm	-2.48	2775	33.6	9	22.6	74.4	79	883	269
OK	McCurtain	2.08	454	33.7	10.1	37.5	70.2	77.5	632	193
ME	Piscataquis	1.20	732	33.7	8.6	23.5	74.3	80.5	1073	327

ST	COUNTY	USDA	AMEN	OBES	DIAB	INACT	M AGE	W AGE	ALT ft	ALT m
GA	Decatur	1.04	797	33.7	12.5	31.8	70.7	77.8	168	51
KY	Cumberland	0.65	982	33.7	11	32.1	70.2	77.3	762	232
OK	McClain	0.64	991	33.7	9.8	27.8	74.6	79.8	1114	340
LA	Iberia	0.48	1086	33.7	11.3	31	72	78	7	2
KY	Knott	0.07	1388	33.7	13.2	36.5	69.7	77.6	1332	406
OH	Monroe	-0.21	1609	33.7	9.8	30.9	74.4	79.8	1033	315
NY	Oswego	-0.23	1621	33.7	9.2	26.1	74.9	79.3	575	175
MO	St. Louis City	-0.48	1805	33.7	11.8	27.6	69.6	77.7	477	145
KY	Hickman	-0.84	2027	33.7	11.4	32.2	72.6	78.2	375	114
OH	Scioto	-0.97	2112	33.7	10.2	30.3	71.3	78.3	784	239
NE	Polk	-3.13	2933	33.7	8.3	28.4	77.1	81.3	1633	498
IA	Boone	-3.35	2974	33.7	6.8	26.4	76.4	81.5	1058	322
IN	Pulaski	-3.48	3000	33.7	9.7	26.9	73.3	79.3	698	213
KY	Russell	1.33	661	33.8	11	32.6	72.5	78.5	902	275
KY	Livingston	0.75	933	33.8	12.5	34.6	73.8	79.6	428	130
FL	Columbia	0.59	1023	33.8	10.9	28.4	71.8	77.8	109	33
MS	Clarke	0.42	1126	33.8	10.9	37.7	71.2	77.6	325	99
AL	Calhoun	0.22	1282	33.8	12.9	33.3	70.5	77.3	760	232
GA	Calhoun	0.21	1294	33.8	12.6	27.4	67.6	74.7	238	73
WI	Kewaunee	0.17	1327	33.8	7.9	24	76.3	81.6	732	223
KY	Mercer	-0.03	1462	33.8	10.5	33.8	73.2	79.1	846	258
OH	Brown	-0.08	1514	33.8	10.2	32.4	73.5	78.7	879	268
NJ	Salem	-0.20	1600	33.8	9.3	30.6	73.4	78.7	44	13
OK	Roger Mills	-0.28	1656	33.8	9.5	34.2	73.3	79.7	2149	655
TN	McMinn	-0.35	1716	33.8	10.7	32.6	71.9	78.3	913	278
TN	Shelby	-0.44	1780	33.8	11.7	28.6	71.4	77.7	284	87
MS	Pontotoc	-0.45	1787	33.8	10.7	34.3	72.1	79.4	409	125
MD	Prince George's	-0.61	1884	33.8	11	24.9	73.5	79.2	147	45
GA	Taylor	-0.62	1890	33.8	11.9	29.1	70.6	76.6	503	153
KY	Owen	-0.64	1905	33.8	11.4	36.3	72.8	78.6	762	232
AR	Lonoke	-0.79	2001	33.8	11	30.8	73.3	79	233	71
KY	Bullitt	-0.87	2048	33.8	10.9	33.8	75.4	80.2	577	176
MI	Mackinac	-0.95	2104	33.8	9	25.3	75	80.3	733	223
OH	Jackson	-1.28	2275	33.8	11.2	37.5	71.4	78.2	782	238
KY	Marion	-1.32	2288	33.8	10.6	34.7	73.3	79.6	790	241
VA	Cumberland	-1.50	2379	33.8	11	27.8	72.4	78.7	335	102
IA	Louisa	-1.83	2516	33.8	7	26.8	76.4	82	623	190
IA	Des Moines	-2.04	2593	33.8	8.5	28.5	75.9	81.6	691	210
WV	Ritchie	-2.42	2750	33.8	11.3	33.8	73.3	79	939	286
KY	Graves	-2.48	2774	33.8	10.5	31	72.6	78.2	465	142
TX	Potter	2.60	360	33.9	9.4	30.8	71.7	77.4	3389	1033
AL	Autauga	0.78	920	33.9	11.7	31.9	72.9	78	365	111
OK	Creek	0.58	1031	33.9	10.1	32.4	72.1	78.2	832	254
VA	Halifax	0.53	1052	33.9	11.8	31.3	70.6	78	461	140
TX	Harrison	0.52	1056	33.9	10.2	32.9	72.3	78.3	312	95
PA	Armstrong	0.36	1176	33.9	8.6	26	74.8	79.7	1208	368
GA	Lowndes	0.27	1237	33.9	11.9	27.6	72.2	77.9	192	59

HEALTHIEST PLACES TO LIVE

ST	COUNTY	USDA	AMEN	OBES	DIAB	INACT	M AGE	W AGE	ALT ft	ALT m
VA	Prince George	0.26	1251	33.9	11.8	28.4	74.9	79.3	88	27
NC	Craven	0.19	1317	33.9	10.5	26.3	74.4	79.2	27	8
WV	Fayette	-0.13	1551	33.9	12.1	33.4	71.1	77.8	1957	596
MS	Webster	-0.32	1688	33.9	11.5	34	71.1	77.3	418	127
NC	Columbus	-0.39	1746	33.9	11.3	27.8	69.4	76.8	70	21
MO	Lewis	-0.40	1755	33.9	8.6	29	74	80.2	631	192
OH	Hocking	-0.68	1931	33.9	10.9	27.3	73.4	79	907	277
WV	Preston	-0.84	2033	33.9	9.6	32.1	73.4	79.8	2020	616
WV	Wetzel	-0.91	2078	33.9	10.6	30.5	73.7	79.7	1125	343
IN	Lake	-1.14	2210	33.9	11	29.8	72.6	78.6	656	200
NC	Johnston	-1.16	2221	33.9	10.5	27.7	73.2	79.4	204	62
NE	Dixon	-1.71	2476	33.9	6.7	30.3	74.8	79.6	1406	429
OH	Union	-3.50	3005	33.9	8.9	26.4	75.3	79.8	982	299
OH	Crawford	-3.71	3037	33.9	9.6	27.1	73.8	79.6	1001	305
AL	Coosa	1.59	570	34	12.8	33.7	70.4	77.3	647	197
TN	Monroe	1.51	598	34	10.4	31	72.5	78.7	1439	438
TX	Runnels	1.18	738	34	8.8	26.5	73.2	78.8	1828	557
OK	Cotton	0.88	870	34	9.7	35.7	71.7	78.1	1005	306
WV	Mineral	0.68	969	34	10.8	30.8	73.8	79.3	1281	390
TN	Houston	0.56	1038	34	10.4	29.3	72.4	78.3	564	172
NC	Perquimans	0.50	1073	34	9.7	26.6	73	78.8	12	4
LA	Plaquemines	0.30	1214	34	12.3	30.9	72.8	79.1	4	1
PA	Bradford	0.29	1228	34	8.1	27.7	75.2	80.6	1368	417
LA	Catahoula	0.08	1377	34	11.3	33.6	70.1	76.8	67	21
AL	Henry	0.07	1383	34	12.8	30.1	70.5	77.2	328	100
KY	Hart	-0.07	1500	34	10	35.6	72.4	78.2	707	216
GA	Dooly	-0.12	1538	34	11.5	29.4	69.2	76.2	333	101
WV	Raleigh	-0.13	1553	34	11.9	34.4	72.4	78.6	2241	683
MS	Stone	-1.13	2208	34	11.4	30.6	70.4	77	177	54
KS	Sumner	-1.15	2214	34	9.1	27.3	75	79.7	1225	373
AL	DeKalb	-1.60	2423	34	10.3	27	71.9	78.1	1216	371
MO	Vernon	-1.60	2424	34	9.4	30.5	73.2	78.6	824	251
MI	Wayne	-1.73	2479	34	11.6	27.6	71.9	78	642	196
MI	Ogemaw	-1.89	2542	34	9	29.2	73.1	78.6	1033	315
KS	Pawnee	-2.07	2607	34	8.8	28.7	75.2	80.6	2089	637
MI	Gladwin	-2.23	2661	34	8.8	26.7	74.2	79.6	792	242
IN	Cass	-3.04	2910	34	9.3	27.9	74.5	79.4	731	223
IN	Fayette	-3.35	2976	34	9.2	30.4	72.9	79.2	974	297
OR	Umatilla	1.64	559	34.1	8.7	24.2	75.6	80.5	2632	802
OK	Jefferson	1.29	683	34.1	10.2	34.4	71.7	78.1	900	274
AR	Clark	1.15	748	34.1	10.7	30.5	72.9	78.5	317	97
TN	Benton	1.13	762	34.1	11.2	30.3	70.6	77.8	470	143
SC	Colleton	0.67	972	34.1	12	32.6	69.7	77.4	50	15
GA	Crisp	0.36	1174	34.1	11.4	31.3	69.8	76.6	326	99
GA	Thomas	0.29	1220	34.1	12.2	28.4	72	78.8	210	64
WV	Barbour	0.22	1291	34.1	10.8	28.1	72.8	79.2	1668	508
GA	Turner	0.11	1358	34.1	12.4	32.4	70.8	76.6	356	109

ST	COUNTY	USDA	AMEN	OBES	DIAB	INACT	M AGE	W AGE	ALT ft	ALT m
VA	King & Queen	-0.13	1550	34.1	10.6	27.7	73.3	79	87	26
AL	Bibb	-0.15	1559	34.1	11.2	36.8	69.8	77.1	413	126
AL	Montgomery	-0.28	1650	34.1	13.5	29.5	71.7	78	270	82
GA	Mitchell	-0.45	1784	34.1	11.6	30.2	69.8	76.7	217	66
TN	Bedford	-0.55	1846	34.1	11.8	30.5	71.9	79	842	257
KY	Logan	-0.75	1971	34.1	10.3	33.5	72.5	78.1	597	182
SD	Jackson	-0.75	1975	34.1	10.9	30.8	71	78.3	2525	770
VA	Greensville	-0.78	1999	34.1	12	29.9	70.5	75.4	147	45
MS	Prentiss	-0.79	2003	34.1	11.6	32.1	71.3	78.9	445	136
TN	Lincoln	-1.20	2238	34.1	9.2	33.6	72.8	79	848	258
KS	Greeley	-1.80	2505	34.1	8.5	28.6	75.9	81.2	3661	1116
IN	Howard	-3.61	3023	34.1	9.7	31	73.8	79.3	814	248
FL	Levy	2.47	375	34.2	10.6	31.4	71.5	78.7	40	12
FL	Jefferson	2.00	469	34.2	11.6	27.9	72.5	78.3	88	27
TN	Franklin	1.68	549	34.2	9.4	33	73.5	78.9	1158	353
OK	Murray	1.34	659	34.2	10.1	31.2	71.6	78.1	1046	319
TN	Rhea	1.33	663	34.2	10.2	30.6	71.1	78	1146	349
KY	Trigg	0.99	819	34.2	9.7	33.5	73	79.3	484	147
OK	Choctaw	0.29	1227	34.2	11.1	33.4	71.3	77.3	492	150
LA	Claiborne	0.08	1378	34.2	12.3	32.7	71.1	76.7	265	81
OK	Noble	-0.04	1477	34.2	9.9	31.3	74.7	80.3	1015	309
KS	Jewell	-0.20	1596	34.2	8.6	24.7	75.7	82	1664	507
KS	Saline	-1.03	2149	34.2	8	24.2	75.5	80.1	1332	406
OH	Ross	-1.10	2191	34.2	10.1	28.8	73.3	78.6	840	256
VA	Lee	-1.36	2303	34.2	10.6	33.2	70.4	77	1776	541
NC	Franklin	-1.43	2343	34.2	9.8	28.1	72.4	78.8	314	96
AR	Woodruff	-1.47	2360	34.2	10.6	33.9	70.9	77.3	198	60
WV	Roane	-1.66	2449	34.2	12.9	32.2	72	78	939	286
AR	Dallas	-1.85	2522	34.2	10.7	32.8	70.8	77.4	276	84
KY	Lyon	1.51	595	34.3	10.1	29.8	72.3	77.9	433	132
TN	Meigs	1.30	681	34.3	11.5	33.6	71.1	78	812	248
KS	Greenwood	0.66	978	34.3	7.8	30.4	74.7	80.4	1175	358
KS	Phillips	0.15	1335	34.3	8.3	24.6	76.3	81.5	2024	617
MS	Choctaw	-0.16	1567	34.3	12	29	71.1	77.3	475	145
MI	Iosco	-0.17	1573	34.3	8.3	22.9	73.5	79.5	737	225
NC	Northampton	-0.65	1913	34.3	12.1	31.9	68.9	77	97	30
KY	Shelby	-0.71	1948	34.3	10.9	28	75.4	80.2	783	239
KS	Lane	-0.90	2068	34.3	8.3	24.8	75.9	81.2	2757	840
MS	Smith	-1.23	2252	34.3	11.3	35	69.6	77	384	117
TN	Madison	-1.44	2348	34.3	10.9	28.8	72.7	78.9	434	132
LA	Washington	-1.57	2409	34.3	13.5	34.7	68.8	75.7	204	62
WV	Mercer	-1.67	2456	34.3	11	33.6	71	77.5	2462	750
WV	Boone	-1.90	2548	34.3	13.8	40.2	69.9	76.7	1340	408
VA	Lunenburg	-2.17	2643	34.3	11.3	31.4	71.1	78.1	431	131
IN	Jay	-3.98	3064	34.3	9.6	31.2	74.2	79.5	905	276
FL	Calhoun	1.12	764	34.4	11.6	29.7	72	77.7	97	29
AL	Tuscaloosa	0.50	1069	34.4	11.8	28.8	71.9	77.8	361	110

HEALTHIEST PLACES TO LIVE

ST	COUNTY	USDA	AMEN	OBES	DIAB	INACT	M AGE	W AGE	ALT ft	ALT m
VA	Roanoke City	0.01	1438	34.4	10.5	26.5	71.2	78.8	1038	316
WV	Braxton	-0.55	1849	34.4	12.5	33.6	71.9	78.3	1186	361
MS	Union	-0.85	2037	34.4	10.8	31.9	72.3	78.4	422	128
LA	Lincoln	-0.99	2122	34.4	10.8	30.8	74	78.9	229	70
MO	Scott	-1.44	2345	34.4	10	32.7	73	79	345	105
MO	Scotland	-1.56	2406	34.4	7.9	27.9	74	80.2	759	231
AR	Greene	-2.00	2580	34.4	10	27	72.7	78.5	302	92
TN	Crockett	-2.21	2659	34.4	11.9	32.2	70.7	77.4	339	103
OH	Auglaize	-3.25	2957	34.4	9.1	25.4	75.8	80.9	918	280
OK	Latimer	0.89	866	34.5	10.7	34.3	72.3	78.8	876	267
VA	Surry	0.79	918	34.5	11.7	26.2	72	77.8	77	24
KY	Hancock	0.48	1085	34.5	9.7	30.8	72.8	78.9	504	154
OK	Pottawatomie	0.26	1249	34.5	9.8	34.5	72.7	77.9	1024	312
KY	Carter	0.12	1353	34.5	11.4	42.8	70.8	77.5	860	262
OK	Jackson	-0.05	1485	34.5	11.4	32.7	73.7	78.1	1393	425
GA	Washington	-0.21	1604	34.5	12.7	27.3	70.1	77	371	113
SC	Florence	-0.56	1853	34.5	11.8	32.9	70.7	77.1	85	26
LA	Calcasieu	-0.67	1923	34.5	11.6	29.4	71.2	78.1	17	5
KS	Barton	-0.88	2057	34.5	9.4	26.4	75.6	81.9	1891	576
AR	Cross	-0.95	2102	34.5	10.6	35	70.7	77.2	234	71
WV	Jefferson	-1.12	2204	34.5	10.6	27.5	74.6	79.1	512	156
KS	Barber	-1.28	2272	34.5	8.9	32.4	75.3	80.1	1639	500
MI	Newaygo	-1.30	2280	34.5	11.5	25.2	75	79.8	885	270
AR	Calhoun	-1.35	2299	34.5	10.5	35.2	70.8	77.4	171	52
KS	Marshall	-1.38	2312	34.5	8.1	25.3	76.3	81.7	1305	398
KS	Allen	-1.43	2339	34.5	9	26.2	74.7	79.4	1018	310
NC	Duplin	-1.51	2383	34.5	11.5	33.1	71.3	78.3	89	27
MI	Bay	-1.53	2394	34.5	9.2	24.7	74.7	80.4	632	193
NE	Dakota	-1.76	2494	34.5	9.3	30.9	74.8	79.6	1227	374
OH	Van Wert	-3.60	3021	34.5	9.9	23.5	75.2	80.5	766	233
IN	Randolph	-3.72	3038	34.5	10.2	36.5	74.2	79.5	1083	330
FL	Hendry	4.22	185	34.6	10.7	31.2	71.8	77.8	21	6
FL	DeSoto	2.74	337	34.6	11.2	30.7	74.2	80.1	55	17
WA	Garfield	2.31	412	34.6	10.7	24.5	77.1	80.8	2721	829
TN	Hawkins	1.21	730	34.6	11.3	31.5	72.6	78.6	1416	432
VA	Northumberland	1.19	736	34.6	9.7	26.7	73	79.5	54	16
KY	Estill	0.55	1040	34.6	11.7	36.8	70.3	76.9	900	274
AR	Lawrence	-0.10	1522	34.6	10.7	32.5	71.6	78.6	311	95
SD	Brule	-1.54	2399	34.6	6.5	32.3	75	80.8	1663	507
KS	Edwards	-3.01	2908	34.6	8.5	26.7	74.9	80.1	2173	662
IL	Logan	-3.89	3053	34.6	8.3	28.9	74	79.8	599	183
WA	Lewis	3.40	258	34.7	9	21.2	75.1	79.8	1900	579
TN	Carter	2.93	319	34.7	10.8	31.7	72.4	78.6	2655	809
OK	Carter	1.18	737	34.7	9.1	34.8	71.7	77.7	914	279
GA	Talbot	1.10	776	34.7	13	28.6	69.4	76	620	189
MO	Madison	1.01	809	34.7	9.4	28.6	72.7	78.7	809	247
AR	Howard	0.99	816	34.7	11.6	32.8	72	78	584	178

ST	COUNTY	USDA	AMEN	OBES	DIAB	INACT	M AGE	W AGE	ALT ft	ALT m
WV	Summers	0.67	977	34.7	11	33.1	72.6	79.2	2147	654
AR	Hot Spring	0.49	1076	34.7	10.2	33.9	72.7	78.4	455	139
GA	Sumter	0.23	1275	34.7	13	29.7	70.9	77	385	117
MS	Rankin	0.16	1331	34.7	10.7	27.9	74.8	80.9	360	110
TN	Henry	0.06	1400	34.7	10.6	32.3	71.6	77.9	469	143
OK	Ottawa	0.03	1414	34.7	11.2	34.8	72.2	78.4	839	256
SC	Greenwood	-0.11	1536	34.7	10.1	30.4	72.5	78.5	535	163
MO	Shannon	-0.23	1620	34.7	10.1	30.9	71.9	78.7	981	299
SC	Allendale	-0.27	1649	34.7	14	34.7	68.7	76.2	148	45
GA	Dougherty	-0.31	1679	34.7	13	27.5	70.8	77.6	203	62
GA	Clayton	-0.32	1686	34.7	12.4	29.9	73.5	78.8	886	270
MI	Muskegon	-0.40	1754	34.7	9.9	25.8	74.3	79.3	667	203
KY	Fleming	-0.86	2043	34.7	10.6	34.6	71	77.5	862	263
NC	Gates	-1.00	2132	34.7	11.2	29.4	72.9	78.2	28	9
MS	Carroll	-1.02	2144	34.7	10.9	31.6	70.7	77.9	312	95
MI	Monroe	-1.43	2342	34.7	10.1	27	74.6	79.7	635	194
OK	Craig	-1.49	2372	34.7	10.9	32.7	73.2	79	803	245
MO	Caldwell	-2.83	2868	34.7	9.2	30.2	74.5	80.4	895	273
NE	Clay	-3.36	2980	34.7	8.4	30.3	75.9	80.7	1772	540
AR	Franklin	2.05	459	34.8	10	29.5	73.3	79.3	852	260
FL	Wakulla	1.95	483	34.8	10.5	27.3	74.5	79.8	33	10
LA	Red River	1.11	768	34.8	11.3	32.4	70	76.1	161	49
WV	Pendleton	0.82	906	34.8	10.8	30.8	73.3	78.6	2567	783
FL	Baker	0.65	980	34.8	12.7	32.6	68.1	77.7	126	38
AL	Clay	0.21	1292	34.8	12.7	36.2	71.8	78	1023	312
GA	Johnson	-0.01	1443	34.8	12.8	29.4	70.6	76.1	332	101
GA	Taliaferro	-0.13	1548	34.8	12.7	30.1	70.8	76.8	535	163
MO	Randolph	-0.22	1614	34.8	10.3	31.6	73.7	79.9	794	242
OK	Beckham	-0.40	1757	34.8	9.9	33.3	72	77.9	1953	595
KS	Crawford	-1.00	2128	34.8	9.4	27.7	73.9	79.6	938	286
KS	Linn	-1.53	2393	34.8	8.8	28.8	74.7	79.4	931	284
NC	Jones	-1.59	2419	34.8	12.1	31.4	71.3	78.3	45	14
KS	Bourbon	-1.85	2524	34.8	7.9	26.1	74.6	79.4	919	280
IN	Huntington	-2.34	2705	34.8	10.3	29.8	75.7	81	804	245
WV	Webster	-2.35	2713	34.8	11.5	35.6	72	78.5	2404	733
MT	Roosevelt	-2.45	2763	34.8	12.1	32.4	73.6	79.5	2288	697
OK	Marshall	2.54	368	34.9	9.7	31	73	78.8	741	226
FL	Dixie	2.42	385	34.9	10.6	33.2	71.3	78.8	27	8
TN	Campbell	1.87	506	34.9	11.4	34.5	70.9	77.4	1561	476
WV	Grant	1.46	611	34.9	12.1	28.9	73.9	79.3	2076	633
MO	Jefferson	0.96	833	34.9	10.1	30.9	74.1	78.4	614	187
NC	Washington	0.31	1210	34.9	12	28.4	71.6	77.6	15	4
OK	Mayes	0.21	1300	34.9	10.8	37	73.1	79.7	712	217
GA	Treutlen	0.02	1418	34.9	10.7	28.3	71.3	76.5	269	82
SC	Chesterfield	-0.38	1736	34.9	11.4	32.5	69.7	76.8	326	99
MS	Simpson	-0.80	2008	34.9	11.7	32.2	70.3	76.4	384	117
KS	Coffey	-0.95	2103	34.9	9.2	23.4	75.2	80.6	1106	337

ST	COUNTY	USDA	AMEN	OBES	DIAB	INACT	M AGE	W AGE	ALT ft	ALT m
TN	Warren	-1.45	2356	34.9	10.1	30.8	71.4	78	1111	339
LA	East Feliciana	-1.46	2358	34.9	11.9	27.6	69.9	76.7	197	60
KS	Wilson	-1.75	2488	34.9	9	25.3	74	79.6	919	280
MO	Dunklin	-2.10	2617	34.9	10.6	40.7	69.8	76.6	267	81
NE	Merrick	-2.29	2688	34.9	7.8	26.8	75.6	80.5	1712	522
WV	Calhoun	-2.37	2727	34.9	10.5	30.8	72.1	78.7	966	295
GA	Warren	1.04	798	35	12.3	27.3	68.4	75.4	502	153
TN	Jackson	0.86	884	35	11.6	32.5	71.3	77.6	756	231
KY	Lewis	0.78	921	35	12.2	34.8	69.8	77.2	867	264
MS	Neshoba	0.61	1017	35	13.6	33.7	71.1	77.3	455	139
AL	Walker	0.51	1059	35	13	36.9	68.3	75.9	472	144
GA	Muscogee	0.08	1376	35	12.4	27.8	70.9	77.5	389	119
KY	Caldwell	-0.52	1823	35	10.4	31.7	73	79.3	507	155
WV	Marion	-0.52	1832	35	10.9	32.1	73.9	79	1218	371
IN	Owen	-0.76	1977	35	9.7	29.5	73.6	79	672	205
ND	Mountrail	-1.35	2301	35	8.3	33.3	75.7	81.4	2190	668
IA	Warren	-2.16	2638	35	7.6	26.6	77.1	81.8	906	276
KY	Bourbon	-3.18	2941	35	11.8	35.3	74	79.2	891	271
NE	York	-4.05	3075	35	7.4	28.1	76.9	81.8	1642	500
FL	Bradford	1.34	656	35.1	12.1	29.8	71.8	78.9	144	44
MS	Itawamba	1.01	810	35.1	12.2	35.6	71.6	77.3	394	120
WV	Hampshire	0.69	963	35.1	9.9	30.3	73.3	79.2	1201	366
MO	Bollinger	0.49	1079	35.1	8.9	31.5	72.7	78.7	596	182
ME	Somerset	0.47	1093	35.1	9.8	26.4	74.8	79.8	1180	360
KY	Morgan	0.39	1148	35.1	12.6	34.4	70.8	76.9	976	297
OK	Pawnee	0.01	1432	35.1	12.4	37.2	74	79	888	271
MT	Rosebud	-0.34	1701	35.1	9.1	29.3	76.1	81	3092	943
KY	Henry	-0.46	1792	35.1	11.4	32.4	73	78.9	775	236
IA	Jasper	-3.19	2943	35.1	8.3	23.5	76.9	80.9	902	275
IN	Shelby	-3.76	3046	35.1	10	32.4	74.4	79.6	771	235
SC	McCormick	0.81	911	35.2	11.9	25.3	72	78.1	411	125
OH	Morgan	0.28	1233	35.2	10.4	29.7	73.2	79.8	885	270
PA	Fayette	0.27	1238	35.2	11.4	32.9	73.4	80	1488	453
MI	Oceana	0.26	1246	35.2	9.6	24.9	75.4	80.9	763	233
TN	Lake	-0.36	1726	35.2	11.9	37.3	71.8	77.9	277	84
MI	Arenac	-1.04	2158	35.2	8.6	24	74.1	79.6	683	208
MS	Jefferson Davis	-1.10	2189	35.2	11.5	31	69.9	76.9	390	119
MS	Tippah	-1.17	2225	35.2	11.7	39.4	70.6	77.9	517	158
TN	Macon	-2.11	2620	35.2	11.5	28.8	71	77.4	858	262
MI	Barry	-2.15	2635	35.2	8.3	25.7	75.4	80.7	878	268
TN	Sullivan	1.27	694	35.3	12	29.4	72.6	79	1688	515
KY	Greenup	0.62	1009	35.3	13.3	31.7	73.3	78.5	758	231
AL	Chilton	0.38	1155	35.3	11.1	30.4	70.4	77.3	528	161
SD	Sully	0.20	1312	35.3	6.4	27	76.6	81.5	1799	548
MT	Blaine	0.19	1316	35.3	10.9	32.4	74.4	80.2	3070	936
GA	Stewart	0.01	1429	35.3	13.7	29	69.6	75.8	417	127
LA	Tangipahoa	-0.28	1652	35.3	10.6	31.4	70.2	76	118	36

ST	COUNTY	USDA	AMEN	OBES	DIAB	INACT	M AGE	W AGE	ALT ft	ALT m
KY	Anderson	-0.45	1785	35.3	11	34.5	75	79	776	237
OK	Okmulgee	-0.87	2052	35.3	9.9	33.2	70.8	78.1	722	220
MS	Chickasaw	-0.98	2117	35.3	11.7	33.1	69.8	77.5	335	102
KS	Osage	-1.17	2223	35.3	9.2	27.3	75.3	80.4	1095	334
TN	Fayette	-1.18	2228	35.3	11.9	30.4	72.3	78.3	397	121
KY	Metcalfe	-3.16	2937	35.3	10.9	33.7	71.9	77.9	850	259
AZ	Greenlee	5.18	103	35.4	8.7	25	74.6	79.5	5710	1740
FL	Taylor	2.32	408	35.4	11	30.7	72.5	78.3	41	12
MS	Lauderdale	1.31	670	35.4	13.2	29.8	70	77.1	383	117
TN	Roane	1.22	726	35.4	11.3	33.9	73.2	79.4	909	277
KY	Rowan	0.97	825	35.4	10.3	30.6	72.4	79	992	302
MO	Lincoln	0.37	1169	35.4	10.1	26.8	73.7	79	607	185
MS	Hancock	0.25	1253	35.4	10.9	28.9	73.9	79.7	59	18
VA	Wise	0.25	1260	35.4	10.2	37.5	71.1	77.1	2296	700
MO	Callaway	-0.06	1493	35.4	10.4	28.7	73.9	80.1	765	233
KY	Hopkins	-0.21	1606	35.4	10.7	33.4	72.3	78.1	445	136
LA	Tensas	-0.47	1800	35.4	12.4	33.3	69.9	76.7	61	18
MI	Sanilac	-1.23	2251	35.4	8.8	27.8	75.2	79.5	765	233
KY	Powell	-1.28	2274	35.4	12.8	40.4	70.8	77.6	915	279
SD	Sanborn	-3.47	2999	35.4	6.9	33.2	75.8	81.4	1295	395
AL	St. Clair	1.39	635	35.5	12.5	34.7	71.8	77.7	699	213
MS	Monroe	0.86	883	35.5	12.1	35.7	71.2	78.3	283	86
NC	Anson	0.06	1399	35.5	12.3	29.5	70.9	77.1	336	102
KY	Monroe	-0.10	1526	35.5	10.5	32.4	71.5	77.9	833	254
KS	Ellsworth	-0.19	1586	35.5	8.7	24.2	75.2	80.7	1675	511
WV	Wayne	-0.19	1592	35.5	11.8	31	72.3	77.9	856	261
MS	Perry	-0.28	1654	35.5	12.4	35.8	70.7	76.6	175	53
AL	Chambers	-0.34	1695	35.5	14.2	35	70.2	77.2	750	228
LA	St. Martin	-0.34	1700	35.5	11.7	29.7	71.6	77.5	8	2
MS	Tate	-0.70	1943	35.5	12.4	32.2	72	77.2	302	92
MS	Wayne	-0.79	2004	35.5	10.2	32	71.1	77.2	253	77
MS	Yazoo	-0.91	2075	35.5	12.8	35.2	69.9	75.9	210	64
NC	Hertford	-1.25	2264	35.5	12	33.6	69.8	75.8	40	12
MI	Calhoun	-2.73	2848	35.5	10.3	27.3	73.1	79.1	938	286
WI	Menominee	-3.38	2984	35.5	12.4	30.8	75.1	80.9	1051	320
AR	Johnson	2.37	393	35.6	9.8	30.7	72.5	78.7	1035	316
FL	Putnam	2.35	399	35.6	11.8	30.9	70.9	78	54	16
FL	Washington	1.95	484	35.6	12.3	29.6	71.3	77.6	103	32
KY	Meade	0.76	927	35.6	11.6	31.8	74.4	79.6	640	195
MO	Texas	0.45	1103	35.6	8.2	31.9	72	78.5	1253	382
MD	Dorchester	0.20	1305	35.6	11.1	29.8	72.5	78.7	12	4
TN	Fentress	-0.05	1487	35.6	11.7	32.7	69.5	77.1	1484	452
OH	Columbiana	-0.25	1636	35.6	11.4	28.1	74.2	79.4	1136	346
SC	Edgefield	-0.25	1640	35.6	10.1	25.6	72	77.6	432	132
TN	Tipton	-0.38	1737	35.6	11	32.4	72.2	78	320	98
AL	Dale	-0.47	1798	35.6	12.6	31	72.9	79	314	96
SD	Charles Mix	-1.23	2254	35.6	9.6	29	75	80.9	1567	478

HEALTHIEST PLACES TO LIVE

ST	COUNTY	USDA	AMEN	OBES	DIAB	INACT	M AGE	W AGE	ALT ft	ALT m
KY	Knox	-1.49	2368	35.6	13.2	35.6	69.9	76.4	1238	377
NC	Pitt	-1.74	2485	35.6	9.3	25.3	72.9	78	46	14
KS	Doniphan	-2.07	2606	35.6	8.5	27.6	75.2	79.9	985	300
AR	Nevada	-2.12	2622	35.6	12	33.6	70.2	77.1	292	89
FL	Gadsden	1.65	556	35.7	12.6	31.1	70.1	77.9	202	62
FL	Union	1.60	568	35.7	12.9	31.7	68.1	77.7	124	38
AL	Monroe	1.27	692	35.7	12.2	31.2	71.1	77.2	269	82
AL	Clarke	1.26	703	35.7	12.9	37.1	72.1	77.6	228	69
LA	Webster	0.71	951	35.7	11.7	30.8	70.7	77.1	228	70
LA	Natchitoches	0.39	1150	35.7	11.6	33.1	70.9	77.2	166	51
SC	Darlington	0.28	1234	35.7	12.6	33.4	69.9	76.8	176	54
LA	Union	0.22	1286	35.7	12.2	34.7	71.7	77.6	148	45
LA	Lafourche	0.11	1359	35.7	12	31	73.1	79.3	4	1
PA	Columbia	-0.05	1486	35.7	8.6	27.4	74.9	80.8	972	296
AR	Randolph	-0.32	1685	35.7	11.1	31.7	72.6	79.1	407	124
OK	Kingfisher	-0.77	1993	35.7	10.3	30.5	73.6	79.4	1121	342
KS	Cherokee	-0.98	2115	35.7	9.1	25.5	73.2	78.9	867	264
LA	St. James	-1.12	2202	35.7	11.5	32.6	71.3	78.3	6	2
AR	Grant	-1.77	2497	35.7	9.2	33.1	73.7	79.6	252	77
IA	Cass	-1.79	2501	35.7	6.5	25.3	77	81.6	1270	387
IN	Wabash	-2.05	2598	35.7	9.3	25.2	74.9	80.5	779	237
IN	Clay	-2.56	2801	35.7	9.2	28.6	73.7	78.7	610	186
KY	Union	0.72	943	35.8	10.4	33.2	72.8	78.8	401	122
TX	Kaufman	0.63	1004	35.8	9.3	31.8	72.7	77.6	430	131
FL	Liberty	0.36	1173	35.8	11.5	31.7	72.4	78.5	75	23
GA	Dodge	-0.08	1506	35.8	12.6	30.1	70.7	76.4	300	92
WV	Jackson	-0.08	1516	35.8	11.7	28.7	74.2	79	806	246
KS	Seward	-0.21	1605	35.8	7.7	29.6	73.3	79.2	2809	856
TN	Sequatchie	-0.44	1779	35.8	9.6	30.7	72.7	79.1	1649	503
SC	Union	-0.80	2010	35.8	11.9	33.6	69.3	77.1	499	152
WV	Wyoming	-1.37	2311	35.8	14.3	40.9	69.5	76.6	1898	579
NC	Sampson	-1.63	2440	35.8	10.9	28.4	70.9	77.6	124	38
WI	Dodge	-1.83	2520	35.8	7.4	23.7	76.1	80.8	920	280
NC	Martin	-2.93	2892	35.8	12	27.8	69.5	76.4	45	14
FL	Glades	5.15	106	35.9	10.2	33	74.2	80.1	29	9
NM	McKinley	3.39	259	35.9	12.4	25.9	71.5	79.5	6942	2116
SC	Georgetown	1.49	601	35.9	11	29.6	73.7	79	21	6
MS	Leake	0.72	944	35.9	13	38.7	68.4	76.2	406	124
KY	Menifee	0.46	1098	35.9	11.9	31.6	70.8	77.6	1059	323
KY	Boyd	0.28	1232	35.9	13.1	32.6	72.5	78.2	727	221
KY	Bell	0.12	1352	35.9	13.9	32.3	69.3	75.9	1659	506
GA	Laurens	0.01	1428	35.9	11.3	28.4	71.4	77.2	284	87
AL	Escambia	-0.03	1461	35.9	12.1	37	71.5	77.6	242	74
MS	Panola	-0.06	1494	35.9	12.6	36.7	68.8	75.7	287	88
AR	Newton	-0.26	1641	35.9	11	31.5	73.1	79.2	1557	475
AL	Geneva	-0.51	1814	35.9	12	34.2	71.6	78.4	212	65
KY	Pendleton	-0.74	1967	35.9	10.1	31.6	72.3	78.5	729	222

ST	COUNTY	USDA	AMEN	OBES	DIAB	INACT	M AGE	W AGE	ALT ft	ALT m
AR	Drew	-1.24	2255	35.9	11	32.8	71.8	77.4	190	58
MI	Genesee	-1.90	2546	35.9	10.6	29.7	73.2	78.6	787	240
SD	Spink	-3.62	3026	35.9	7	30.7	74.9	81.2	1314	400
MS	Harrison	1.00	813	36	11.3	29.5	71	78.6	77	23
TN	Lauderdale	0.05	1407	36	10.9	34.8	69.8	76.4	304	93
IN	Crawford	-0.20	1594	36	9.8	30.2	73.5	78.9	638	195
TN	Dyer	-0.39	1748	36	10.8	34.2	71.2	77.7	292	89
NC	Scotland	-0.69	1935	36	13.4	28.4	70.5	76.9	252	77
MS	Copiah	-1.08	2180	36	12.2	37.1	69.6	76.7	325	99
MS	Hinds	-1.21	2242	36	12.4	35.2	71.1	79	259	79
KY	Lawrence	-0.19	1587	36.1	12	35.7	70.2	77.3	812	247
GA	Randolph	-0.49	1808	36.1	13.4	31.9	67.6	74.7	386	118
MS	Lincoln	-0.99	2123	36.1	11.8	34.1	71.8	77.9	418	127
MI	Roscommon	-1.20	2235	36.1	9.7	30.3	73.8	79.9	1169	356
LA	Sabine	1.63	562	36.2	12.5	31.6	72.8	78.9	254	77
KY	Spencer	0.39	1149	36.2	10.3	29.9	75	79	654	199
NC	Beaufort	0.02	1421	36.2	10.4	28.4	73	78.5	23	7
WV	Nicholas	0.02	1426	36.2	11.2	32.9	73	78.5	2051	625
KY	Leslie	-0.41	1764	36.2	14	37.5	69.2	76.1	1419	433
OH	Jefferson	-0.77	1992	36.2	12	31.5	72.6	78.3	1073	327
AR	Lincoln	-1.24	2256	36.2	10.6	31.3	71.8	77.4	200	61
LA	East Carroll	-1.24	2257	36.2	13.4	32.8	70.1	76.2	87	26
LA	Franklin	-1.35	2300	36.2	10.6	36	70	76.6	66	20
VA	Brunswick	-1.44	2349	36.2	12.2	28.9	69.9	76.6	279	85
AR	Yell	1.63	561	36.3	12.2	28.6	71.6	78.3	608	185
MT	Big Horn	1.38	640	36.3	11.8	27.1	74.6	80.3	3982	1214
FL	Madison	1.30	676	36.3	12.2	31.1	70.2	76.5	104	32
WV	Brooke	0.38	1161	36.3	13	34.1	73.8	78.8	1003	306
MS	Marion	0.04	1411	36.3	12	28.9	68.7	76.2	246	75
PA	Cambria	-0.23	1622	36.3	11.5	29.7	74.3	80.1	1931	588
GA	Elbert	-0.34	1696	36.3	12.2	30	71.7	78.1	553	169
AL	Washington	-0.49	1806	36.3	11.4	32	72.9	78.5	148	45
KS	Neosho	-1.01	2135	36.3	10	30	74	79.6	945	288
TN	Haywood	-1.70	2473	36.3	12.1	32.6	68.8	77	333	101
LA	Richland	-1.75	2489	36.3	10.4	29.1	69.3	75.3	71	22
OK	Sequoyah	2.55	367	36.4	12.6	38.1	71.7	78.8	695	212
OK	Cherokee	2.39	390	36.4	10.6	31.2	73.2	78.6	855	261
LA	Vernon	0.20	1304	36.4	11.3	28.9	73.8	79.3	251	77
MS	Montgomery	0.05	1403	36.4	13.7	36.1	70.7	77.9	379	115
MS	Forrest	-0.03	1464	36.4	12	32.7	71.9	77.5	217	66
AR	Hempstead	-0.65	1911	36.4	12.4	31.6	71.5	77.2	343	105
MS	Benton	-1.04	2159	36.4	11.8	33.3	70.6	77.9	503	153
TN	Chester	-2.01	2588	36.4	11.1	28.3	72.9	78.2	492	150
LA	St. Helena	-2.02	2589	36.4	13	33.9	69.9	76.7	210	64
MI	Jackson	-2.45	2761	36.4	9.4	27	74.4	79.3	983	300
OK	Adair	1.00	815	36.5	13.1	32.5	71.3	77.7	1068	325
AL	Winston	0.88	867	36.5	10.3	32.4	70.9	77.6	722	220

HEALTHIEST PLACES TO LIVE

ST	COUNTY	USDA	AMEN	OBES	DIAB	INACT	M AGE	W AGE	ALT ft	ALT m
KY	Adair	0.24	1263	36.5	12.1	37.5	72.6	78.1	848	258
MS	Lawrence	-0.08	1511	36.5	14.2	34	69.9	76.9	311	95
KY	Rockcastle	-0.35	1713	36.5	10.7	37.3	71.1	77.2	1154	352
AR	Arkansas	-0.87	2047	36.5	11.3	35.6	71.5	78.5	177	54
TN	Giles	-1.46	2359	36.5	9.9	30	72.2	78.9	831	253
KY	Casey	-1.97	2572	36.5	12.2	35.6	71.1	78.2	1008	307
LA	De Soto	0.37	1166	36.6	11.8	30.9	70.5	77.3	240	73
OH	Allen	-2.37	2726	36.6	9.7	26.2	74.9	79.7	842	257
WV	Gilmer	-2.64	2826	36.6	11.5	34.2	72.1	78.7	1004	306
IN	Madison	-3.47	2998	36.6	11	32.8	74.1	79.1	864	263
VA	Hampton	1.27	697	36.7	11.8	27.6	74.4	79.1	4	1
SC	Sumter	0.45	1110	36.7	12.8	31.7	71.6	78.5	162	49
AR	Lee	-0.42	1769	36.7	12	37.1	69.5	76.3	194	59
LA	Madison	-0.68	1929	36.7	12.6	34.5	69.3	75.3	72	22
SD	Mellette	-0.76	1984	36.7	12.8	33.1	71	78.3	2219	676
SD	Lyman	-1.28	2276	36.7	9.3	32.1	76.2	81.5	1765	538
SD	Tripp	-2.25	2672	36.7	9.1	30.9	75	80.8	2096	639
KS	Brown	-2.64	2824	36.7	9.2	28.9	75.1	80.9	1091	333
GA	Hancock	1.52	591	36.8	14.5	28.5	68.4	75.4	486	148
MS	Winston	0.49	1080	36.8	14.2	34.1	70.4	78.6	456	139
SC	Newberry	0.18	1321	36.8	10.7	30.4	71.7	78.5	433	132
KY	Floyd	0.04	1409	36.8	14.6	39.9	69.7	76.2	1031	314
WV	Mason	-0.05	1488	36.8	10.7	32.3	71.9	78.6	721	220
NC	Warren	-0.25	1634	36.8	12.6	29.8	70.4	76.9	301	92
LA	Iberville	-0.56	1852	36.8	12.2	32.6	69.4	76.3	8	3
AR	Monroe	-1.13	2206	36.8	11	35.2	69.5	76.3	171	52
WA	Adams	-1.34	2298	36.8	10.4	26.7	74.2	79.4	1590	485
SD	Roberts	-1.68	2464	36.8	9.5	29.2	74.9	81.2	1320	402
AL	Talladega	1.34	655	36.9	13.3	34.6	70.5	77.2	613	187
TN	Cocke	1.31	672	36.9	11.4	33.4	69.9	76.7	1725	526
OK	McIntosh	1.21	729	36.9	9.7	34.8	72.2	79.4	660	201
SD	Bennett	0.50	1074	36.9	11.7	28.7	71	78.3	3168	966
AL	Pickens	0.13	1347	36.9	13.9	32.5	70.3	76.7	273	83
OK	Kay	0.05	1405	36.9	10.9	31.3	73	78.7	1069	326
KY	Pike	-0.18	1582	36.9	13.9	38.1	68.7	76.3	1297	395
AL	Fayette	-0.38	1733	36.9	12.2	31.8	70.5	78	487	148
LA	Avoyelles	-0.50	1813	36.9	11.2	36.1	69.4	76.3	47	14
AR	Poinsett	-2.26	2676	36.9	10.4	37.3	69.3	76.6	231	71
KY	Webster	-2.30	2692	36.9	11.6	33.8	72.4	78.9	436	133
WA	Cowlitz	4.54	159	37	8.8	22.3	74.6	79.3	1345	410
KY	Laurel	1.25	709	37	12.9	35.7	72	77.7	1138	347
SC	Clarendon	1.15	751	37	12.3	32	70.8	77.4	103	31
OK	Pontotoc	1.04	800	37	10.4	34.7	72.9	78.2	971	296
OK	Seminole	0.58	1032	37	10.3	34.6	71.3	78.2	927	283
GA	Burke	-0.77	1987	37	11.4	30.7	68.3	75	255	78
AL	Pike	-0.93	2085	37	15	32.3	71.7	77.1	430	131
AL	Barbour	0.19	1314	37.1	13.2	33.8	71	76.9	374	114

ST	COUNTY	USDA	AMEN	OBES	DIAB	INACT	M AGE	W AGE	ALT ft	ALT m
KY	Marshall	-0.24	1630	37.1	9.5	25.8	73.8	79.6	414	126
NC	Bladen	-0.31	1681	37.1	12.2	30	69.3	76.7	86	26
NE	Thurston	-1.96	2569	37.1	12.9	34.2	74.2	79.8	1345	410
AL	Covington	-0.17	1569	37.2	10.9	36	71.4	77.9	299	91
SC	Barnwell	-0.21	1610	37.2	11.8	31	70.4	76.5	232	71
SC	Laurens	-0.35	1715	37.2	10.9	31.8	71.2	77.7	605	184
AR	Crittenden	-1.05	2160	37.2	13.1	33.1	69.6	75.9	207	63
SD	Hyde	-2.39	2735	37.2	8	30	76.3	82.4	1849	564
MS	Lowndes	-0.07	1501	37.3	13	33.5	72.5	78.4	222	68
GA	Terrell	-0.21	1603	37.3	12.5	29.7	67.6	74.7	336	102
WV	Wirt	-0.34	1707	37.3	12.7	28.1	72	78	866	264
GA	Jefferson	-0.46	1790	37.3	12.4	29.7	67.9	75.2	335	102
WV	Clay	-0.51	1821	37.3	13.4	33.2	71.9	78.3	1167	356
TN	McNairy	-1.69	2469	37.3	11	32.1	71.4	78.4	490	149
TN	Gibson	-1.86	2530	37.3	11	37.3	70.3	77.5	371	113
OK	Grady	-0.25	1637	37.4	8.4	28	73.1	78.9	1220	372
MO	Buchanan	-0.47	1801	37.4	10.3	30.1	73.8	79.6	923	281
AR	Ouachita	-0.88	2055	37.4	11.6	34.2	71.1	76.9	185	56
AL	Crenshaw	-0.91	2072	37.4	12.2	32.5	69.9	76.4	422	129
KS	Rice	-1.62	2434	37.4	9	23.8	74.9	80.1	1694	516
LA	Caldwell	0.35	1185	37.5	11.1	31.4	70.1	76.8	119	36
KS	Jefferson	-1.06	2170	37.5	9.4	22.8	75.4	80	1026	313
MO	Linn	-1.26	2268	37.5	8.8	32.9	74.2	80.2	815	248
TN	Carroll	-1.91	2551	37.5	11.1	33	70.1	77.2	469	143
FL	Hardee	2.25	423	37.6	12.2	31.2	73.2	78.9	87	26
MS	Grenada	1.78	526	37.6	12.3	35	68.8	76.7	253	77
KY	Elliott	0.29	1223	37.6	10.6	37.5	70.2	77.3	914	279
MS	Jones	-0.38	1735	37.6	12.3	32	71.8	77.9	247	75
MS	Tallahatchie	-0.92	2083	37.6	12.8	33.5	68.6	76.3	187	57
KY	Grant	-0.93	2086	37.6	10.4	36.7	72.6	78.7	809	247
AL	Tallapoosa	2.19	432	37.7	12	30	71.7	78.2	631	192
SC	Berkeley	0.71	954	37.7	12.3	30.1	73.9	79.2	45	14
NC	Bertie	-0.30	1668	37.7	13	29.9	68.8	76.2	38	12
MI	Gratiot	-3.92	3056	37.7	9.1	27.9	75.2	79.6	735	224
MS	Adams	0.12	1355	37.8	12.5	38.8	70.8	77.6	170	52
MS	Issaquena	-0.89	2063	37.8	13.2	33.8	69.9	75.9	90	27
MS	Amite	-1.01	2137	37.8	11.9	32.3	69.3	76.1	351	107
WV	Logan	-1.03	2152	37.8	13.6	42.7	68.9	76.4	1355	413
AR	St. Francis	-1.28	2271	37.8	12.1	39.8	69.4	75.3	215	65
VA	Petersburg	-1.34	2297	37.8	13.5	32.5	66.9	76.2	95	29
LA	Morehouse	-1.85	2525	37.8	11.6	35.7	69.5	75.6	90	28
LA	St. Mary	0.85	888	37.9	11.6	32.2	70.3	78	4	1
KS	Wyandotte	-0.17	1572	37.9	11.7	32.5	71.1	77.5	882	269
AR	Miller	-0.30	1664	37.9	12.3	35	73.3	79	261	80
MS	George	-0.81	2015	37.9	10.1	33	70.4	77	134	41
AR	Desha	-1.04	2153	37.9	12.1	31.9	69.4	75.8	141	43
ND	Grant	-1.79	2503	37.9	7	29.8	75.7	81.6	2239	682

HEALTHIEST PLACES TO LIVE

ST	COUNTY	USDA	AMEN	OBES	DIAB	INACT	M AGE	W AGE	ALT ft	ALT m
AL	Lawrence	0.54	1043	38	12.4	35.3	71.5	77.7	678	207
MS	Scott	-1.15	2215	38	13.6	35	69.3	77.8	422	128
MS	Clay	-0.36	1724	38.1	12.9	36.8	71	77.8	242	74
MS	Kemper	-0.60	1879	38.1	14.3	32.9	68.9	76.5	344	105
LA	St. Landry	-0.71	1949	38.1	12.6	32.5	70.7	77.2	34	10
KY	Johnson	0.64	988	38.2	11.7	34.5	69.7	77.4	891	272
SC	Lee	-1.00	2133	38.2	13.1	34.9	68.3	75.4	217	66
MS	Washington	-1.03	2151	38.2	11.6	36.1	68.1	75.3	109	33
AR	Jefferson	-1.08	2178	38.2	12.9	34	70.4	77.2	216	66
MO	Pemiscot	-1.16	2220	38.2	10	35.8	68.5	76.5	261	79
FL	Hamilton	0.58	1028	38.3	13.3	33.3	70.2	76.5	108	33
SC	Marion	-0.15	1561	38.4	13.3	33.6	68.8	76	55	17
WV	Lincoln	-1.05	2167	38.4	10.7	37.7	70.6	76.6	911	278
LA	Allen	-2.38	2729	38.4	12.2	33.8	73.1	78.7	77	24
AR	Polk	1.08	780	38.5	9.4	30.9	73.1	79.3	1180	360
LA	St. John Baptist	-0.34	1699	38.5	11.5	32	71.3	76.8	4	1
MS	Attala	0.02	1419	38.6	12.7	35.2	68.2	77.3	403	123
AR	Chicot	-0.45	1782	38.6	12.8	35.1	69.4	75.8	113	34
KY	Martin	-0.92	2080	38.6	12.6	38.1	69.7	77.4	943	288
TN	Hardeman	-1.05	2165	38.6	11.4	33.8	70.7	77.2	459	140
SC	Dillon	-0.68	1932	38.7	11.9	37.3	67.9	75.4	101	31
NC	Halifax	-1.30	2282	38.7	12.6	33.3	69.5	76.9	153	47
AL	Choctaw	0.92	850	38.8	14.3	34.1	70.4	77	197	60
MS	Yalobusha	0.53	1051	38.8	13.4	34.5	68.6	76.3	327	100
KY	Perry	-0.19	1588	38.8	13.1	39.2	68.4	76.6	1261	384
MS	Marshall	-1.00	2131	38.8	14.7	37.5	68.5	76	438	134
AR	Mississippi	-1.76	2491	38.8	12.1	42	68.7	76.2	234	71
LA	Terrebonne	0.50	1071	38.9	12.4	32.5	71.8	78.6	3	1
KY	Letcher	-0.74	1966	38.9	15.2	36.1	69.4	76.8	1717	523
MS	Franklin	-1.29	2278	39	12.6	37.9	70.8	77.6	322	98
MS	Leflore	-1.41	2325	39	13.8	35.2	68.5	75.5	122	37
SC	Fairfield	0.67	973	39.1	14	35.1	69	76.8	406	124
VA	Portsmouth	0.48	1092	39.1	12	29	70.7	76.9	8	2
MI	Cheboygan	0.08	1379	39.1	9.1	26.7	75.8	80.6	744	227
LA	Bienville	-0.03	1463	39.1	11.2	29	70	76.1	241	73
MS	Warren	-0.14	1558	39.1	12	30.9	71.1	77.3	156	48
MS	Bolivar	-0.57	1861	39.2	13.3	31.4	67.9	75.2	136	42
AL	Bullock	-1.08	2177	39.2	15.6	30.9	68.4	75.3	415	126
SD	Edmunds	-2.68	2835	39.2	6.5	27.1	74.1	80.3	1696	517
AR	Ashley	-1.12	2199	39.4	10.4	37.4	72.4	77.4	134	41
AL	Russell	-0.24	1627	39.5	12.5	36.5	69.3	76.3	339	103
OH	Lawrence	-1.08	2184	39.5	11.3	35.4	71.7	77.4	756	230
MS	Jasper	-1.11	2195	39.5	14.4	35.5	70.5	77.2	404	123
ND	Rolette	-2.21	2656	39.5	13.3	35.4	74.4	80.2	1799	548
SC	Calhoun	0.20	1311	39.6	12.9	32.8	71.9	78.1	214	65
MS	Walthall	-0.87	2050	39.6	12.4	34.9	69.9	76.9	355	108
KY	Breathitt	-1.36	2302	39.6	14.7	33.7	68.2	76.1	1045	318

ST	COUNTY	USDA	AMEN	OBES	DIAB	INACT	M AGE	W AGE	ALT ft	ALT m
SC	Jasper	0.59	1024	**39.7**	12.9	30.2	71.1	77	31	9
MS	Greene	0.02	1420	**39.7**	12.1	32.7	70.7	76.6	170	52
MD	Somerset	-0.04	1474	**39.7**	11.4	32	72	77.4	11	3
MS	Wilkinson	-0.09	1518	**39.7**	14.9	35.3	69.3	76.1	214	65
AR	Phillips	-0.68	1927	**39.7**	13.2	37.8	66.8	75	174	53
NC	Edgecombe	-2.13	2630	**39.7**	12.1	30.4	68.9	75.6	71	22
MS	Noxubee	0.39	1152	**39.9**	13.7	33.4	68.9	76.5	230	70
MS	Pike	-0.29	1662	**39.9**	13.7	35.2	69.9	76.5	347	106
MI	Saginaw	-3.33	2970	**39.9**	9.8	30.2	73.5	79.1	624	190
KY	Lincoln	-1.25	2262	**40.1**	11.7	37.8	71.7	78.2	1060	323
MS	Quitman	-1.97	2573	**40.1**	15.1	34.8	66	74.1	156	48
MS	Tunica	-0.40	1756	**40.2**	14.2	39.1	66	74.1	181	55
MS	Sharkey	-1.34	2295	**40.2**	13.3	35.2	66.5	74.1	92	28
AL	Marengo	-0.72	1957	**40.4**	14.8	34.8	69.9	76.3	181	55
AL	Perry	0.84	891	**40.5**	17.8	34.1	69.3	75.5	277	84
MS	Covington	-1.11	2194	**40.7**	12	30.8	69.2	77	323	98
MS	Holmes	-0.92	2082	**40.8**	14.1	35.3	65.9	73.5	246	75
SD	Shannon	-0.10	1531	**40.9**	16.8	32.4	71.1	78.5	3101	945
NC	Robeson	-1.52	2389	**40.9**	13.3	38.5	68.7	76.8	150	46
SC	Orangeburg	0.25	1256	**41**	13.5	32.2	69.4	76.9	183	56
SD	Todd	-0.98	2119	**41**	14.4	31.5	71	78.3	2697	822
SC	Hampton	-0.69	1937	**41.1**	14.3	30	69.9	76.7	82	25
SD	Buffalo	-1.59	2422	**41.2**	17.2	36.8	75.8	81.4	1650	503
AL	Butler	-1.16	2218	**41.3**	14.6	35.9	69.6	77.2	385	117
MS	Humphreys	-1.17	2224	**41.4**	13.6	33.4	66.5	74.1	101	31
MS	Sunflower	-1.47	2363	**41.4**	14.4	34.6	67.1	73.6	122	37
SC	Bamberg	-0.75	1974	**41.5**	12.6	33.1	68.7	76.2	159	48
MS	Claiborne	-0.35	1714	**41.6**	14.5	39.9	67.8	74.5	177	54
AL	Macon	-0.56	1850	**41.7**	14.2	31.1	68.4	75.3	328	100
SD	Corson	-0.71	1953	**41.7**	13	31.6	72.9	79.9	2088	636
ND	Sioux	-0.96	2109	**41.8**	13.5	32.3	74.6	80.6	2029	618
AL	Dallas	-0.18	1581	**41.9**	14.2	33.3	68.5	75.3	195	59
SC	Williamsburg	-0.88	2060	**41.9**	13.4	31.4	67.8	75.6	53	16
SD	Dewey	0.62	1011	**42.3**	15.5	33.9	72.9	79.9	2004	611
AL	Sumter	-0.48	1803	**42.4**	16.8	32.3	67.9	76.6	173	53
SC	Marlboro	0.27	1240	**42.7**	12.7	33.1	68.1	75.3	147	45
SD	Ziebach	-0.55	1845	**43.3**	14.1	34.5	72.9	79.9	2278	694
AL	Hale	1.43	623	**43.5**	14	35.2	69.3	75.5	211	64
AL	Wilcox	1.58	573	**43.6**	15.5	34.4	69.9	76.3	198	60
MS	Coahoma	-0.65	1912	**44.3**	14.7	36.1	66.8	75	158	48
AL	Lowndes	-0.41	1761	**44.7**	16.4	37.5	69.9	76.4	251	76
MS	Jefferson	-0.71	1950	**44.9**	15.3	37.2	67.8	74.5	256	78
AL	Greene	-0.04	1469	**47.9**	16.2	37.3	67.9	76.6	167	51

ACKNOWLEDGMENTS

The following government agencies, education institutions, and individuals are acknowledged for providing critical data. Without their information, this book could not have been written.

- **United States Department of Agriculture Economic Research Service**
  Natural Amenities Scale map and data. http://www.ers.usda.gov/data-products/natural-amenities-scale.aspx

- **Centers for Disease Control and Prevention**
  County-level maps and data for rates of obesity, diabetes, and leisure-time physical inactivity. http://www.cdc.gov/diabetes/atlas/countydata/atlas.html

- **University of Washington Institute for Health Metrics and Evaluation**
  "Falling behind: life expectancy in US counties from 2000 to 2007 in an international context." Published in Population Health Metrics 2011, 9:16 doi:10.1186/1478-7954-9-16. http://www.pophealthmetrics.com/content/9/1/16

- **United States Geological Survey**
  Procedure for obtaining mean county elevations by extracting an elevation for the centroid of each county polygon. http://www.usgs.gov/faq/categories/9865/7021

- **Generosity of a Bright Young Man**
  The mean county elevations calculation was done free of charge by a young man named Steven Jay. He has a master of science degree in Land Resources and Environmental Science and he used USGS and ESRI data and software.

NOTES

INTRODUCTION

1. *It's lean times for the diet industry.":* J. Kell, Lean times for the diet industry, Fortune.com, accessed on Sept. 30, 2015, http://fortune.com/2015/05/22/lean-times-for-the-diet-industry.

2. *A 2015 Marketdata report says the value of the US weight loss market actually declined in 2014 by 1.1 percent, to $59.8 billion.:* Marketdata Enterprises, Inc., accessed on Sept. 30, 2015, https://www.bharatbook.com/healthcare-market-research-reports-467678/healthcare-industry-healthcare-market-research-reports-healthcare-industry-analysis-healthcare-sector1.html.

3. *The graph below is a five-year weight loss chart... WEIGHT REDUCTION MAINTAINED OVER TIME:* J.W. Anderson et al., Long-term weight-loss maintenance: a meta-analysis of US studies, American Journal of Clinical Nutrition, 2001. 74. pp. 579-584, accessed on Nov. 11. 2015, http://ajcn.nutrition.org/content/74/5/579.long.

4. *For the 78.6 million adult Americans who are obese...:* Centers for Disease Control and Prevention, accessed on Nov. 9, 2015, http://www.cdc.gov/obesity/data/adult.html.

5. *What are natural amenities? As defined by the 1999 USDA Natural Amenities Scale, they are: warm winter, winter sun, temperate summer, low summer humidity, topographic variation, and water area.:* USDA Economic Research Service, accessed on Oct. 15, 2015, http://www.ers.usda.gov/data-products/natural-amenities-scale.aspx.

CHAPTER 1: How High Natural Amenities and Altitude Help You Lose Weight

1. *By the time I turned fifty-two, I was diagnosed with insulin resistance (a physiological condition in which the natural hormone insulin becomes less effective at lowering blood sugars).*: Wikipedia, accessed on June 22, 2012, https://en.wikipedia.org/wiki/Insulin_resistance.

2. *A 1999 United States Department of Agriculture (USDA) Natural Amenities Scale... The six measures are warm winter, winter sun, temperate summer, low summer humidity, topographic variation, and water area.*: USDA Economic Research Service, accessed on October 15, 2015, http://www.ers.usda.gov/data-products/natural-amenities-scale.aspx.

3. *The Centers for Disease Control and Prevention (CDC) data...running, calisthenics, golf, gardening, or walking for exercise.*: CDC, accessed on Nov. 9, 2015, http://www.cdc.gov/diabetes/pdfs/data/calculating-methods-references-county-level-estimates-ranks.pdf.

4. *Falling behind: life expectancy in US counties from 2000 to 2007 in an international context.*: S. Kulkarni et al., Population Health Metrics 2011, 9:16, accessed on Nov. 9, 2015, http://www.pophealthmetrics.com/content/9/1/16.

5. *This correlation with health is especially true for diabetes...about 1.5 times higher among adults aged 18 years or older with diagnosed diabetes than among adults without diagnosed diabetes.*: Centers for Disease Control and Prevention. National Diabetes Statistics Report: Estimates of Diabetes and Its Burden in the United States, 2014. Atlanta, GA: U.S. Department of Health and Human Services; 2014, accessed on Nov. 11, 2015, http://www.cdc.gov/diabetes/pubs/statsreport14/national-diabetes-report-web.pdf.

6. *Obesity prevalence in the United States is inversely associated with elevation and urbanization, after adjusting for temperature, diet, physical activity, smoking and demographic factors.*: J.D. Voss, et al., International Journal of Obesity (2013) 37, 1407-1412; doi:10.1038/ijo.2013.5, accessed on Nov. 9, 2015, http://www.nature.com/ijo/journal/v37/n10/full/ijo20135a.html.

7. *Recently, we've identified a strong association between obesity prevalence and altitude within the US… after controlling for diet, activity level, smoking, demographics, temperature, and urbanization.*: T. Saunders, Public Library of Science, Obesity Panacea, Obesity and Altitude, accessed on Nov. 9, 2015, http://blogs.plos.org/obesitypanacea/2013/04/10/obesity-and-altitude/.

8. *Physical activity can improve health…About 1 in 5 (21%) adults meet the 2008 [CDC] Physical Activity Guidelines.*: CDC, accessed on Sept. 22, 2015, http://www.cdc.gov/physicalactivity/data/facts.htm.

9. *So in the fall of 2004…joined the nearby Copper Mountain Over the Hill Gang for fifty-plus-year-old skiers.*: Copper Mountain – Over the Hill Gang (OHG), accessed on Nov. 9, 2015, http://www.coppercolorado.com/winter/ski_and_ride_school/adult_seasonal_programs/over_the_hill_gang.

10. *After adjustment, altitude had a beneficial association…Men and women who lived in counties at a higher altitude in the USA had a longer life expectancy.*: M. Ezzati et al., Journal of Epidemiology and Community Health (2011). doi:10.1136/jech.2010.112938, accessed on Nov. 11, 2015, http://www.ncbi.nlm.nih.gov/pubmed/21406589.

11. *Persons with asthma do better at high altitude…than at sea level.*: Institute For Altitude Medicine, accessed on Sept. 18, 2015, http://www.altitudemedicine.org/altitude-and-pre-existing-conditions/.

12. *Studies in the United States have shown that 30–40% of all asthmatics and the majority of patients with hay fever are allergic to dust mites…Dust mites cannot survive when the relative humidity falls below 40% or at very high altitudes (greater than 9,000 feet elevation) or when it is too cold.*: The Asthma Center, Allergic Disease Associates, P.C., accessed on Sept. 19, 2015, http://www.projectallergy.com/medical-information/allergy-medical-information/dust-mite-allergy-avoidance.cfm.

13. *It…took about twenty-five years for Barry Marshall and Robin Warren to be awarded the Nobel Prize for their discovery that peptic ulcer disease is caused by bacteria, not excess stomach acid.*: Wikipedia, accessed on Aug. 21, 2015, https://en.wikipedia.org/wiki/Timeline_of_peptic_ulcer_disease_and_Helicobacter_pylori.

14. *While it is always important to remember correlation does not prove causation…* *additional research will help clarify the mechanisms and long term health effects of* *either high altitude residence or normobaric hypoxia [simulated altitude].*: T. Saunders, Public Library of Science, Obesity Panacea, Obesity and Altitude, accessed on Nov. 9, 2015, http://blogs.plos.org/obesitypanacea/2013/04/10/ obesity-and-altitude/.

15. *This is not the first time humans have leveraged Mother Nature…Photograph* *courtesy the Colorado Springs Pioneers Museum.*: Nicola, Edible Topography, accessed on Nov. 9, 2015, http://www.ediblegeography.com/edible-topography/.

16. *According to the CDC, tuberculosis was once the leading cause of death in the* *United States.*: CDC Division of Tuberculosis Elimination, accessed on Oct. 15, 2015, http://www.cdc.gov/tb/.

17. *The graph below is a five-year weight loss chart…WEIGHT REDUCTION* *MAINTAINED OVER TIME*: J.W. Anderson et al., Long-term weight-loss maintenance: a meta-analysis of US studies, American Journal of Clinical Nutrition, 2001. 74. pp. 579-584, accessed on Nov. 11. 2015, http://ajcn.nutrition. org/content/74/5/579.long.

CHAPTER 2: Altitude is NOT the Bad Guy We Think He Is

1. *The human body can adapt to high altitude through both immediate and long-term* *acclimatization… The upper altitude limit of this linear relationship has not been* *fully established.*: Wikipedia, accessed on Aug. 16, 2015, https://en.wikipedia.org/ wiki/Effects_of_high_altitude_on_humans.

2. *Each motor/engine/furnace will react differently…anything combustion loses* *approximately 3 percent of its power.*: M. Harley, Speedy Daddy, accessed on Aug. 20, 2015, http://speedydaddy.com/the-effect-of-altitude-on-a-car-or-truck-engine/.

3. *AMS feels like a bad hangover.*: Institute For Altitude Research, accessed on Oct. 15, 2015, http://www.altitudemedicine.org/altitude-illness/.

4. *Symptoms can include headache, queasiness, tiredness, and trouble sleeping.*: Altitude Research Center, accessed on Sept. 2, 2015, http://www.altituderesearch. org/traveling-to-altitude/fast-facts.

5. *According to the National Institutes of Health (NIH)… You have had the illness before*: NIH MedlinePlus Acute mountain sickness, accessed on Aug. 19, 2015, https://www.nlm.nih.gov/medlineplus/ency/article/000133.htm.

6. *According to the NIH, severe cases may even result in death due to lung problems or brain swelling, called cerebral edema.*: NIH MedlinePlus Acute mountain sickness, accessed on Aug. 19, 2015, https://www.nlm.nih.gov/medlineplus/ency/ article/000133.htm.

7. *The scientific community has been hard at work to tease out…research continues to fit more puzzle pieces together.*: F. Jabr, Scientific American, Mountain Maladies: Genetic Screening Susses Out Susceptibility to Altitude Sickness, accessed on Aug. 19, 2015, http://www.scientificamerican.com/article/genetic-tests-for-altitude-sickness/.

8. *Cows also get AMS…ranchers would like nothing more than to strip the responsible genes from the breeding population.*: F. Jabr, Scientific American, Mountain Maladies: Genetic Screening Susses Out Susceptibility to Altitude Sickness, accessed on Aug. 19, 2015, http://www.scientificamerican.com/article/genetic-tests-for-altitude-sickness/.

9. *In fact, healthy older folks are actually a little less susceptible to AMS than younger people are.*: Altitude Research Center, accessed on Sept. 2, 2015, http://www.altituderesearch.org/traveling-to-altitude/fast-facts.

10. *However, if folks are already suffering from certain chronic conditions like COPD, heart failure, arrhythmias, congenital heart problems, emphysema, pulmonary hypertension, and cystic fibrosis, a lower altitude may be in order.*: Institute For Altitude Medicine, accessed on Oct 15, 2015, http://www.altitudemedicine.org/altitude-and-pre-existing-conditions/.

11. *And the Institute for Altitude Medicine in Telluride, Colorado, recommends "an overnight stay at an intermediate altitude such as Denver or preferably a bit higher prior to further ascent into the mountains."*: Institute For Altitude Research, accessed on Oct. 15, 2015, http://www.altitudemedicine.org/altitude-illness/.

CHAPTER 3: A Case Study: Why Leadville, Colorado, is #1 in the United States

1. *Historic Leadville, Colorado, with a population of 2,602*: Wikipedia, accessed on Aug. 6, 2015, https://en.wikipedia.org/wiki/Leadville,_Colorado.

2. *The majority of Lake County's 7,290 residents live near the city of Leadville.*: United States Census Bureau, accessed on Aug. 31, 2015, http://quickfacts.census.gov/ qfd/states/08/08065.html.

3. *Fifteen miles south of Leadville is the rural enclave of Twin Lakes, with a population of 171.*: Wikipedia, accessed on Oct. 15, 2015, https://en.wikipedia.org/wiki/ Twin_Lakes,_Lake_County,_Colorado.

4. *Obesity prevalence in the United States is inversely associated with elevation and urbanization, after adjusting for temperature, diet, physical activity, smoking and demographic factors.*: J.D. Voss et al., International Journal of Obesity (2013) 37, 1407-1412; doi:10.1038/ijo.2013.5, accessed on Nov. 9, 2015, http://www.nature. com/ijo/journal/v37/n10/full/ijo20135a.html.

5. *According to 2013 US Census Bureau numbers,…and 47.7 percent of all residents have a bachelor's degree or higher.*: United States Census Bureau, accessed on Aug. 31, 2015, http://quickfacts.census.gov/qfd/states/08/08065.html and http:// quickfacts.census.gov/qfd/states/08/08117.html.

6. *According to the AARP, only about 10 percent of advertising dollars are currently being directed at baby boomers because Madison Avenue remains youth obsessed.*: S. Vranica, AARP Launches Baby Boomer Ad Firm Despite Marketers' Obsession with Millennials, The Wall Street Journal, Aug. 13, 2015 2:29 PM ET, accessed on Sept. 21, 2015, http://blogs.wsj.com/cmo/2015/08/13/aarp-launches-baby- boomer-ad-firm-despite-marketers-obsession-with-millennials/.

7. *Here are the AARP numbers.*: M. Bradbury, Huffpost's The Blog, The 7 Incredible Facts About Boomers' Spending Power, accessed on Nov. 10, 2015, http://www. huffingtonpost.com/mark-bradbury/the-7-incredible-facts-about-boomers- spending_b_6815876.html.

8. *According to a March 11, 2015, report published by the Center for Western Priorities (CWP),:* Center for Western Priorities, The Golden Rush: How Public Lands Draw Retirees and Create Economic Growth, March 11, 2015, accessed on Nov. 10, 2015, http://westernpriorities.org/2015/03/11/release-study-finds-retirees-are-drawn-to-counties-with-protected-public-lands/.

9. *This nonlabor income is one of the fastest-growing sources of income in the western United States.:* Center for Western Priorities, The Golden Rush: How Public Lands Draw Retirees and Create Economic Growth, March 11, 2015, accessed on Nov. 10, 2015, http://westernpriorities.org/2015/03/11/release-study-finds-retirees-are-drawn-to-counties-with-protected-public-lands/.

10. *According to an analysis by the University of Georgia, it takes only 1.8 in-migrating retirees to create one job; in other words, for every 100 retirees relocating to a new community, about 55 new jobs are generated.:* Golden Rules, Evaluating Retiree-Based Economic Development in Georgia, Aug. 2013, accessed Nov. 10, 2015, http://www.terry.uga.edu/media/documents/selig/golden-rules-2013.pdf.

11. *Thus, seniors relocating to western states created nearly 300,000 jobs between 2000 and 2010.:* Center for Western Priorities, The Golden Rush: How Public Lands Draw Retirees and Create Economic Growth, March 11, 2015, accessed on Nov. 10, 2015, http://westernpriorities.org/2015/03/11/release-study-finds-retirees-are-drawn-to-counties-with-protected-public-lands/.

12. *In the sweepstakes to attract relocating retirees, America's spectacular public lands, with their high natural amenities, provide a unique and enduring competitive advantage to western towns and cities.:* Center for Western Priorities, The Golden Rush: How Public Lands Draw Retirees and Create Economic Growth, March 11, 2015, accessed on Nov. 10, 2015, http://westernpriorities.org/2015/03/11/release-study-finds-retirees-are-drawn-to-counties-with-protected-public-lands/.

13. *According to the US Census Bureau, between 1990 and 2000, Summit County, with 180.3 percent growth, experienced the largest increase in residents age 65+ in the United States. Eagle County was number five in the nation, with 135.2 percent growth.:* United States Census Bureau. The Older Population: 2010, Issued Nov. 2011, accessed on Nov. 10, 2105, https://www.census.gov/prod/cen2010/briefs/c2010br-09.pdf.

14. *Frisco Population Growth by Age Sector 1990-2000.*: The Summit Foundation, Trends Affecting Summit County, June 10, 2009, accessed on Nov. 10, 2015, http://www.surveyvsr.com/sf.pdf.

15. *Compared with Highways 24 and 91 into Leadville, the Interstate 70 corridor in Summit and Eagle Counties is a nightmare, especially during the winter…In contrast, Highway 24 (between Leadville and Minturn) had six closures. Highway 91 (between Leadville and Copper Mountain) had two closures.*: Colorado Department of Transportation e-mail sent on June 3, 2015, under CORA.

16. *In Eagle, Summit, and Pitkin Counties, these younger populations are even referred to as "the lost generation."*: The Summit Foundation, Trends Affecting Summit County, June 10, 2009, accessed on Nov. 10, 2015, http://www.surveyvsr.com/sf.pdf.

17. *Plans are currently under way for a $94 million luxury hotel and resort a mile north of Leadville. With rooms in the $300/night range, an indoor water park, three restaurants, and a convention center for 250 people,…gentrified.*: M. Martinek, The Herald Democrat, posted Aug. 19, 2015, accessed on Aug. 21, 2015, http://www.leadvilleherald.com/news/article_9ddf5da6-4692-11e5-8fda-b703e50a6063.html.

CHAPTER 4: Altitude Facts and Figures

1. *At this time, the United States Geological Survey (USGS) website does not post mean elevation by county. However, the website does provide a procedure to extract an elevation for the centroid of each county polygon using Environmental Systems Research Institute (ESRI) ArcGIS software.*: United States Geological Survey, accessed on Oct. 2, 2015, http://www.usgs.gov/faq/categories/9865/7021.

2. *This calculation was done by a bright young man named Steven Jay. He has a master of science degree in Land Resources and Environmental Science and he used USGS and ESRI data and software.*: E-mail communication on Sept. 22, 2015.

3. *"Go West young man, go West and grow up in the country."*: Wikipedia, accessed on Oct. 4, 2015, https://en.wikipedia.org/wiki/Go_West,_young_man.

4. *Recently, we've identified a strong association between obesity prevalence and altitude within the US... after controlling for diet, activity level, smoking, demographics, temperature, and urbanization.*: T. Saunders, Public Library of Science, Obesity Panacea, Obesity and Altitude, accessed on Nov. 9, 2015, http://blogs.plos.org/obesitypanacea/2013/04/10/obesity-and-altitude/.

5. *It's called the finger-pulse oximeter. This little contraption measures your blood oxygen saturation level and pulse rate. Just clip it on your finger sort of like a clothespin.*: Picture from healthcare-manager.com, accessed on Oct. 31, 2015, http://healthcare-manager.com/products/fingertip-pulse-oximeter-contec.

6. *Currently, the portable pulse oximetry market is estimated at $200 million, with 9 to 11 percent compound annual growth.*: Oxitone Medical by Gefenbiomed on 7 Feb. 2015, accessed on Oct. 6, 2015, http://www.gefenbiomed.com/oxitone-medical.

7. *There's even a new pulse oximeter being developed that can be wrapped around the wrist like a watch.*: Oxitone Wearable Platform, accessed on Nov. 10, 2015. http://oxitone.com/products/.

8. *The United States Olympic Committee has an Altitude Factsheet that discusses "sleep high, train low.".*: accessed on Nov. 10, 2015, http://webcache.googleusercontent.com/search?q=cache:GXTNJeKyXAcJ:www.teamusa.org/~/media/TeamUSA/Nutrition/Altitude%2520Fact%2520Sheet%25202015.pdf+&cd=2&hl=en&ct=clnk&gl=us.

9. *The air Phelps slept in was the equivalent of the air at 8,500–9,000 feet.*: J. Rosen, The Baltimore Sun, May 7, 2012, accessed on Oct. 7, 2015, http://articles.baltimoresun.com/2012-05-07/features/bal-michael-phelps-bed-20120507_1_michael-phelps-chamber-high-altitude.

10. *(Michael Phelps Twitter pic)*: J. Rosen, The Baltimore Sun, May 7, 2012, accessed on Oct. 7, 2015, http://articles.baltimoresun.com/2012-05-07/features/bal-michael-phelps-bed-20120507_1_michael-phelps-chamber-high-altitude.

11. *So, to borrow a phrase from NASCAR, "Ladies and gentlemen, start your engines.".*: C. Ramotar, Feb. 19, 2015, accessed on Oct. 15, 2015, http://www.genre.com/knowledge/blog/ladies-and-gentlemen-start-your-engines-nascar-history-and-risks.html.

12. *Elevation States – State Information*: Wikipedia, accessed on Nov. 3, 2015, https://en.wikipedia.org/wiki/List_of_U.S._states_by_elevation.

13. *Elevation States – County Information*: This calculation was done by a bright young man named Steven Jay. He has a master of science degree in Land Resources and Environmental Science and he used USGS and ESRI data and software.: E-mail communication on Sept. 22, 2015.

CHAPTER 5: Alphabetical Listing of 3,108 Lower Forty-Eight Counties

1. *Natural Amenities Scale map and data.*: USDA Economic Research Service, accessed on Oct. 15, 2015, http://www.ers.usda.gov/data-products/natural-amenities-scale.aspx.

2. *County-level maps and data for rates of obesity, diabetes, and leisure-time physical inactivity.*: CDC, accessed on Nov. 9, 2015, http://www.cdc.gov/diabetes/pdfs/data/calculating-methods-references-county-level-estimates-ranks.pdf and http://www.cdc.gov/diabetes/atlas/countydata/atlas.html.

3. *Falling behind: life expectancy in US counties from 2000 to 2007 in an international context.*: S. Kulkarni et al., Population Health Metrics 2011,9:16, accessed on Nov. 9, 2015, http://www.pophealthmetrics.com/content/9/1/16.

CHAPTER 6: Natural Amenities Ratings for 3,108 Lower Forty-Eight Counties

1. *The natural amenities scale is a measure of the physical characteristics of a county area that enhance the location as a place to live…data are available for counties in the lower 48 States.*: USDA Economic Research Service, accessed on Oct. 15, 2015, http://www.ers.usda.gov/data-products/natural-amenities-scale.aspx.

2. *The six measures used in the natural amenities composite score were selected on the basis of a conception of the environmental qualities most people prefer, availability of measures, simplicity, nonredundancy, and the correlation to population change…. Implicit in the transformation is the assumption that a difference between 5 percent and 10 percent in water surface area improves the*

attractiveness of an area as much as a difference between 10 and 20 percent.: USDA Economic Research Service, accessed on Nov. 10, 2015, http://www.ers. usda.gov/data-products/natural-amenities-scale/documentation.aspx.

CHAPTER 7: Obesity Ratings for 3,108 Lower Forty-Eight Counties

1. *There is no data on weight loss when you go to a health club, either.*: C. Lagorio, CBS/AP/Jan. 3, 2005, quote from Thomas Wadden, a University of Pennsylvania weight-loss expert and the study's co-author (Annals of Internal Medicine), accessed on Nov. 10, 2015, http://www.cbsnews.com/news/diet-plan-success-tough-to-weigh/.

2. *Knowing which proteins regulate brown fat is significant because brown fat is not only important for thermogenesis, but…could possibly lose more weight even if eating the same amount of food.*: S. Yang, To trigger body's energy-burning brown fat, just chill. Quoting Professor Hei Sook Sul, of the U of C Berkeley, accessed on Nov. 10, 2015, http://news.berkeley.edu/2015/01/08/energy-burning-brown-fat-protein/.

www.ingramcontent.com/pod-product-compliance
Lightning Source LLC
Chambersburg PA
CBHW081146270326
41930CB00014B/3058